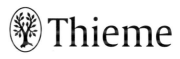

Shonishin: Japanese Pediatric Acupuncture

Second Edition

Stephen Birch, PhD
Associate Professor
Norwegian School of Health Sciences
Kristiania University College
Oslo, Norway

168 illustrations

Thieme
Stuttgart • New York • Delhi • Rio de Janeiro

Library of Congress Cataloging-in-Publication Data

Names: Birch, Stephen, author.

Title: Shonishin : Japanese pediatric acupuncture / Stephen Birch.

Description: Second edition. | Stuttgart ; New York : Thieme, [2016] | Includes bibliographical references and index.

Identifiers: LCCN 2015040232 | ISBN 9783131500625 (alk. paper)

Subjects: | MESH: Acupuncture—methods. | Acupuncture Therapy. | Child. | Infant.

Classification: LCC RJ53.A27 | NLM WB 369 | DDC 615.8/92–dc23 LC record available at http://lccn.loc.gov/2015040232

© 2016 by Georg Thieme Verlag KG

Thieme Publishers Stuttgart
Rüdigerstrasse 14, 70469 Stuttgart, Germany
+49 [0]711 8931 421, customerservice@thieme.de

Thieme Publishers New York
333 Seventh Avenue, New York, NY 10001 USA
+1 800 782 3488, customerservice@thieme.com

Thieme Publishers Delhi
A-12, Second Floor, Sector-2, Noida-201301
Uttar Pradesh, India
+91 120 45 566 00, customerservice@thieme.in

Thieme Publishers Rio, Thieme Publicações Ltda.
Edifício Rodolpho de Paoli, 25° andar
Av. Nilo Peçanha, 50 - Sala 2508
Rio de Janeiro 20020-906 Brasil
+55 21 3172 2297 / +55 21 3172 1896

Cover design: Thieme Publishing Group
Typesetting by DiTech Process Solutions, India

Printed in Germany by Grafisches Centrum Cuno, Calbe (Saale)   5 4 3 2 1

ISBN 978-3-13-150062-5

Also available as an e-book:
eISBN 978-3-13-162612-7

Important note: Medicine is an ever-changing science undergoing continual development. Research and clinical experience are continually expanding our knowledge, in particular our knowledge of proper treatment and drug therapy. Insofar as this book mentions any dosage or application, readers may rest assured that the authors, editors, and publishers have made every effort to ensure that such references are in accordance with the state of knowledge at the time of production of the book.

Nevertheless, this does not involve, imply, or express any guarantee or responsibility on the part of the publishers in respect to any dosage instructions and forms of applications stated in the book. Every user is requested to examine carefully the manufacturers' leaflets accompanying each drug and to check, if necessary in consultation with a physician or specialist, whether the dosage schedules mentioned therein or the contraindications stated by the manufacturers differ from the statements made in the present book. Such examination is particularly important with drugs that are either rarely used or have been newly released on the market. Every dosage schedule or every form of application used is entirely at the user's own risk and responsibility. The authors and publishers request every user to report to the publishers any discrepancies or inaccuracies noticed. If errors in this work are found after publication, errata will be posted at www.thieme.com on the product description page.

Some of the product names, patents, and registered designs referred to in this book are in fact registered trademarks or proprietary names even though specific reference to this fact is not always made in the text. Therefore, the appearance of a name without designation as proprietary is not to be construed as a representation by the publisher that it is in the public domain.

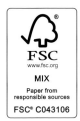

Contents

Section I   Overview and History

Section II   Treatment Principles and Tools of Treatment

Section III   Root Treatment Approaches and Techniques

Contents

Appendix

Video Contents

Foreword

Traditional East Asian medicine (TEAM) boasts a rich variety of literary genres. The medical discourse (*yi lun* 醫論), the case record (*yi an* 醫案), and the modern textbook are just a few of the most prominent styles of TEAM writing today. Stephen Birch's Shonishin: *Japanese Pediatric Acupuncture* certainly qualifies as a textbook, and it is to some extent a medical discourse and a collection of case reports. But it also belongs to another venerable genre of the TEAM literature that is still in its infancy in the West. In many ways, this is a "clinical insights" memoir.

An entire generation of TEAM practitioners in the West have now fully matured as master clinicians. With 30 or more years' experience in adapting this medicine to practice in the West, members of this generation have begun sharing their clinical insights with the rest of us. The present volume is a rich and very personal expression of this process of transmission by an eminent member of this generation. In this, it also represents the full blossoming of *shonishin's* development and assimilation into TEAM in the West. It is ample evidence that we have truly made this medicine our own.

As much and perhaps more than any other specialty of TEAM practice, *shonishin* rewards knack over theory. It is easy to learn but difficult to truly master. Each practitioner must ultimately "get" the technique in his or her hands. A skilled teacher, however, knows how to effectively communicate that knack to others. Steve brings the sensibilities of a professionally trained clinical researcher to the task of unpacking the *shonishin* practice with consummate skill. This is evident both in his writing and in the materials provided at the MediaCenter. thieme.com website. The book and website combine to bring the techniques vividly to life.

Children are remarkably responsive to therapeutic influence, making them much more prone to overtreatment than their adult counterparts. Though questions of optimal therapeutic dosage are familiar territory for all experienced clinicians, Steve has thought this issue out and articulated it with an unprecedented depth and clarity. The clinical ramifications of his dosing model extend far beyond pediatrics and into medical practice as a whole, almost regardless of the modality being used.

Nowhere in clinical practice is the demand for fluid adaptability to changing circumstances more pressing than in pediatrics. Steve discusses this often unspoken aspect of the therapeutic encounter as the "dance of treatment." Once again, one's sensitivity to optimum dosing lies at the heart of the matter. It is a dance that embraces moment-to-moment decisions concerning which technique to use, what tool to administer that technique with, precisely how much of that technique to administer, and with what degree of force. Then too, it is a dance largely choreographed by a squirming, sometimes squawking partner, and one typically overseen by a pensive parent hovering in the wings.

The themes of therapeutic dose and the fluid dance of treatment run throughout the text. A brief glance at the table of contents reveals the comprehensive discussions of pediatric needling techniques, and expositions on individual diseases accompanied by prescriptive treatment strategies requisite for a textbook on a pediatric specialty.

But the entire book is constructed around case examples. Many of these are from Steve's own practice illustrating his personal approach to both the topic at hand, and its relationship to the dose and the dance. Many other case records are those of colleagues, illustrating a variety of creative approaches to treatment. It is a technique that is best transmitted within the context of specific examples as opposed to theoretical abstractions, though both are necessary for a full understanding.

In some ways, *shonishin* isn't much to look at. It is an unassuming technique that can easily leave one wondering how a bit of stroking, a little tapping, and perhaps even a touch of tickling could have any real therapeutic value. Yet experienced *shonishin* practitioners know how almost miraculously effective it can be. It can work where biomedical, naturopathic, and other TEAM modalities have fallen short, and it combines easily with all of them. In this book, Steve has shown us what a potent tool of efficacy and thing of beauty the *shonishin* dance can be.

Charles Chace
Boulder, Colorado

Preface to the Second Edition

It is only a few years since this book was first published. In this second edition I have updated some of the treatment descriptions and expanded them with newer case histories of my own and of colleagues. I have added a new chapter on the treatment of headaches. I have expanded the chapter dealing with emotional and affective problems. With the help of my colleague and friend Manuel Rodriguez I have also expanded the section on combining the treatment methods in this book with the treatment systems of Bach flowers and Chinese herbal medicine. Here we have focused on the processes of selecting these methods as additional treatments rather than describing how to practice each. I have also expanded the descriptions of how to use the techniques of *shonishin* and the Meridian Therapy root treatment. For these practical expansions I have described a series of exercises to help readers improve their skills and double-check the techniques. It would have been difficult to do this without the creative input and contributions of Manuel, who is great at thinking outside the box for issues like these. The second edition has more treatment information and examples as well as more practical skill development information to help readers develop their clinical skills so that they can perform their treatments better.

Stephen Birch
Amsterdam, June 2015

Preface to the First Edition

I have been treating patients with acupuncture for almost 30 years. I first applied treatment to children over 25 years ago. My practice, since finishing acupuncture school, has been to use Japanese acupuncture and moxibustion methods exclusively. I have studied in Japan numerous times, mostly with practitioners who have more than 40 years of experience (some with 55 to 60 years of experience) and often with practitioners who have extensive experience treating babies and children. In this book I have tried to pull together these experiences and the insights and genius of my teachers. It represents the accumulation of many practical experiences and treatment ideas. I hope I have done these lineages justice.

Over the years I have taught and come across many acupuncturists who hardly if ever treat babies and children. Sometimes this is because of the interests or focus of the practitioner, they specialize in fertility or pain, for example; but more often it is because acupuncture treatment of children, and especially babies, is too scary. Many acupuncturists are not exposed to such treatment in school, never developing the confidence to try. Many are afraid that what they have learned is not suitable for the treatment of babies and children. The child is suffering enough, how can we cause more suffering with our needles? This is a great pity. We sometimes see very inspiring results when we treat children, especially the younger child. It is as though the potential for acupuncture is more strongly expressed in treatment of children compared to treatment of adults. Sometimes the results when we treat children are completely amazing, even shocking. The child who has been diagnosed with a genetic anomaly and is unable to digest food properly suddenly starts digesting food following treatment; the child with a cardiac disorder who has been so tired that she has not been able to play like other children is suddenly running around tirelessly after the first treatment! What is going on? How can this be? Why don't more practitioners try treating children? The answers to these questions lie in how we approach the child and what we think acupuncture is supposed to be.

Many acupuncturists are afraid of treating children because they are afraid of using on children the needling techniques they have learned in school. I know I was, and most people I have talked to have expressed the same fears and concerns. I feel that this is because most people have been trained in only the modern Chinese needling methods, which use relatively thick inserted needles that are manipulated until the sensations called 'de-qi' are obtained. It seems most acupuncturists think that this is acupuncture. While it seems to be the more commonly found form today, it is by no means the only form of acupuncture. Many styles of acupuncture have developed over the centuries, and, for various reasons, relatively gentle techniques have developed in Japan. Recognizing the sensitivities and needs of babies and children, a specialized style of acupuncture for treatment of children called *shonishin* developed in Japan over 300 years ago. This not only survived but, in the second half of the twentieth century has flourished in Japan. This style applies various surface stimulation methods using specialized treatment tools. Inserted needling is not always needed and often is unnecessary. It is neither painful nor scary. Practitioners who have learned it, patients who have received it, and parents who have observed and experienced it no longer feel afraid of the idea of acupuncture for children.

Another issue that makes it difficult for many acupuncturists to treat children lies in the belief that the kind of acupuncture treatment that they use on adults can be adapted simply by modifying the techniques to some degree (make them softer) but that the same theoretical basis of diagnosis and treatment can be used as with adults. I feel that this is an unreasonable assumption. There is not a lot of published literature in European languages about differences between children and adults based on traditional East Asian medical (TEAM) literature. The historical TEAM literature is not so detailed either; instead we have hints about what those differences may be. Of course the basic physiology must be the same or very similar; children breathe, eat, drink, digest, excrete, sleep, move, etc. with the same organs that adults use. They require the same basic functional systems in order to do these things. But there are some fundamental differences about how things occur, the rate and quality of changes that make children fundamentally different from most adults when it comes to how they respond to treatment and thus how treatment can be applied.

By focusing on those differences and highlighting the characteristics of children, namely that they are very sensitive and thus can be influenced by very little input (the "less is more" model), it is possible to develop a practical approach to the treatment of children that is much less theoretically complex. In this book I have tried to explain and highlight these issues to show how, regardless of how complex a model or pattern another system might construe for a pediatric patient, especially one with complex problems, we can find adaptable, practical solutions with a simpler model of practice. This is key to understanding the treatment approach for babies and children.

For a number of years I have wanted to write a practical book about the treatment of children using the unique treatment approaches from Japan called *shonishin*. I kept delaying, in part because of being busy and in part because I was not quite ready; I needed time to work out a strategy for making the book both practical and realistic. This text and its accompanying DVD are the product of those desires, plans, and strategies. I also resisted writing a *shonishin* book before because I did not want to write the same type of book that is often found in the field. Many books focus on telling the reader what points to treat for which symptoms or patterns. Once the correct points have been selected, then everything is supposed to right itself, so we almost never find descriptions in these books of what to do if it doesn't work. I find this approach rather unhelpful, even when such books are based on a traditional system of diagnosis and matched treatments. I find many of these books so theoretically driven that they are not typically rooted in clinical practice and are not structured to help the reader easily adapt to changing circumstances, ineffective chosen treatments or matching to the individuality of each patient. I wanted to avoid falling into the same trap with the book I wanted to write. I have also been concerned that too many practitioners think they can learn practical skills just from reading books. I know from my own ex-

perience that this is not realistic. Imagine learning to play the piano from reading books! Thinking about these problems I was delighted to find that my colleague Rayén Antón had worked in the media of film and editing before, so I found I was able to start this project with the plan that we could at least let people look at what is to be done, which is definitely better than simply reading about it. I believe the old adage "a picture is worth a thousand words" starts to cover this idea. Working with Rayén I have been able to complete this project. We both hope that the format and content of this text and DVD will sidestep the limitations I have worried about, will help to get more practitioners started in the treatment of babies and children, and will enhance the effectiveness of those who already treat them.

The first section deals with the origins and nature of the *shonishin* approach. It explores the origins of its approaches in the historical early Chinese literature and shows how these were adapted and adopted into Japanese traditional medicine several centuries ago.

The second section explores the nature of the physiological and treatment response differences of children with most adult patients. Principally it focuses on their innate increased sensitivity and the clinical implications of this in terms of dose and regulating the dose of treatment. It also describes how one can practically grasp and attend to these differences and, through palpatory feedback, continuously adapt treatment as it is being given to ensure proper clinical applications. It also describes the various treatment tools. Here I have focused on showcasing my private collection of *shonishin* tools organized along traditional ideas of treatment method.

The third section describes two basic forms of applying "root treatment" (Chinese "*zhibenfa*"), the principle purpose of which is to strengthen the body's natural healing abilities by helping regulate physiology. The first of these is the "non-pattern-based root treatment" system which is the core of the *shonishin* treatment method. This method, regardless of the child's symptoms and any "traditional patterns" of diagnosis, applies light stimulation in set patterns to the body surface using the tools described in the previous section. This approach targets an improvement of the vitality and mood of the child and through this a strengthening of the natural healing abilities. The second root treatment system is the "pattern-based root treatment" approach, a simplified form of traditional Japanese acupuncture called *Keiraku Chiryo* or Meridian Therapy. First I outline the use of this approach on adults and then its diagnostic and treatment modifications for children. This method focuses on regulating the *jingluo* (Japanese "*keiraku*") or channels while at the same time strengthening the child's vitality and natural healing ability. In actual clinical treatment, one can use only the Meridian Therapy root treatment approach, only the "non-pattern-based" *shonishin* treatment approach, or a combination of these two. It is also possible to teach the parent to do a simplified form of the core *shonishin* non-pattern-based treatment at home regularly. This is also described in this section and can greatly enhance treatment effects and speed up recovery time.

The fourth section describes symptomatic treatment approaches, the use of normal acupuncture treatment methods strictly adapted to the unique needs of children. This covers adapted forms of needling, moxa, retained dermal stimulation methods such as press-spheres, press-tack needles and intra-dermal needles, cupping and bloodletting. Point locations are also covered as needed both for the main root and extra symptomatic treatment points.

The fifth and final section of the book describes how to use all of the diagnostic skills and methods and treatment methods carefully selected in adaptable and evolving treatments for a number of different health problems. Most importantly I wanted this to be practical, thus many case histories are described. I received help from colleagues around the world who sent me some of their most inspiring cases. For each condition I give clinical example(s) of how the systems are used and a range of treatment ideas and suggestions for each condition, with details of how to select between them and what to do if they are not working. In this section I also describe treatment of underlying issues as well as specific symptoms. For example, there is a chapter on constitutional diagnosis and treatment, which is important when dealing with children with severe and complex health problems. Similarly there is a chapter on strengthening the vitality, which is the principle reason for applying a "root" treatment to begin with. But in some children, one can only focus on treating to improve the vitality so as to strengthen the natural healing ability, for example prior to surgery, so as to improve recovery afterward.

Nothing works on everyone. No system of treatment is ever fool proof. No single individual practitioner is free of limitations. We must start with these axiomatic truths to build a practical, adaptable, and responsive system of treatment. It has been my hope and intention in the writing of this book to keep these limits in mind while laying out strategies that allow the reader to develop a practical system that they can make work for them. I have placed a practical palpatory based understanding of qi at the heart of the treatment approach, which is natural given my teachers and training in Japan. I hope you find the book useful and stimulating.

Stephen Birch

Acknowledgments

As always, writing a book is not possible without the help and support of others. First, thanks to my family and friends for their support and understanding.

Second, this project is as good as it is because of the work and talents of my colleague and friend Rayén Antón who helped me with the structure of the project, all illustrations, and video work. Her assistance and collaboration have been invaluable. I feel fortunate to have worked with her and look forward to future projects.

Third, the contributions of my friend and colleague Manuel Rodriguez have been really helpful in this second edition. His creative thinking and down-to-earth approach is invaluable.

Fourth, thank you goes to a number of other people: Junko Ida for helping me with translations of the Japanese materials that provide the background for the materials organized and presented in the book; Josephine Haworth for help with editing of the text; my editor Angelika Findgott for her support and encouragement of the project, and her team at Thieme Publishers for their care and assistance; my colleagues Brenda Loew and Paul Movsessian, for their support and encouragement of the project, and Manuel Rodriguez for giving an extra hand; thanks to Michael Blanz of mb Film & Video and David Ferrando Navarro of Xochipilli Producciónes for their technical help with the video materials; to David Ferrando Navarro also for photography; to my teachers who helped me improve and deepen my skills, in particular Yoshio Manaka, Toshio Yanagishita, Akihiro Takai, Shuho Taniuchi, Koryo Nakada, Yukata Shinoda; to a number of colleagues listed here alphabetically who agreed to send me their cases to be included in the book: Rayén Antón (Spain), Mourad Bihman (Germany), Joke Bik-Nwee (Holland), Zoe Brenner (US), Marian Fixler (UK), Bhavito Jansch (Switzerland), Brenda Loew (US), Paul Movsessian (Australia), Diana Pinheiro (Portugal), Sue Pready (UK), Bob Quinn (US), Manuel Rodriguez (Spain), Dan Zizza (US)—their contributions add much to the book; to Hitoshi Yamashita who helped track down pictures in Japan, and to the Harikyu Museum, Osaka for permission to use these pictures; to Sayo Igaya for help tracking down historical information about *kanmushisho*; to Wolfgang Waldmann and the European Institute of Oriental Medicine, Munich for permission to videotape my workshop there in November 2008; to Stefan Maegli of Liestal, Switzerland and Hamid Montakab of the Academy of Chinese Healing Arts, Winterthur, Switzerland for permission to videotape my workshop there in February 2009; to the various children, parents, and students who participated in the workshops at these acupuncture schools, especially those who appear in the video; to Elias and his mother Hetty for agreeing to star in the video; to the original practitioners of *shonishin* in Japan several centuries ago who created this wonderful system; and finally to my patients for teaching me about healing and to their parents for helping with the treatments.

Finally, I dedicate this book to my son Nigel, for living this with me, and to my mother for making it all possible.

Section I   Overview and History

1 Introduction

The term *shonishin* (小兒鍼) is a Japanese rendering of the older Chinese term *erzhen* (兒鍼). It literally means "children's needle" or "children's needling." Acupuncture has been used for a long time on both adults and children; hence we find the term *erzhen* in the early Chinese literature. However, today the Japanese term *shonishin* refers to a tradition that dates from the 17th century. Although there is speculation about its precise origins and its development, its widespread use appears to have started in the late 20th century in Japan. Several practitioners, such as Yoneyama and Mori, who wrote a text entitled *Shonishin Ho—Acupuncture Treatment for Children* (1964), and Shimizu, who wrote an extended section on *shonishin* in a well-known Japanese acupuncture journal, *Ido no Nippon (Journal of Japanese Acupuncture and Moxibustion)* (1975), helped set the stage for a more widespread adoption of this method within the acupuncture community in Japan. This was further reinforced by the publication of articles about *shonishin*, pediatric acupuncture, by various other authors. Today, many acupuncturists treating children use these methods or variations of them in Japan. These methods started spreading outside Japan to the West by the 1980s, where further modifications began to appear.

I have used these methods in the treatment of children since 1982 and have played a role in introducing these methods in various regions in the United States, Europe, and Australasia over the past 20 years. This book is a culmination of having used and adapted these methods to a modern Western-based acupuncture practice over the past 30 years. This book is primarily a practical guide for using these methods to treat children, but it also briefly covers the history of and theoretical justifications for these methods.

In the West, the common styles of acupuncture are Chinese based and Western anatomically based. Both styles consider acupuncture to involve *only* the use of inserted needles. I have found that, because the methods of *shonishin* often do not involve the use of inserted needles, it is conceptually foreign to the acupuncturist trained in both Chinese and Western styles; thus it is not yet well known among the acupuncture community in the West. I have also found that many acupuncturists in the West are afraid to treat babies and small children because they have to insert needles, which makes pediatric acupuncture less popular overall than it could be. This is unfortunate because it is very effective, and children generally respond more quickly to treatment than adults. After teaching *shonishin* to acupuncturists in the West, especially in Europe, I have found that it often has a transformative effect on how those acupuncturists practice. Many feel able for the first time to treat babies and children, where before they had been afraid to. Sometimes remarkable results can be seen. In the United Kingdom, there is a saying, "The proof of the pudding is in the eating." Knowing that the reader will not take this at face value without evidence, I have consulted with several colleagues in Europe, the United States, and Australasia and asked them to submit their cases. The evidence will speak for itself. It is hoped that, after reading this book and going through the online content available on MediaCenter.thieme.com, so as to properly grasp the methods, readers will try the *shonishin* method themselves and understand the power of the system.

The treatment works, and it works well and quickly in many cases. This book focuses on practical, reproducible methods. The content available on MediaCenter.thieme.com also makes the materials covered more practical and reproducible. A more detailed description of conceptual and theoretical explanations will have to wait until a later time. This is a pragmatic system, the practice of which requires minimal theory. Readers are encouraged to think about how the treatment works after they have practiced it for a while and seen the often surprising results.

The historical, theoretical, and associated diagnostic sections are consequently relatively simple, short, and easy to understand. The bulk of the text is more practically oriented. It includes discussions on how to work with children, how to modify what one usually does as an acupuncture practitioner to treat babies and children, how to use the unique methods that arose in the *shonishin* tradition, and how to combine all of these to match the needs of each individual patient.

This book does not take a typical textbook approach by describing which points and techniques are good for which diseases or symptoms; rather, through varied case histories, it illustrates how to use the tools and methods described within to help patients. These cases are taken mostly from my own experience, but a number of them have been provided by colleagues worldwide who have been using the *shonishin* methods for their pediatric patients. To successfully treat infants and children, we have all found that it is necessary to be very flexible and adaptable. This material has been selected and presented in a manner that best illustrates and encourages such flexibility and adaptability.

The basic *shonishin* treatment method takes a very practical approach to treating babies and children, using a basic treatment methodology that does not require differential diagnosis according to traditional principles and methods. It does not have to differentiate the types of patterns that are found in, for example, traditional Chinese medicine (TCM) acupuncture using the language of *qi, zang fu*, channels, and so on. The characteristic treatment of *shonishin* is a "non-pattern-based root treatment." It is a simple, easy-to-apply general treatment on the surface of the body that is used for all babies and small children and many older children. This general treatment helps restore and stimulate the body's natural healing mechanisms, which is the goal of a "root treatment."

When treating adult patients, I mostly use the Japanese system of *Keiraku Chiryo* or Meridian Therapy (Shudo 1990), especially the Toyohari approach (Fukushima 1991) and the methods of Manaka (Manaka, Itaya, and Birch 1995) along with miscellaneous Japanese methods (Birch and Ida 1998). When treating children and babies it is hard to put all this information aside. Rather, it is natural to integrate aspects of these approaches along with the *shonishin* approach. For almost 25 years I have routinely combined selected aspects of these treatment approaches with the *shonishin* methods to treat babies and children. In particular, I combine a simplified form of Meridian Therapy and Japanese acupuncture methods along with the *shonishin* methods. This allows the application of a simple form of "pattern-based root treatment" according to the principles of Meridian Therapy and the addition of an expanded range of treatment methods to target symptoms. Thus this book will cover sufficient information to describe how to use these additional approaches and will give examples of the integrated approach that I use. I have taught this integrated approach for over 10 years throughout Europe and have found it is easily learned and adopted. My colleagues and I find it to be a very effective and flexible combination of treatment approaches.

Readers will naturally seek to integrate the new *shonishin* treatment system into their own practice, using at least some of the ideas and methods that have been learned on adults. Therefore, it is important to show how to do this. However, I do not use the common styles of acupuncture found in the West, such as some forms of Chinese needling or some forms of the Western anatomical approach, and so cannot illustrate specifically and through experience how to integrate *shonishin* with these methods. But, having taught many acupuncturists who primarily practice these styles (**Fig. 1.1**), it is my experience that, by illustrating the principles of treatment of children and babies and giving examples of how to integrate adapted forms of my usual (adult) acupuncture methods with the *shonishin* methods, this will be a useful guide for others on how to integrate their methods of acupuncture with *shonishin*.

Because there are several other texts available on pediatric treatments within the field of Traditional East Asian Medicine (TEAM) that describe the standard information on normal development, growth, and physiology of children, I will not repeat this information here; rather, the reader is referred elsewhere for that standard

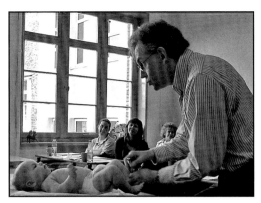

Fig. 1.1 Treating Pim in class.

information (in English, see Scott and Barlow 1999; in Spanish, see Rodriguez 2008). There are also many acupuncture books describing point locations, pathways of the *jing mai* (channels), functions, and so on of the *zang fu* (organs). For this basic acupuncture information, readers are referred to an appropriate text, such as Ergil and Ergil (2009) *Pocket Atlas of Chinese Medicine* and Hempen and Wortman Chow (2006) *Pocket Atlas of Acupuncture,* both also published by Thieme. For the most part, the system of *shonishin* is very practical and not very theoretical; thus it is not necessary to use so much of the information available in other texts. The history and diversity of acupuncture practices dictate the need for flexibility. Acupoints, for example, are not fixed anatomical structures; they are instead related to movement of *qi* in the body,[1] which means that they are found within a small region rather than at a fixed point. Further, the different traditions of practice have located many acupoints in different locations (Birch and Felt 1999). For the reader unfamiliar with Japanese traditions of acupuncture practice, some of the point locations in this book will, however, be new. Where appropriate, point locations are described.

---

[1]   This is discussed by Sivin (1987:51), Lo (2003:31), Lu and Needham (1980:14), and Birch (2014:193–202).

2 History and Theory

Shonishin for babies and very small children does not use regular acupuncture needles; rather, it uses a variety of tools that are tapped, rubbed, or pressed onto the body surface in a very gentle, noninvasive treatment approach. **Fig. 2.1** shows several typical tools used today, and **Fig. 2.2** shows photograph of tools in Hidetaro Mori's historical collection.

These tools do not incorporate needles; they are not inserted into the skin and thus not into acupuncture points. In fact many tools are applied over areas of the body surface rather than targeted to acupuncture points. **Fig. 2.3** shows areas of the body that are typically stimulated.

So what is the history of this method and what are the precedents for such ideas and methods? It is believed that *shonishin* began as a medical family treatment method in the Osaka area around 350 years ago. It takes little imagination to understand that the practitioners of that time would

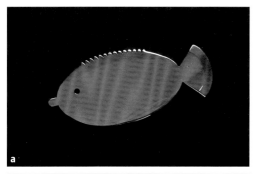

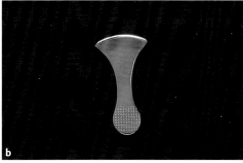

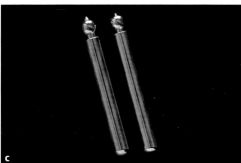

Fig. 2.1(a–c) Examples of modern treatment tools.

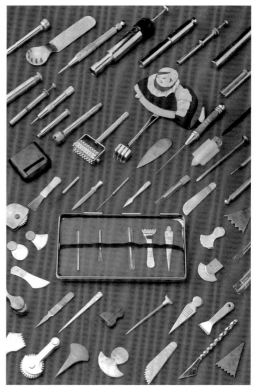

Fig. 2.2 Collection of modern and historical tools from Hidetaro Mori's collection at the Harikyu Museum, Osaka. (Courtesy of Mori H, Nagano H. *Harikyu Museum. Museum of Traditional Medicine.* Vol 2. Osaka, Japan: Morinomiya Iryougakuen Publishing; 2003. Special thanks to the editor Ms. Oda and to Hitoshi Yamashita for his assistance.)

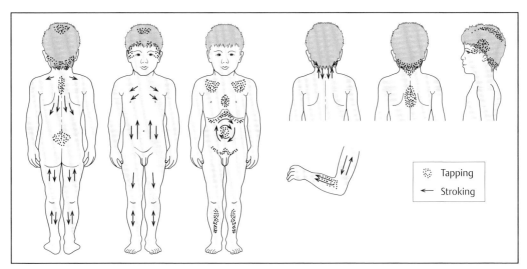

Fig. 2.3 The basic treatment map from Yoneyama and Mori (1964). Apply tapping techniques where there are dots and stroking techniques where there are arrows.

have had the same or greater problems than we have today, trying to insert needles into emotional, frightened, unhappy, resistant, restless, moving children. I say *greater* problems because needle technology was not at all as it is today; the needles available in the 1600s were significantly thicker and had a rougher surface than what is available now. Nobody enjoys treating children when they are crying, screaming, and resisting treatment. Thus, it is easy to understand why the developers of *shonishin* would have sought a different approach; one that would be more comfortable for the child and less stressful for the parents. The motivations for developing the system are clear.

Given this kind of motivation it is still necessary to understand how this approach developed by briefly discussing historical trends within the larger context of Traditional East Asian Medicine (TEAM). The term *TEAM* refers to all those therapies and approaches that arose in East Asia and were strongly influenced by the early Chinese medicine *qi*-based theory of systematic correspondence. It thus includes diverse practices, such as herbal medicine, acupuncture, moxibustion, cupping, bloodletting, and massage (Birch and Felt 1999). TEAM started in China and evolved there into many different strands and approaches. After spreading to neighboring countries, such as Japan, Korea, and Vietnam,

adaptations and new interpretations emerged from those countries. Today TEAM embraces the multitude of practice styles and treatment approaches that can be found throughout China, Taiwan, Japan, Korea, and their offshoots outside Asia, such as in Europe, the United States, and Australasia (Birch and Felt 1999). The commonly used system of traditional Chinese medicine (TCM) is a subset of the larger field of TEAM, representing a unique and broad combination of historical and modern methods and ideas.

Historically in Japan, medical texts were written in Chinese; thus literate medical practitioners in Japan read Chinese source texts for information about medical practice. When *shonishin* was developed (17th century) there were many texts and traditions of medical practice available to a literate practitioner. The first specialized pediatric texts in China and thus in Japan were, however, exclusively herbal medicine texts (Gu 1989). Given the fear that can be encountered using acupuncture on children, it is not surprising that the trend in China might have been toward using herbal medicines rather than acupuncture in pediatrics. This is not to imply that acupuncture, moxibustion, massage, and other such methods were not also used, but the dominant trend in Chinese pediatric treatments has been herbal medicine. The evidence for this is found in many modern TCM texts on pediatrics (Cao, Su, and Cao 1990). We can imagine that those who developed *shonishin* were not much influenced by these pediatric herbal texts: but why?

Before the sixth century, Japan was isolated and had little knowledge of China. After embracing Chinese ways, the Japanese of the day began a wholesale import of everything Chinese. The first medical texts were brought to Japan in 562 CE by Chiso (or Zhi Cong in Chinese), a Korean Buddhist monk (Birch and Felt 1999). At the time of this first appearance, Japanese practitioners were content to study and copy what these older Chinese traditions could teach them. Because the first medical texts from China were, by and large, acupuncture related or herbal medicine related rather than a combination of both, (though some early texts did combine them), it seems clear that the Japanese at that time began imitating this older tradition. From early on, acupuncture and moxibustion were taught and learned separately from herbal medicine (which one can say is a kind of homage to the ancients, who for the most part worked the same way). The first Imperial Colleges established in 702 CE taught acupuncture and herbal medicine separately in 7-year programs (Birch and Felt 1999, p. 23). This tendency for separation thus became the tradition.

Most acupuncturists in Japan have worked very little with herbal medicine, if at all, and vice versa. Although there were sections in earlier Chinese texts dealing with pediatric care, such as Sun Simiao's *Bei Ji Qian Jin Yao Fang (Thousand Golden Essential Prescriptions)* (ca. 652 CE), the first text devoted to pediatric treatment was the herbal text *Lu Cong Jing (The Fontanel Classic)* of the mid-10th century (Gu 1989). Additionally, the primary pediatric texts were dominantly herbal medicine texts, including the important and very influential *Xiao Er Yao Zheng Zhi Jue (The Correct Execution of Pediatric Medicinals and Patterns)* of 1107 (Gu 1989). Given these facts, it is highly probable that the literature specializing in pediatrics from China would have provided no assistance to those who developed the *shonishin* system. Not only because its treatment methods were inaccessible, but also because the diagnostic

methods and the theories of physiology and pathology needed for safe and effective herbal prescription would likely have had little utility as well. For example, tongue diagnosis developed within the domain of herbal medicine practices, and to this day, many acupuncturists in Japan do not use tongue inspection because it is thought of as being a tool used by herbal medicine practitioners.

Are there other ideas in the acupuncture-related literature that could provide a basis for treating children? After reading various texts and sources over the years I believe that the answer to this question is yes. I have found several ideas and descriptions that may well have provided the ideas and precedents influential for those who developed *shonishin*. Although it is not possible to provide a definitive answer to this question, the information described following here represents a potential, or at least a partial, explanation. To answer this question, my speculations are based on small pieces of evidence found in various sources.

First, the *Huang Di Nei Jing Ling Shu (The Yellow Emperor's Inner Classic Spiritual Pivot,* originally called the *Zhen Jing* [鍼經] or *Needle Classic)*, specifically Chapter 1, describes nine kinds of needles, only one of which is the regular thin filiform needle widely used today (**Fig. 2.4**).[1] Of these nine needle, two were explicitly described as round-headed "needles" that were to be pressed onto the body or rubbed along the surface of the body (the book *Japanese Acupuncture: A Clinical Guide* by Birch and Ida 1998, pp. 39–57, summarizes the historical descriptions from the *Ling Shu* and some modern ideas about the nine needles and how to use them).

The *yuanzhen* (Japanese *enshin*) was described as having a round head and was to be used by rubbing on the body—**Fig. 2.5** shows a modern form of the *enshin* from Japan; **Fig. 2.6** shows a historical image from East Asia of the *yuanzhen*. In each case one can see a similar image of the *yuanzhen* or *enshin* as having a rounded end. Likewise, the *shizhen* (Japanese *teishin*)

---

[1]   See the illustrations on page 40 of *Japanese Acupuncture* (Birch and Ida 1998) for various interpretations of what these nine needles look like.

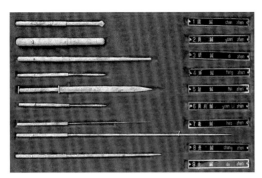

Fig. 2.4 The "nine needles" of the *Ling Shu*. From Hidetaro Mori's collection at the Harikyu Museum, Osaka. The filiform needle is number 7, third from bottom. (Courtesy of Mori H, Nagano H. *Harikyu Museum. Museum of Traditional Medicine.* Vol 2. Osaka, Japan: Morinomiya Iryougakuen Publishing; 2003. Special thanks to the editor Ms. Oda and to Hitoshi Yamashita for his assistance.)

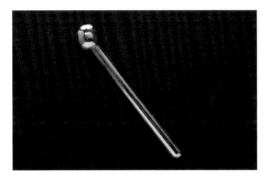

Fig. 2.5 Modern form of the *enshin* from Japan.

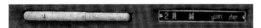

Fig. 2.6 Historical form of the *enshin* (*yuanzhen*). (See also different images in Birch and Ida 1998, p. 40.)

was described as a thicker needle with a rounded point, reminiscent of a millet seed, used for pressing the body surface. **Fig. 2.7** shows two modern *teishin* from Japan and **Fig. 2.8** a different historical image.

Another of the nine needles, the *chanzhen* (Japanese *zanshin*—literally the "arrow-headed needle") was described as having a sharp edge and was used for lightly cutting the skin (much like a paper cut). It does not penetrate the body; rather, it breaks the skin only. **Fig. 2.9** shows the arrow-headed point of the *chanzhen*. Although this instrument was intended originally to break the skin, various modern forms of it are used for

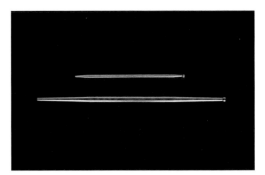

Fig. 2.7 Modern forms of the *teishin* from Japan.

Fig. 2.8 Historical form of the *teishin* (here called *dizhen*). (See also different images in Birch and Ida 1998, p. 40.)

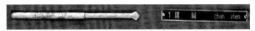

Fig. 2.9 Historical form of the *zanshin* (*chanzhen*). (See also different images in Birch and Ida 1998, p. 40.)

rubbing or scratching on the skin surface rather than breaking it. Today the *zanshin* has taken on a variety of forms in Japan. **Fig. 2.10** shows a typical shape for the *zanshin,* and **Fig. 2.11** shows a conically shaped version.

From this one can easily see a clear precedent for the idea of using hand-held instruments (interestingly called *zhen* [鍼], "needles") that could be used for rubbing, pressing, or scratching on the body surface, rather than penetrating the body (like the needles we commonly use today). It therefore seems likely that those who developed *shonishin* were influenced by these old ideas about needle types and needle methods and started experimenting with different constructions and surface stimulation applications.

What about the acupuncture points? Why is it that much of the therapy is targeted to regions of the body rather than the usual acupuncture points (as we tend to find in the treatment of adults)? Here it is easy to speculate, so I shall keep it short and simple. There is a very clear statement in the *Huang Di Nei Jing* (*Ling Shu,* Chapter 10) about how *qi* does not start moving and circulating in the *jing mai,* or channels (meridians),

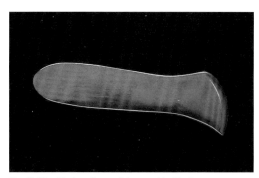

Fig. 2.10   Modern form of the *zanshin*-like instrument.

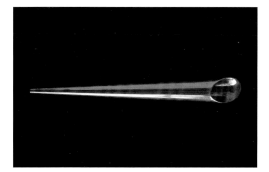

Fig. 2.11   Modern conically shaped form of the *zanshin*.

until after birth. *Ling Shu,* Chapter 10, describes the development thus:

> The Yellow Emperor said "[after] the person's conception, the jing is first composed. The jing composes the brain and bone marrow. The bones become the stem [the spinal column forms?]. The vessels become the ying [nourishment]. The muscles become firm. The flesh becomes [like a] wall. The jing is hard, and then the hair and body hair grow. [After labor when the] gu [grains] come into the stomach, the vessel-meridian pathways are [all] connected, the blood and qi [begin to] move."

This, of course, makes sense when one is familiar with historical ideas about the circulation of *qi*. One of the most important early ideas in acupuncture that has remained influential is that the *qi* circulates through the 12 *jing mai* or channels in a continuous circuit. It is propelled through the *jing mai* by breathing, moving 3 *cun* with each inhalation and 3 *cun* with each exhalation (*Ling Shu,* Chapter 15, and *Nan Jing*

[*Classic of Difficulties*], Chapter 1, are quite clear on this point [Matsumoto and Birch 1988, pp. 77–78]; see also Birch 2014, pp. 188–190). The lungs were seen as a kind of pump for the *qi* as a parallel to the heart as a pump for the blood. Since the *jing mai* have thus not yet started circulating the *qi* before birth—this circulation beginning only with the first breath after birth—one can imagine that this is not yet a well-developed system and could reasonably be thought of as being different from that found in an adult. Thus, in a newborn, the *jing mai* can be thought to be in an immature state. Further, we know that each *jing mai* was described as having intimate relationships with at least two internal organs, often being "branches" of those organs (Matsumoto and Birch 1988, p. 50). At birth, several of these organs have functioned little as well and exhibit considerable changes over the next few years as the child grows and matures. Thus the evidence about acupuncture points shows that they were not mentioned before the system of *jing mai* or channels had been described (Birch 2014). Rather, they were first described at the same time that the theory of *qi* circulation in the channels was proposed, and they are related to the movements of the *qi*, rather than to the underlying anatomical structures. Based on this, one can easily imagine that the acupoints start forming out of the developing *jing mai* or channel system. *Ling Shu,* Chapter 1, describes the nature of the acupoints thus: "At the articulations within the body there are 365 points of communication . . . 'articulations' refers to where the divine *ch'i* [sic] travels freely and moves outward and inward, not to skin, flesh, sinews, and bones." The translator of this passage, Nathan Sivin, continues: "A modern Westerner expects these points of communication, where the physician's needles can affect the circulation, to be places in tissue, but here we find them related instead to processes" (Sivin 1987, p. 51).

It is very easy to continue speculating here, but the point I am trying to make is that it is not unreasonable to think of the channels and their acupoints as being in less-well-developed states in babies and small children, and that at some time in the child's development they reach a state of development that makes them similar to those found in adults. There are other ideas and sources that support this idea. Li Shizhen is famous as the author of the seminal herbal medicine text, the *Ben Cao Gang Mu* (*Materia Medica*). He also wrote a small treatise on the extraordinary vessels, the *Qi Jing Ba Mai Gao* (*The Eight Extraordinary Vessels Examined*), ca. 1578. This places the text as predating the development of *shonishin*, but it is important for us here because Li Shizhen was a considerable scholar of older ideas. This text has been translated by Charles Chace and Miki Shima (2010). Of interest here is a short passage in a discussion on the origin of the extraordinary vessels. A Japanese colleague drew my attention to this passage as evidence for the immature state of the channels in babies and children and thus a theoretical reason that could have contributed to the development of *shonishin* (Kurita, personal communication, 1989). My crude translation of this passage renders it thus: "All people have these eight vessels. They belong to the *yin shen. They close and do not open.* Only the [Daoist] adepts can push them open with their *yang qi.* Therefore [by this means] they are able to grasp the *dao*" (Anon 1970; Wang 1990). Chace's more refined translation does not contradict the interpretation my colleague explained to me: "All people have these eight vessels but they all remain hidden spirits because *they are closed and have not yet been opened.* Only divine transcendents can use the *yang qi* to surge through and open them so that they are able to attain the way" (Chace and Shima 2010, p. 110). I have italicized the relevant line. *The eight extraordinary vessels are closed in adults.* My Japanese colleague speculated that, since before birth the 12 *jing mai* are similarly not functioning or are closed, instead, something else—the extraordinary vessels—had the function of helping regulate *qi* movement in utero. After birth the 12 *jing mai* start to function, and then, gradually, as they mature, they take over and replace the functioning of the extraordinary vessels. At a certain point (in most people) the extraordinary vessels would become closed while the 12 *jing mai* would take over the function of helping regulate *qi* movements in the body.

I am not saying this is correct, but rather that important historical ideas and passages have been interpreted as showing precedents to the notion that the channels and their acupoints are immature at birth and thus temporarily of a different nature until they reach a more mature state. Nor should the reader interpret that I am suggesting or supporting the use of the extraordinary vessels as a specialized treatment in pediatric conditions. First, there is almost no literature supporting this (i.e., there is little or no published experience of this idea). Second, Li Shizhen's notions and treatments of the extraordinary vessels differ greatly from the typical ones learned in the study of acupuncture using the eight treatment points (Chace and Shima 2010).

The foregoing ideas can be seen as purely abstract and speculative, but I describe them because they account for clinical experience treating children and seeing some of the different responses between children and adults. With adults it can be very important to be right on the point for the treatment to work. However, with babies and small children, it is usually enough to be at least in the right area using the right techniques timed appropriately. In this sense, I feel that acupuncture points in babies and small children are more likely to be very open spheres of influence rather than sharply defined loci.

It may well have been this kind of straightforward thinking about the nature of the acupoints, channels, and *qi* movements, coupled with experiments using different-shaped hand-held instruments found to have different effects, that guided those who developed *shonishin*. In the end we will probably never know, but this seems reasonable given the historical evidence and precedents.

There is one other historical influence on the development of *shonishin* that is relevant, at least for a part of its practice. In modern *shonishin* practice we still find the diagnosis and treatment of *kanmushisho*, related primarily to behavioral problems. What is this and where does it come from? There is an interesting history related to the development of diagnostic categories for children in China and ideas in Japan about normal development and problems before modern concepts of physiology had penetrated Eastern thinking, and the fusion of these two traditions.

Kanmushisho (疳虫証) or *Kannomushisho* (疳の虫証)[2]

The term *kanmushisho* or *kannomushisho* refers to a class of problems that manifest in childhood. The term comes out of a historical period when the concepts of different medical traditions were fused in the development of medical practices.

The term *mushi* (虫) refers to a kind of worm or insect that was thought to inhabit the body. There were thought to be many different *mushi* in the body, which influenced both normal and abnormal physical and mental functioning. An example of the "liver *mushi*" (肝虫) is seen in **Fig. 2.12**.[3]

The *mushi* concept comes from Japanese history several centuries ago, and had both lay and medical uses. Many older societies have had different concepts about entities inside the body that influence health and disease. Pictures of some of these *mushi* give them the appearance of different parasites, but others are more anthropomorphic; thus we cannot say they were based on observing parasites in the body. The text *Shin Bun Sho* (*The Book to Understand Acupuncture* [針聞書]) from the 17th century explains their use in a medical context, but they had lay uses as well, and various rites or ceremonies conducted by Buddhist monks were developed, some of which can still be found today.[4]

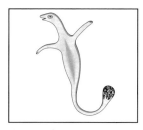

Fig. 2.12   Redrawing of the *kan no kanmushi* (liver *mushi*).

The term *kan* (疳) comes from the Chinese medicine tradition: the Chinese term is *gan*. It refers to a disease of childhood characterized by "emaciation, dry hair, heat effusion of varying degrees, abdominal distention with visible superficial veins, yellow face and emaciated flesh, and loss of essence-spirit vitality" (Wiseman and Feng 1997, p. 236–237). There are as many as 22 different *gan* associated with the internal organs and other structures and symptoms (Wiseman and Feng 1998), such as "spleen *gan*," "liver *gan*," "lung *gan*," and so on. Each has a different manifestation.[5] The concept of *gan* developed within the Chinese medicine tradition and came to be useful in pediatrics. As this tradition was absorbed into Japanese medical practices, it encountered the concept of *mushi*, which was in vogue at the time. The term *kan no mushi* (疳の虫) represents a fusion of these two different concepts of disease. At first there were several concepts in this fusion tradition, but the term *kan no mushi sho* (疳の虫証) is the only one that has survived and come down to us today. The term *sho* (証) means pattern.

The term *kannomushisho* has therefore come to mean the pattern of *kannomushi* disturbance. It is particularly associated with behavioral problems in children. In the infant the *kannomushisho* manifests as irritability, crying, screaming, and poor sleep. In the toddler the child has poor sleep, irritability, angry outbursts, and tantrums. In the older child the behavioral problems manifest usually as hyperactivity, but can also be the distracted child who has poor concentration at school. Shimizu describes his belief that in Japan the term *kan* came to represent children's diseases in a more general sense, and that the term *kanmushi* took on both a medical sense referring to earlier stages and more easily responding medical problems, as well as a lay understanding about stages of normal development in children. Hence, *shonishin* has also been used as a tool to assist in normal development of the child by

---

[2]   Thanks to Sayo Igaya for her assistance with this section. Ms. Igaya conducted research to investigate *kannomushisho* for her thesis as a student at the Toyo Shinkyu Senmon Gakko acupuncture school in Tokyo and offered invaluable help with this section.

[3]   For more examples see http://www.kyuhaku.com/pr/collection/collectionJnfo01–2.html; last accessed 14 October 2015.

[4]   Ms. Igaya showed me a short video of a ceremony she witnessed and the intriguing effects of the ceremony.

[5]   Reflecting Japanese uses and understanding of the concept of *gan* (Japanese *kan*), Shimizu (1975) describes how *kan* is commonly associated with bad mood, sleep problems, night crying, poor appetite, diarrhea, and cough, and the association of the five organ *kan* are listed as follows: "heart *kan*"—surprise *kan*; "liver *kan*"—wind *kan*; "lung *kan*"—*qi kan*; "spleen *kan*"—food *kan*; "kidney *kan*"— hasty *kan* (Shimizu 1975).

parents that followed this way of thinking (Shimizu 1975).[6]

Shonishin Today

In the modern period the practice of *shonishin* uses many tools. As we will see in Chapter 6, they can be largely classified around different stimulation techniques (tapping, rubbing, pressing, scratching), but they are also used based on personal experience and preferences. Each of us who practices *shonishin* has our preference for which instruments we commonly use. For the most part the instruments are made of metal, but there are precedents for the use of other tools, such as the claws of a mole (Yoneyama and Mori 1964, p. 15), and the plastic presterilized disposable *shonishin* tools that were created by Seirin. Some practitioners have had specific tools constructed, such as the *daishi hari* of Masanori Tanioka of Osaka (Tanioka 2001a, 2001b) (see **Fig. 2.13**). In this way, *shonishin* has exhibited changes over time, as new instruments are used. One of these developments began in the United States in the 1980s. It was here that I helped contribute to another new usage of *shonishin*.

Before World War II, there were several *shonishin* specialists, acupuncture practitioners who exclusively treated children with *shonishin*. Since the war, the relative number of such specialists has dropped considerably, and most acupuncturists who use *shonishin* do so as part of their practice (Shimizu 1975), some obviously more than others. In Japan the typical practitioners who use *shonishin* do so in their clinic, where they apply the treatment periodically on the child, who must return for additional treatments. Many practitioners in Japan tend to work from their home, living upstairs while working downstairs. Their clinics are often in or very near residential areas. As such, many of their patients will come from the local part of town where they live. In many clinics I visited in Japan, most patients lived nearby and walked to the clinic or arrived by a short ride. Thus a practitioner can ask the parent to bring the child back for daily treatment over the next few days, or regularly several times a week. This has been reinforced by the fact that in Japan many mothers stop going to work once they have children and are thus available to bring the child in for frequent treatments as needed.

Working in Boston in the United States in the 1980s I encountered an entirely different set of circumstances. For many pediatric patients both parents were working, the child was in day care, and the family lived within driving distance of the clinic. Scheduling the child for treatment involved dealing with two or three people's schedules (four if you added mine). I found early on that most parents were simply unable to bring their children in for treatment more than once a week, and even that could create a burden that made continuing treatment difficult. Thus I was faced with the problem of not being able to treat frequently or regularly enough. As we will see in the following chapters, it is important to make the clinical setting as easy and emotionally calm as possible for the child in order for the treatment to be most effective. When parents are very stressed, trying to coordinate short clinic visits, it can create the opposite effect. Thus I had to consider how best to deal with the need for frequent treatment.

The solution first offered itself when a mother called me from New York. Her daughter was almost 3 years old and had a problem with cerebral palsy. She had been looking for acupuncture treatment for her child and was willing to fly to Boston. Not only did the travel distances and costs make regular treatments unfeasible, but I

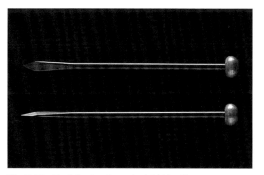

Fig. 2.13   Tanioka-family-style *daishi hari* instrument.

---

6   Wolfgang Michel, a medical historian writing in Thomas Wernicke's recent English language text on *shonishin*, gives useful additional information in an interesting historical overview of pediatric treatments in Japan (Wernicke 2014, pp.:12–30).

was about to leave for the summer for my first studies in Japan. My solution was to schedule to see the child, and to teach the parent an acceptable short form of the *shonishin* therapy to be performed daily at home. This was an immensely successful strategy (the case is reported in detail in Chapter 25, Case 1 Catherine). Then over the next few years, when I began seeing many 2- to 5-year-olds with ear infections (otitis media) that would recur upon completion of a round of antibiotics, I found I had to offer an alternative approach to allow for more frequent treatments. Weekly treatments were not frequent enough for this kind of recurrent problem. Thus I began routinely teaching parents to do some form of *shonishin* treatment, preferably daily, at home. With the success of these experiences, I have routinely taught home therapy as an additional component of *shonishin*. Many acupuncturists in Europe, the United States, and Australasia are familiar with this model. It is now being used by some practitioners in Japan as well. Home therapy approaches and rationales are covered in Chapter 8 and represent a very powerful addition to the whole *shonishin* treatment approach. My colleagues in Barcelona have written a book for parents about child care containing recommendations for home treatment. This includes simple *shonishin*-style treatments (Rodriguez and Anton 2008).

This concludes my very brief introduction to the history and development of *shonishin*. Much more can be said but the purpose of this book is to explain how to treat patients, thus I shift gears here and move to things of more clinical relevance.

Section II   Treatment Principles and Tools of Treatment

3 General Considerations in the Treatment of Children

Children are generally more sensitive to acupuncture treatment than adults; thus greater care is required as to choice of treatment, regulation of dosage, and method of application. Also, given their sensitivity, children respond very quickly to treatment, and assessment techniques are required to minimize the risk of overtreatment. Successful acupuncture treatment of children requires a thorough understanding of these issues. This may be one of the main reasons why many, if not most, acupuncturists do not treat children, or find it difficult.

To properly address these important issues, we need to examine the following:
- Ascertaining the appropriate dose for patients—and a model for doing so
- Understanding how treatment manifests in babies and children (0–18 years)
- Modifying treatment methods, so as to be able to regulate the dose of treatment delivered
- Continuously assessing changes in the patient to determine when sufficient treatment has been delivered, both regionally and globally
- Recognizing and correcting treatment overdose

Estimating the dosage and tailoring the treatment to individual patients involve several important diagnostic and therapeutic considerations. Selecting the correct root treatment pattern and the correct acupuncture points for treatment is important, as is obvious in any traditionally based system of acupuncture. Likewise, it is important to match the choice and application of treatment techniques to the diagnosis.

It is also important to understand the goals of root treatment: are they to effect a cure, or to help patients manage their problems? In some cases acupuncture treatment may be used primarily to help patients through a difficult process or to help them deal with difficulties, rather than being used to eliminate those difficulties. For example, if we are treating a patient with a complex condition, such as terminal cancer, our role

is primarily one of palliation and support of the patient. Likewise, if you treat a child who is about to undergo a complex surgical procedure so that the child can recover more easily and quickly from the surgery, there are no symptoms to focus on. Treatment focuses on supporting the patient through the process, using only some form of root treatment. However, given the fact that most acupuncturists work in ambulatory care private practice, most of our patients are not so ill and so we generally attempt to cure those problems that we see. The pattern chosen, the treatment points, and the treatment methods are fundamental parts of any traditionally based root treatment (this is discussed in Chapters 9 and 10 in relation to pattern recognition and treatment in Meridian Therapy). Additionally, it is important to select appropriate branch treatment or symptom control treatment methods and apply the techniques properly at the correct locations (point location is covered in Section 4 of the book). But an aspect of the clinical individualization of treatment that is not usually discussed, if at all, in most acupuncture textbooks is the issue of choosing the correct treatment dose.

It is very important to tailor treatment to match the needs of each individual patient. The descriptions in the following chapters are based on my studies with Yoshio Manaka, and especially Toyohari Association instructors, such as Kodo Fukushima, Toshio Yanagishita, Akihiro Takai, Shuho Taniuchi, Koryo Nakada, Shozo Takahashi, and Yutaka Shinoda, and refining these ideas through clinical practice. I hope in a later text to describe these same issues in more detail as they relate to the treatment of adults, where the issues can become more complex. It is essential to be able to adapt and apply the acupuncture treatment approaches described in this book on children who come to you for treatment. *If you do not understand the issues of dosage you are better off not treating babies and children at all.* The material described in the following chapters makes it possible for you to adjust your treatment to every child you encounter in clinical practice, and to arrive at effective treatments.

Chapters 4 and 5 focus on clinical issues involved in determining the correct treatment dose. This includes a discussion of reasons for lowering the dosage, requirements for particular patients, and reasons why some patients are more sensitive than others. This discussion also provides an overview of dosage judgment and how to modify and select appropriate treatment approaches and treatment techniques so as to match the dose to the needs of each patient. The chapters also discuss how to identify when a reaction to treatment might be due to a misapplication of the dose or the application of an inappropriate technique. These are often the same or related issues. If a child has a reaction to treatment due to overdose or application of less than optimal techniques, the child or parents may begin to lose their trust in you as their practitioner, and treatment may be stopped. Dealing with patient reactions to your treatment requires many levels of skills. First, you must be grounded and able to react through controlled emotions without defensive responses. Then you must also be practical enough and patient focused enough to recognize and correct the treatment so that the patient will continue receiving treatment without resistance (Yanagishita 2003). When correctly applied, the appropriate treatment is clinically more effective. Although this book outlines several useful ideas, understanding the correct treatment dose can be a lifetime endeavor (Kasumi 2003).

Chapter 6 describes the *shonishin* treatment tools, their methods of application, ways of adjusting dose in their application and finally some simple practice methods to help train the very light methods we use to adjust the doses of treatment.

4 A Model for Judging the Dosage Needs of Patients

The Therapeutic Dose—A Conceptual Model

In mainstream medicine, it is generally well understood that there is an optimal dosage range for a particular drug to be effective. The concentration of the drug in the blood should lie roughly between two values for it to be effective. Below the lower value, the drug is less effective or ineffective, and above the upper value the drug is in too high a concentration and can cause unwanted side effects or lead to a treatment overdose. This general idea is quantitatively based, where the optimal dosage range is often based on body mass and the upper and lower dosage ranges are numerical values. But it is possible to extend this idea to a more qualitative illustration of dosage needs—qualitative because there is no laboratory value to measure. We can make qualitative estimates of need only. The following ideas are extensions of explanations that Yoshio Manaka made about treatment dose in relation to the intensity of stimulation delivered (Manaka, Itaya, and Birch 1995, pp. 118–119). My teacher Dr. Manaka explained this to me as an argument for why one could say that "Japanese acupuncture" approaches were generally better than "Chinese acupuncture" approaches because Japanese needling approaches tend to be much gentler and milder than modern Chinese approaches.

Upon reaching the therapeutic dose threshold (TDT), a therapy starts having its expected therapeutic effects. If the treatment dose exceeds the maximum therapeutic dose (MTD), the patient may experience unwanted side effects due to overtreatment.

With a medication, the dose taken and the intervals between doses are often coordinated so that the medication's concentration in the blood remains in the optimal range—between TDT and MTD (**Fig. 4.1**). For an acupuncture treatment, this figure is interpreted differently. Two treatments, Y and Z, are charted. Both treatments start from point X. Treatment Y has a relatively high-intensity stimulation, the dose buildup is quicker than that for treatment Z, which delivers a stimulation of milder intensity. Y1 and Z1 are the times that treatments Y and Z cross the TDT, respectively, and Y2, Z2 are the times that treatments Y and Z cross the MTD, respectively. The time that the practitioner of treatment Y has to judge the correct dose of treatment is T1 (the distance between Y1 and Y2), whereas the time that the practitioner of treatment Z has to judge the correct dose of treatment is T2 (the distance between Z1 and Z2). Because T2 is larger than T1, we can say that the risk of reaching treatment overdose is less with treatment Z than with treatment Y. It is therefore easier and safer to administer treatment Z. Hence, Dr. Manaka argued, the milder needling approaches represented by Z are better than the heavier needling approaches

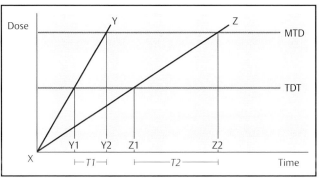

Fig. 4.1 Dose levels for normal sensitivity patient with different intensities of treatment (Y, Z). TDT, therapeutic dose threshold; MTD, maximum therapeutic dose.

represented by Y, where Y, figuratively speaking, represents modern Chinese needling methods and Z modern Japanese needling methods.

This model is an oversimplification. For example, in homeopathy the lower the physical dose of treatment (the more diluted), the higher the therapeutic dose (energetic). Manaka hinted at these things with his X-signal system model of acupuncture (Manaka, Itaya, and Birch 1995, pp. 118–119). A lower intensity form of acupuncture (as physical stimulus) is not necessarily a lower treatment dose because, at very low energy content (very low intensity stimulus treatment), the more the treatment's energy level approaches or approximates the energy level content of the physiological systems, the more it could be therapeutically active (i.e., the less the physical stimulus, sometimes the stronger the signal system mediated therapeutic effects). See Manaka et al (1995) for a detailed discussion of this idea. But, for the purposes of the model here, if we assume that within the context of a particular treatment model the foregoing graphical representation of the treatment doses is applicable, then it is possible to illustrate what happens with sensitive patients.

After learning this basic model from Manaka I gradually extended it to incorporate patients with different dosage needs. The following is a model that I developed and that appears to work well for understanding what happens with "sensitive" patients.

The Sensitive Patient

A sensitive patient will typically show two characteristic differences compared with the typical patient. First, the TDT drops and can be very low, meaning that it takes very little to trigger change. Second, the width of the optimal dose range narrows considerably; once the TDT is crossed a very slight increase in therapeutic treatment can cross the MTD. Of course, it is possible that the sensitive patient may be very healthy, in which case the TDT is very low and the MTD is high, so that the optimal therapeutic range remains very wide. These are the ideal patients, for whom very little treatment is required to trigger healthful effects and for whom one can do a lot more without any adverse effects. These patients are, in my experience, very rare. Most sensitive patients who show the lowered TDT also show a lowered MTD and thus have a low optimal dose range. This can be seen graphically in **Fig. 4.2**.

If treatment Y from **Fig. 4.1** were administered on this sensitive patient, the time to judge proper dose, T1, is very small, and an overdose of treatment is hard to avoid. Even treatment Z, which has a lower intensity of treatment, would be difficult because T2 is also very small. One has to administer a treatment that is extremely low dose, has a very low intensity, and is mild and gentle: treatment A, if one wants to have any chance of avoiding overdose of treatment on this patient. Here the time to judge treatment dosage (distance from A1 to A2), A3, is much larger than T1 or T2. The use of a very low intensity treatment allows the dose to build up much more slowly, so that one has more time (T3) to make the clinical judgment to stop treatment. This idea is important and is clinically very helpful.

It is necessary to assume that *all* children, even teenagers, fit this profile of the sensitive patient. Certainly, all babies and smaller children fit this profile, but even older children can.

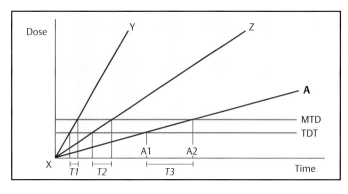

Fig. 4.2 Dose levels for the very sensitive patient (child) with different intensities of treatment (Y, Z, A). TDT, therapeutic dose threshold; MTD, maximum therapeutic dose.

Thus, at least until one has evidence to the contrary, one should approach even older children as being more sensitive. The next section discusses how to adjust techniques to increase or decrease dose and how to match this judgment to each individual child.

Explanations of Increased Sensitivity

There is a long-standing tradition in Asia that addresses the need to regulate one's emotions. This is an important theme in Confucian, Daoist, and Buddhist thinking. The early medical literature in China followed this theme when it discussed how all emotional expressions represent some kind of disorder of *qi* movement or function in the body, and classified several common emotions in relation to the primary organs (*zang*) in the body (Chiu 1986; Matsumoto and Birch 1988; Unschuld 2003; Birch, Cabrer, and Rodriguez 2014b). These dominant emotions were said to injure their corresponding organ, and each was described in relation to particular *qi* disturbances. The emotions were discussed in relation to health problems. In larger social discourse, the ability to manifest correct behavior and help regulate oneself is necessary to regulate one's emotions. In fact, emotions were not only seen in relation to *qi, all* emotions were defined as or thought to be some *disturbed* movement of *qi*, whether excessively or mildly expressed (Birch et al 2014a). Thus anything that we can do to help control emotional expression can be helpful if our goal is to regulate the *qi* of the patient.

Babies are unable to talk. Instead, they express themselves via their emotions. Of course, we see different manifestations of this: a liver-related expression is an angry one that manifests with a lot of explosive crying and an inability to settle, whereas a kidney-related expression is one of jumpiness, of fearful reactions. But the important issue is that babies and small children have no ability to regulate their emotions. Communication in babies and smaller children is achieved by emotional expression. Thus, in babies and small children, many forms of normal healthy communication can trigger disturbances in *qi* movements and functions in the body. This has immediate consequences: it

tends to make babies and children very sensitive because their *qi* is easily changed involuntarily. Thus one of the goals of treatment is to try not to cause the child emotional distress. As therapists we are trying to help regulate the *qi* of the patient, but if what we do causes emotional distress so that the child starts crying and becomes very upset, this can counter the effects of our treatment and can trigger unexpected reactions. Further clinical implications of this for the treatment of babies and children are discussed in Chapters 17 and 21.

This same issue holds for all children, even teenagers. Sometimes a 4-year-old child can be "very mature," being more in control of his or her emotions than other children of the same age, and it is easier to deal with such a child. Conversely, a 15-year-old may be a physically well-developed child who is emotionally very unregulated and thus "immature." It can be difficult to deal with such a child, who is unable to control his or her responses. The 4-year-old can handle things better than other 4-year-olds, whereas the 15-year-old cannot handle things well in comparison to other 15-year-olds. This becomes apparent in the responsiveness to treatment and how one handles the child.

I will provide various examples of this later, showing how, with a good understanding of this, one can demonstrate treatment effectiveness in how one approaches and deals with the child, and with how one adjusts one's treatment techniques. For example, below the age of 5 we prefer not to have to insert any needles, but beyond the age of 5 we start to think about how and whether we need to insert needles. This is a double-edged idea. On the one hand, needling is frightening, and thus potentially more distressing to a more immature (younger) child. On the other hand, needling is a bigger dosage than the standard *shonishin* techniques described following here; thus it is more difficult to control the treatment. However, there are always exceptions—the emotionally mature 4-year-old can (with good needling techniques) handle being needled better than the immature 15-year-old.

There are several consequences of this for application of treatment with children. First of all, *try not to upset the child during treatment.* This requires attention to several details. Take time over the course of treatment to make sure that the child is comfortable with you and what you are doing. Don't try to force things unless it is necessary. The therapeutic relationship is very important in acupuncture treatment, especially with children. Some children will immediately like you and what you are doing; others take time to develop trust, especially if they have been chronically ill and have seen many health care providers or have had many treatments. It is thus advisable to take the time over the first treatment to make sure that the child is settled, comfortable with you, and not frightened by you. This has to do with your manner and behavior, and also with how you apply your treatment techniques—how you handle the child. Thus we modify how we apply treatment techniques so that they are not distressing, and we try to choose only those techniques that can be applied without upsetting the child. One pediatric specialist in Japan even recommends not making eye contact with the child during treatment because babies and small children can be easily frightened. Although this last idea can be useful with some babies and small children it is not always advisable. There are some with whom it is better to maintain eye contact to help them feel secure and comfortable.

When we apply techniques that could be distressing, such as inserting needles, we do it in such a way that the child does not feel pain or discomfort. Likewise, if one needs to bleed a *jing* point (which is not often required) it needs to be done in such a way that the child feels nothing and sees no blood. This requires the use of needling techniques that are guaranteed to be painless and sensationless. Such methods of needling are discussed in Chapter 15. A consequence of this basic rule is that we have to be careful how we choose to apply some of our treatment techniques. It does not help to try negotiating with a small child who is frightened of needles. First, get discreet permission from the parent, and then needle in such a way that the child cannot feel or see what you have done. With older children this can be trickier. The example of George shows the successful needling of a 6-year-old.

Besides the difficulty with regulation of emotions, there are other causes of the increased sensitivity we see in children. The more ill a patient is the more sensitive he or she becomes.

Example

George had been having problems with repeatedly catching colds and having prolonged periods of bronchitis over the last year. He had tried homeopathy but the current episode of bronchitis was not clearing up, and the symptoms of coughing, congested lungs, and disturbed sleep had been ongoing for a few weeks. He agreed to come to try acupuncture only because he had been promised that "Steve will never insert any needles in you." A typical 6-year-old with these symptoms will usually benefit quickly from a few strategically inserted needles, but this was not an option. For the first visit, the task was to make sure that he liked what was being done and that it was comfortable and not frightening. I applied a simple version of the non-pattern-based root treatment described in Chapter 7. I found hard knots around BL-13 on both sides, and left press-spheres[1] on these points.

He came back a week later and there had been some improvement in his symptoms, albeit slight. He was still very wary about the needles and nervous that I might insert some. I repeated the treatment at a slightly higher dose. He returned a week later, with a further slight improvement in his symptoms, but this time he was more settled with me and less worried that I was going to use needles on him. After doing the basic treatment, I turned my back on him while I prepared a 3 mm-long intradermal needle held with tweezers. I turned to him, putting the tiny needle in front of him and asked "Is it alright if I insert this in your back?" He laughed and replied "You can do what you want with that!" I then inserted two intradermal needles at the knots at left and right BL-13, giving instructions to his mother on how to care for them. When he returned for treatment a week later the coughing, lung congestion, and sleep were much better. He took his clothes off, threw himself onto the treatment bed and said "Needle me!" After this I could

---

[1] There is much more information in Chapter 12 on using press-spheres, but, briefly, the press-sphere, or *ryu*, is a stainless steel ball bearing usually no bigger than 2 mm in diameter. It is secured to a circular piece of tape that can then be pressed onto the skin. In Japan, the press-spheres are placed mostly on body points that are particularly sore and are retained for a maximum of 3 to 4 days.

use a larger variety of treatment techniques to help him fully recover, and to help make sure that the next colds would not linger on as chronic bronchitis.

This means that, in very ill children, it is better to do minimal treatment—even less than usual. Examples given here describe how even the usual low dose of treatment for some children can be too much and can trigger overdose reactions when a child becomes additionally ill with, for example, a cold. I can speculate on why the more ill a patient becomes the more sensitive. Very likely this involves an increased emotional sensitivity. Parents will tend to agree on the observation that when their child is poorly he or she is usually more emotional and more emotionally needy and cries more easily. Thus, when treating a very ill child, it is better to do less. It may seem counterintuitive at times, but it is a better strategy to do less at first while you determine over time what the child can tolerate and what range of dosage is better.

The more run down and weakened a child is, the better it is to do less treatment. Thus, when treating a child after an acute infection like bronchitis, where the child has been ill for 2 weeks with fevers, coughing, antibiotics, poor appetite, poor sleep, and loss of weight, do less treatment at first. Similarly, the child who has had an acute gastrointestinal disturbance with repeated diarrhea will be in an acutely weakened state, so do less treatment.

I would also like to speculate that an additional reason for the increased sensitivity of children, especially smaller children, is that their physiology is accelerated compared with that of adults. Children are continuously growing and require an accelerated physiology to support this. Hence we see a more rapid heart rate, more rapid breathing, and so forth. Because everything is in a more accelerated state we can also see a quicker response to treatment. This makes it necessary to use lower doses of treatment, to do less, to trigger the same degree of change that we trigger in an adults using larger doses of treatment.

5 Assessing Changes, Recognizing and Correcting Problems of Overdose

Traditional texts instruct us to gather information through the primary senses to assess a patient and decide what treatment to apply. The "four diagnoses" are the primary modes of information gathering, and among these some of the information is very malleable and sensitive, showing changes very easily and quickly. The color and complexion of the patient can be observed to change quickly so it is reassessable while you are applying treatment. A lusterless complexion can become visibly more lustrous during treatment. Sometimes this is very clear, and the parent as well as you will notice it. But at other times the changes in complexion are subtle, and the lighting source can make them difficult to observe. A more useful and reliable indicator of change is the palpable texture of the skin. With proper training, one can observe this in adults, and it can be very useful. However, with babies and children it is an essential and indispensable observation because the surface of the child's body changes more easily and quickly than that of an adult, and the changes are literally quite palpable and obvious with only a little training. Besides, we direct much of the treatment on babies and children to the skin, the surface of the body.

Palpating the Skin of Babies and Children

To palpate the surface of the body on babies and children we need to be confident and calm. Use the palm of the hand and the whole palmar surface of the fingers. Touch very lightly so that your hand does not cause a depression in the skin. Apply simple touching and light stroking methods. MediaCenter.thieme.com shows the methods of touching and examining changes in skin condition. In general, the skin texture changes in the area one is working on and should be monitored continuously. When change is seen, move on

to the next area. Touching is applied quickly to match the application of the tapping or stroking techniques (which are also applied quickly—see Chapter 7).

The signs of improvement in the skin condition are evidenced by the following changes in skin texture: it becomes springier, a feeling of soft fullness develops, and it may become slightly warmer. If the skin had been dry, it might feel slightly less dry.

A sign of overtreatment is the skin starting to feel moist. One must pay attention to the earliest signs of increased moisture and not wait until the skin pores are quite open and the skin becomes obviously damp or the area starts sweating.

Reactions to Overtreatment

Sometimes a patient returns to us following a treatment or a parent calls to report that there are difficulties. For example, symptoms are worse, new symptoms have occurred, or the child has been behaving badly or has been much more tired than usual. Our job is to figure out what happened and correct it if possible. Signs of overtreatment must be distinguished from the following:
- Improper treatment
- Healing reaction to treatment
- The natural course of a disease
- Reactions that have little to do with your treatment but are due to lifestyle issues of the patient

As one can imagine, this is sometimes complicated and difficult. To understand when reactions are likely to be due to overtreatment, it is necessary to briefly discuss when reactions are due to these other factors.

The most common sign of overtreatment in children is that the patient is more tired. This tiredness can last for the rest of the day, in which case it is not so bad and may just be a normal healthy reaction to treatment. If it persists into the next day and especially beyond, you can suspect that you overtreated the patient. On a couple of occasions I have seen young babies become "floppy" for a while following treatment, where they were so relaxed the muscles were acutely and temporarily hypotonic. This did not last long, and although it may be distressing to the parent at the time, it is not a bad sign, merely indicating that you should do less treatment next time. The more common reaction is seen while the child is still with you in the treatment room. He or she becomes quieter, less active, even falls asleep. As you observe this process starting, you know to do less and less for the rest of treatment, and possibly less on the next visit. As mentioned, unless this state of lessened activity persists for extended periods, it is not a problem but is an indication of the probable need for more careful dose regulation. On a few occasions, treatment has led to the child falling asleep and having to be carried out of the treatment room, which can be inconvenient for the parent.

Sometimes overtreatment can lead to increased activity. Usually this is not a problem, but on occasion it has been. On two occasions, despite trying to be careful, first-time treatment of young (5- to 6-year-old) hyperactive children has triggered acute bouts of increased hyperactivity, which were not only stressful in the treatment room but created a period of prolonged hyperactivity that was very difficult for the parents to handle. This is not common, but it can happen. Thus I recommend on a first visit with hyperactive children being even more careful than usual about stimulation levels and dose. Sometimes parents will report on a next visit that they had difficulty getting the child to sleep during the week since the last treatment. This is most likely due to overtreatment, and you need to look carefully at what you did and make appropriate modifications as a result. Typical causes of this kind of reaction are the objects that you leave as mild continuous stimulation of points, such as press-spheres (see Chapter 12) and especially intradermal needles. Not using these things on the next treatment, or leaving them in place for much less time, is usually enough to stop the reaction. Sometimes this type of reaction to treatment can take a couple of sessions to adjust your approach sufficiently. These can be very complicated clinical cases to handle.

There are atypical reactions to overtreatment, as may be seen in the example. They usually depend on the condition of the child as to how they manifest. The following is a rather extreme example of overtreatment. It is not at all common to see this, but I describe it to illustrate that reactions can be quite severe, even though you appear to have done an extremely light treatment and find it hard to believe it is possible to cause reactions like this.

Example

Dianne, a 4-year-old girl with Rett syndrome with the main symptoms of autism, mental development problems, structural and postural problems, and instability (see Chapter 25 for her case study), had a severe reaction to overtreatment. Progress had been good and she was handling treatments well. However, she missed an appointment due to a bad cold, and when she came the next week I misjudged her condition (which was weaker than usual due to the cold). Her reaction to overtreatment was a fear reaction that made her unable to take a step. After she was lifted off the treatment table she would not move. It was necessary to lift her to dress her and then to carry her to the car. This persisted for several days, which was very distressing to her mother. After I acknowledged what had happened and explained why, her mother was happy to continue. With appropriate treatment modification, the effects were improved, and this never happened again. Dianne's strong and prolonged reaction was specific to her disturbed neurological condition.

You must always be honest both with yourself and with the parents about these circumstances. Becoming defensive is a sure way to make the parent lose confidence in you. One of my teachers, Toshio Yanagishita, goes so far as to say that you must accept responsibility for anything that happens after the patient leaves your treatment room (Yanagishita 2003). This is not such an extreme idea, but is more about how you present yourself to your patients. It is an expression about your mental attitude and focus.

In the following sections I discuss how to modify the dose of treatment with the root treatment approach, different techniques, and the symptom-targeting treatment techniques. Details of how to avoid and compensate for overtreatment will be covered in each relevant section.

As a general rule, *when you first see a patient for treatment, don't do too much treatment, keep it very light and simple so it is easier to figure out what to change if there is some reaction to your treatment.* If you at all suspect that the child is even more sensitive, then do not leave anything (e.g., a press-sphere, or an intradermal needle) on the first visit.

■ Incorrect Treatment

It can be difficult to distinguish causes of children's bad reactions to treatment. In general, it has been my experience that applying the wrong techniques or wrong treatment (rather than too much of the right treatment) only worsens the child's symptoms. For example, in Chapter 7, where the various surface-stimulating root treatment methods are described, the dominant methods are those of light tapping and light stroking. The stroking technique is contraindicated for patients with skin conditions like eczema or atopic dermatitis. On one child whose main symptoms were asthma, the rubbing techniques that were applied started irritating and increasing the small patches of eczema. As the asthma symptoms improved gradually the mother realized that the skin condition was worsening. This can happen in the atopic patient anyway, but I realized that we should use only tapping instead of rubbing, and I switched techniques. The eczema symptoms immediately started improving, while the asthma remained improved. Although this was a mild, and in the end, quite successful case, it is an example where the technique of treatment was discovered to be inappropriate for the patient.

I have over the years also figured out that the tapping technique is better avoided or minimized on children with problems of hyperactivity. It does not cause problems in many chil-

dren, but it can increase the risk of causing problems, and I feel it better to minimize or avoid the risk. This is discussed in Chapter 21.

■ *Meng Gen*—A Healing Reaction

Chinese medicine has the concept of a healing reaction—the *meng gen*. It doesn't seem to happen very often, and most schools of Traditional East Asian Medicine (TEAM) therapy rarely explore it or mention it only in passing. If this *meng gen* reaction should happen, why does it occur and how would it manifest?

In simple terms we can consider that most patients are in a stable state in which symptoms are occurring. We have an idea about a different state that they could be in, where they would have fewer or no symptoms (our diagnosis and root treatment usually target a return to that more ideal state). Our treatment tries to move the patient's system from the current, not-so-healthy stable state, to a healthier stable state. However, the body of the patient thinks that its current state is normal so it resists this change and tries to maintain the status quo. Sometimes this process of resistance triggers some reaction to treatment, such as a worsening of symptoms. A second explanation is that the treatment succeeds in pushing the patient's system out of its unhealthy stable state, but not yet into the targeted healthier stable state. So it stops for awhile in a different stable state in which new symptoms arise or old symptoms recur.

The typical sign that a *meng gen*–type reaction has occurred is that the worsening of symptoms, occurrence of new symptoms, or recurrence of old *symptoms lasts no longer than 24 hours* and is then *followed by a clear and prolonged improvement in symptoms* compared with the level of symptoms before the treatment was given (**Fig. 5.1**).

Usually this improvement is long-lasting (days, weeks) but sometimes is only short-lived (a couple of days). This short-term worsening followed by improvement can be a clear pattern, but parents can be confused about it, or they may call you as the symptoms develop or worsen. It is not advisable to make any judgments about it too quickly. To understand if this is indeed what has happened requires a longer-term look at the pat-

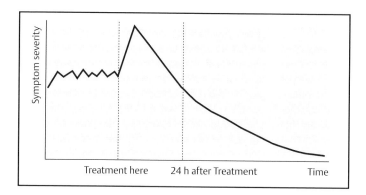

Fig. 5.1 Example of *meng gen* symptom intensity changes following treatment.

tern of changes. If the parent calls on the day of a treatment to say that things are worse, it is often impossible to know what is really going on. It may be better to advise to wait until the next day and see if things have settled down. If the parent calls the next day and things are still bad, with no sign of settling down, and it is more than 24 hours since the treatment, you can start to suspect that it is not a *meng gen* reaction and that something else is going on, perhaps a wrong treatment, or more likely an overtreatment. In that case you may want the patient to return to see if you can help. If, for example, you have left an intradermal needle, press-tack, or press-sphere on the patient you can instruct the parent to remove it. If this triggers an improvement in complaints you can then suspect that the intradermal needle, press-tack, or press-sphere was an inappropriate treatment method (which is occasionally the case) or that it created an overdose of treatment (a much more likely explanation). This helps you to understand that the patient is more sensitive than you had thought, and that you should be more careful about the use of that technique in the future.

However, if a patient returns the next week for treatment and reports a short-term worsening or development of symptoms immediately after the treatment, followed by a clear improvement, without having called you about it, it is easier to understand what may have happened. With the time frame of a week you can see the pattern of changes more clearly.

A cautionary note on this topic: I have had a few patients who have some form of brain damage or neurological problems (such as the 4-year-old girl, Dianne—see earlier example) where the reactions to treatment are more prolonged than 24 hours. It is even more difficult in these cases

to distinguish between *meng gen* and overdose of treatment. My recommendation is to always approach such cases as an overdose reaction, and adjust your treatment accordingly.

Modifying Treatment Methods to Regulate the Dose of Treatment and Deliver Treatment Successfully

If, while you are working on a child, your continuous palpation of the areas you are working on reveals changes, albeit very subtle ones, you can start to understand that the area you are working on may be "done." Once you recognize this, stop working on that area. Sometimes it is hard to feel these changes; they can be very subtle. You may be treating an unusually sensitive child, and things change much more quickly than you imagine they might. In this case, despite your continuous monitoring by touching, you are beginning to overtreat the area. Stop working on that area the moment you notice this, and assume that the child may be more sensitive than you had previously thought. Consequently, when you go to work on other areas with stroking, tapping techniques, and so on, first, you will be even more attentive and focused on feeling change, and, second, you should be automatically applying less treatment to those regions. This is a very interactive process. Many things may be happening during treatment—the child is moving around, resisting, crying; a sibling keeps trying to interfere or play; and you are continuously dancing around the child to stay ahead of his or her reactions arms you would have been less focused on trying to sense or extend your senses, but would have done so either neutrally, not so much focusing on what you feel, or with an idea in your mind that you are trying to change the forearm so that you can feel changes when you repalpate. This exercise is about training your ability to sense or observe subtle differences and subtle changes in skin texture. The next exercise is to help train you to learn how to touch neutrally, trying not to influence or change things. This is important because a very sensitive patient can start responding to your touch even when you didn't mean to create changes so it is important to train this neutral touch to minimize this possibility. Also, when you palpate on babies and young children, they are often not still and your touch is applied not in a static on–off mode but in a moving or sliding mode. This movement, whether applied deliberately by you or as a result of patient movement, has the potential to create change—thus again the importance of training the neutral touch.

Exercise Two

Palpating and trying not to create changes as you palpate requires attention to two additional issues: First, what is your internal difference when you palpate and try not to create change versus when you palpate and try to create change? Second, by what measure can you evaluate this?

You can apply the touching and stroking in the same manner described in the first exercise but we need to look at what you are doing that might or might not create change and what to do to monitor or observe if things change.

Practically speaking, both of these aspects feedback to each other, so I describe two methods together by which you can evaluate what is happening and at the same time monitor what was involved.

Obviously applying touch and feeling whether there is a change or not can be applied, but this is more useful if you have another person also apply the palpation while you do the touching with intention to create change or not. Another less direct, but perhaps more practical, method is to look at how the radial pulses change. In my recent book on *qi* and the channels (Birch, Cabrer, and Rodriguez 2014a) we describe a series of exercises in the last chapters. Palpation of the radial pulses for feedback and two exercises using it are described (Chapter 10, pp. 457–466). You can feel the radial pulse during or after you apply the palpation method or a colleague can feel the radial pulse while you palpate. The key to doing this and getting the more useful feedback is to monitor basic pulse qualities of depth, strength, and speed and see how those change. If there is no or minimal change in the depth, strength, or rate of the pulse as you apply your palpation, you are not creating any meaningful change as you palpate. If, however, the depth or strength or rate of the pulse change as you palpate this tells you that you are creating change with your palpation. By practicing repeatedly and varying your focus, attention, intention, or, more generally, your inner approach as you do the palpation trying to create and trying not to create change, you can see which helps create change or no/minimal change and then try to both remember what was involved and what it felt like. Studying repeatedly with simple techniques like this allows you to accelerate the rate at which you learn to feel the subtle changes in the skin condition that can occur and learn to detect them more easily and quickly. This allows you to refine your diagnostic assessment, your treatment techniques, and your judgments about dose of treatment.

6 Basic *Shonishin* Treatment Tools

Over the centuries many different tools have been developed and used in the practice of *shonishin*. **Fig. 6.1** shows tools in the author's collection.

One can see that there is a wide range of different stimulation methods possible with these tools. There are four types of stimulation techniques:

- Tapping
- Stroking or rubbing
- Pressing
- Light scratching

Some of the instruments seen in **Fig. 6.1**, and in the figures later in the chapter, can be used in the application of more than one of these four methods of stimulation; thus some of the different tools are mentioned in more than one of the technique classifications.

It is natural to wonder why there are so many different tools, even within each of the four categories. There are a few possible explanations:

- A particular tool was developed by an individual and came to be a hallmark of that person's approach. This unique tool then fused into the general trend of *shonishin* practice, possibly inspiring others later to develop tools that look similar or have a similar function.[1]
- Some creative people designed many different tools, and *shonishin* integrated this creative element within its general practice.
- Practitioners have found it useful to have more than one instrument in each category because this can reduce emotional reactions in particular children. For example, after one picks up a tool and the child cries in fear after seeing it, one shows the tool more closely to the child, which does not reduce the fear; one then picks up another tool that does not provoke the reaction in the child; this allows one to proceed with treatment.

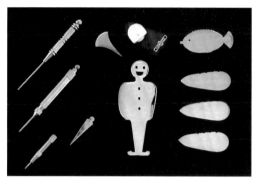

Fig. 6.1 Examples of different *shonishin* treatment tools.

Of course we don't know, but I can easily imagine at least one of these three factors influencing the overall development of treatment tools within the *shonishin* tradition. The last explanation is actually a practical strategy regardless of whether it is a potential explanation for the variety of available tools.

This chapter discusses the different types of tools and how to handle them. Chapter 7, The Core Treatment Model, and Section 5, Treatment of Specific Problems/Diseases, discuss how to use the different tools in the context of the root treatment and the branch treatment.

Tools Used for Tapping

Fig. 6.2 shows a range of tools that are used for applying the tapping technique. **Fig. 6.3** shows the tools that are usually easy to obtain from suppliers and which the author has found easy to use.

One of the characteristics of the tools used for tapping is that they have some kind of a point on them. But some of these pointed surfaces are a little sharp; some are quite sharp. It is thus important to know how to hold the tool so as not to cause pain or injure the child. Generally it is easier to hold the tool out of sight. The pointed end or edge is held between the index finger and thumb of the right hand (if the practitioner is right-handed). The instrument

---

[1] Mr. Tanioka uses such a tool; see Tanioka (2001a) and Wernicke (2009).

Table 6.1   Dose regulation with tapping technique

Dose/factor	Location of pointed end	Number of taps[a]	Weight of tapping
Higher dose	Point held level with or slightly protruding beyond end of finger and thumb	More	Slightly more
Lower dose	Point held slightly behind the level of the finger and thumb	Fewer	Less, barely touching the skin

[a] The number of taps on a body area will also vary depending on whether one is using only the tapping method for the root treatment or using only a little additional tapping along with the rubbing methods for the root treatment, or whether one is targeting symptoms and tapping a whole area or a single acupoint.

be more uncomfortable for the patient, thus provoking unnecessary and unwanted emotional reactions. The methods of holding and applying the tapping technique are discussed further at MediaCenter.thieme.com and in Chapter 7.

After estimating the amount of stimulation you want to apply you should hold the instrument so as to give less (point held slightly retracted) or more (point held slightly protruding) stimulation. You then tap the region you are working on the estimated number of times required, additionally modifying the weight of the tap. The dose is thus adjusted according to the scale outlined in **Table 6.1**.

It is generally a good idea to briefly apply tapping with the instrument on yourself, for example on the back of the hand. This allows you to quickly see how it feels and whether your attempt to adjust the dose through how you hold and tap matches the level you are attempting to use on the child. When it matches you can immediately go on to applying the technique on the child. If not, you can readjust what you are doing.

Tools Used for Stroking/Rubbing

Fig. 6.4 shows the range of tools used for applying stroking or rubbing techniques. **Fig. 6.5** shows the tools that are usually easy to obtain from suppliers and which the author has found easy to use.

The tools used for stroking or rubbing come in two varieties. The first (**Fig. 6.5a**), which is used for stroking or rubbing, has a rounded, ball-like surface. The second (**Fig. 6.5f**) has an elongated flatter surface that is either rounded or straight and smooth, both of which are used only for stroking. I use the term rubbing to refer to a back-and-forth *rubbing* of the skin surface,

whereas *stroking is applied in a single direction*. This is an important distinction because, based on the treatment principles outlined earlier, it is useful to apply stroking only in a downward direction, as this helps direct the *qi* in this direction. In babies and small children this is often a very helpful tactic (see Chapter 7 for an explanation). Not only is stroking very gentle and soft and therefore easily received by the child, the ability to direct the *qi* makes it a very useful technique. Many practitioners, such as my colleague Brenda Loew in Seattle, generally use almost exclusively stroking techniques rather than stroking and tapping.

Like the tapping tools, it is often helpful to keep the instrument out of view of the child, in which case it should be held within the right hand (if right-handed). MediaCenter.thieme.com provides various examples of how to hold these instruments for stroking so that as one strokes or rubs with them they are out of view of the patient.

How one holds the instrument and which instrument one uses can apply different doses to the region worked on. For example, when using the rounded ball instrument, allowing the rounded end to protrude slightly out from the surface of the palm can apply an increased dose. Holding the fingers of the stroking hand in such a way that the instrument is cushioned within them, and then stroking with both fingers and the instrument can apply a lower dose. This is illustrated at MediaCenter.thieme.com.

If one is using the flat surface instrument, such as the *chokishin*, stroking with the long, flat surface generally gives a little more stimulation and thus a higher dose than stroking with the narrower, rounded end.

After estimating the amount of stimulation you want to apply you should hold the

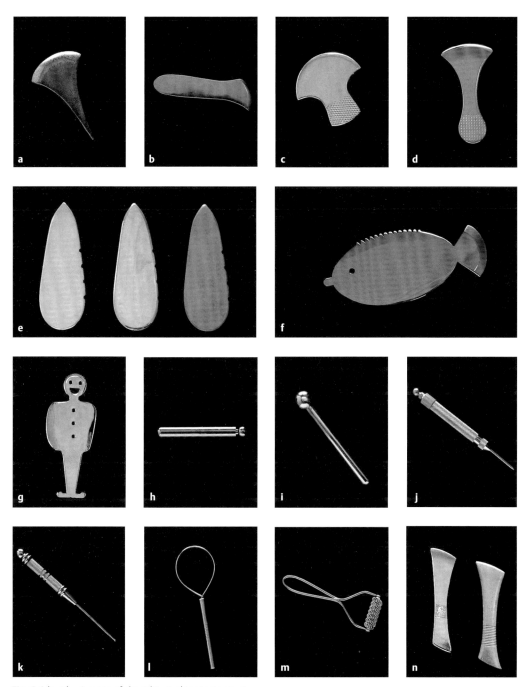

Fig. 6.4 (a–n)   A range of *shonishin* stroking instruments.

instrument so as to give less or more stimulation. You then stroke the region you are working on with the number of required strokes, addition-ally modifying the weight of the contact. The dose is thus adjusted according to the scale in **Table 6.2**.

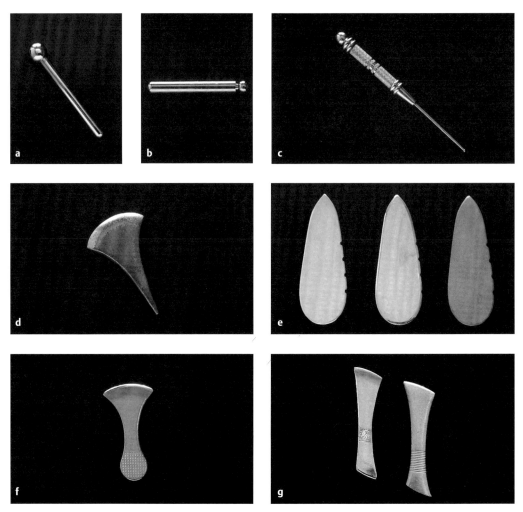

Fig. 6.5   The author's preferred *shonishin* stroking instruments. **(a)** *Enshin*, **(b)** small *enshin*, **(c)** round end of spring-loaded *teishin*, **(d)** *yoneyama*, **(e)** *chokishin*, **(f)** *bachibari*, **(g)** *choto*.

Table 6.2   Dose regulation with stroking/rubbing technique

Dose/factor	Placement, width of the instrument, and angle of contact	Number of strokes	Weight of contact
Higher dose	Rounded-ball instrument held level with the fingers	More	Slightly more
	Long, smooth edge		
	Greater angle to the skin		
Lower dose	Rounded-ball instrument held within fingers	Fewer	Less
	Smaller round edge		
	Smaller angle to the skin		

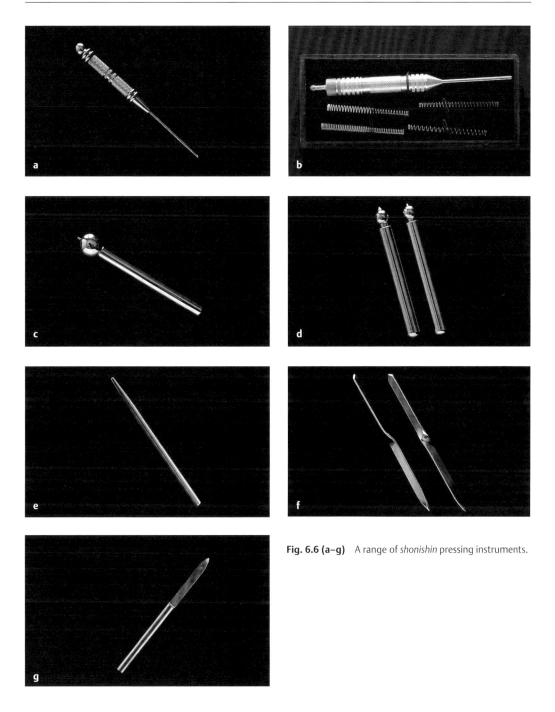

Fig. 6.6 (a–g) A range of *shonishin* pressing instruments.

Tools Used for Pressing

Fig. 6.6 shows the range of tools that can be used for pressing the skin at specific acupoints. **Fig. 6.7** shows the tools that are usually easy to obtain from suppliers and which the author has found easy to use.

Tools that are used for pressing have a small, rounded end that is pressed perpendicularly to the

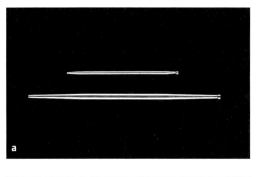

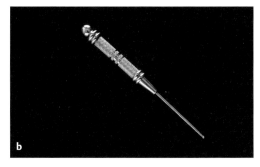

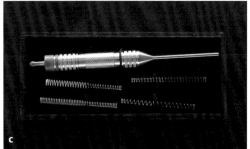

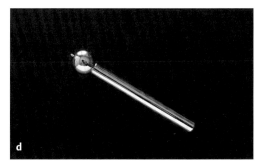

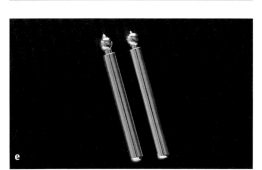

Fig. 6.7   The author's preferred *shonishin* pressing instruments. **(a)** *Teishin*, **(b)** spring-loaded *teishin*, **(c)** *tsumo-shin*, **(d)** small *enshin*, **(e)** *enrishin*.

skin. Usually the pressure applied is light. Although the skin is slightly depressed by the pressure of the instrument, it should not cause discomfort for the child and certainly not pain. If one is using the spring-loaded *teishin*, it is important that the spring inside is not too hard. The author has purchased several different spring-loaded *teishin* over the years: some have extremely stiff springs inside that render the instrument useless for treating children and babies. In such cases, the spring can be replaced with a softer one or it can be cut it in half and elongated; this usually makes the spring softer, but not always. The Japanese spring-loaded *teishin* was invented by Keiri Inoue, one of the founders of *Keiraku Chiryo* (Meridian Therapy). The spring inside this instrument is suitably soft.

A more recent alternative is the *tsumo-shin*, which comes with a variety of springs so that you can adjust the pressure. For babies and children, use the softest spring. If using the spring-loaded *teishin* or *tsumo-shin*, one can either press the point and hold the mild continuous pressure or bounce the instrument slightly, making sure not to let the varying pressure cause discomfort. In Chapter 10, Pattern-Based Root Treatment, I describe how to use the soft spring-loaded *teishin* or *tsumo-shin* for applying the tonification/supplementation technique and the draining technique. For these techniques, the method of using the instrument is somewhat different from when simply stimulating a point to target symptoms (like LI-4 for teething). I will not discuss those differences here.

These are thus very useful instruments to possess if one wants to apply the pattern-based root treatments of Meridian Therapy.

If using one of the other instruments for pressing the point, it can be a good idea to hold the instrument between the index finger and thumb of the right hand (if right-handed) and let the other fingers of the right hand also touch the skin. It is not only easier to keep the instrument out of sight of the child, but the child will often feel your fingers more than the instrument, and this is usually easier for the child to tolerate. See MediaCenter.thieme.com for illustration of this.

Adjusting the dose of stimulation for simple point pressing is brought about through adjusting the pressure applied, the length of time the pressure is applied, and, if using the bouncing method with the spring-loaded *teishin*, the number of bounces, as shown in **Table 6.3**.

The descriptions in **Table 6.3** relate only to the use of pressing on the body surface, usually at specific acupoints, to stimulate that point to help target symptoms. This does not relate to the use of pressing as part of the root treatment.

Tools Used for Scratching

Fig. 6.8 shows a range of tools that are used for applying the scratching technique. **Fig. 6.9** shows the tools that are usually easy to obtain from suppliers and which the author has found easy to use. The scratching technique is a form of stroking but with a greater dose of treatment. When done correctly it is very light and generally does not leave light red marks on the skin. The author does not use this technique so much, and you need to be careful of the following issues if you wish to use the technique:

- Make sure that you are clear about the needs of the child you are treating. If the child is more sensitive, it may be better to avoid the scratching technique. If the child is a more "excess" type and can tolerate stronger stimulation and higher doses, then be careful of the following two points:
- Don't overapply the technique, and especially not until you see strong red lines appearing on the skin. Not only can this be a sign of possibly having given too much stimulation to that region, but sometimes parents complain afterward if the marks don't disappear quickly.
- To understand how well you have applied the technique, pay special attention to monitoring the condition of the skin with touch and visual inspection. Also make sure that the technique does not seem to be causing any distress to the child.

When applying this technique over small areas, such as along the index finger to stimulate the large intestine channel and the points in that area, such as LI-2 and LI-3, it is easier to use, for example, the rough edge of the spring-loaded *teishin*, the *yuko* instrument, or the *kakibari*. When applying the technique over larger areas, such as down the back, the indented surface of the *chokishin* is the easiest to use, and it gives a milder stimulation. Otherwise the rollers and needle brush are good to use.

Needle Sets

In Japan one can purchase sets of *shonishin* tools, usually in sets of seven or nine, in a metal case. **Fig. 6.10** shows an example of these sets. You may find it helpful to have such a set at hand in your practice. The various instruments included in each set cover the range of techniques described

Table 6.3 Dose regulation with pressing technique

Dose/factor	Nature of instrument and number of bounces with spring-loaded instrument	Pressure applied	Length of time applying pressure
Higher dose	Rounded instrument with point More bounces of instrument (e.g., 10–20)	Slightly more	Slightly more (e.g., 10–20 s)
Lower dose	Rounded instrument only Fewer bounces of instrument (e.g., 5–10)	Less	Less (e.g., 5 s or less)

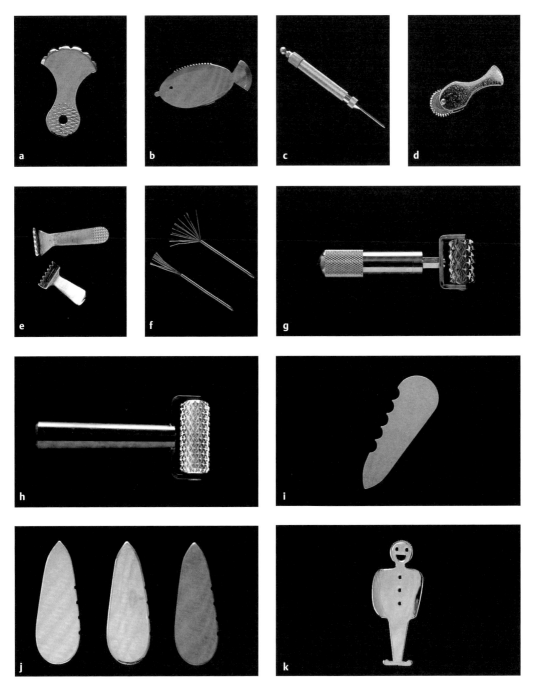

Fig. 6.8 (a–k)   A range of *shonishin* scratching instruments.

here: tapping, rubbing, pressing, and scratching, with more than one instrument that can be used for each technique. Some of the sets include instruments that are difficult to purchase singly, at least outside of Japan. It is not necessary to have such a set, but you may find it useful.

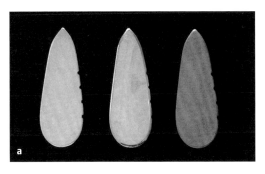

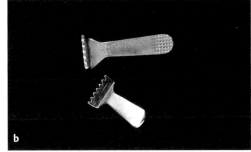

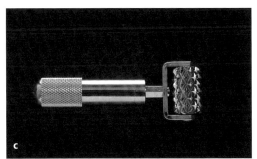

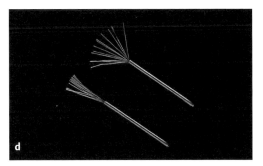

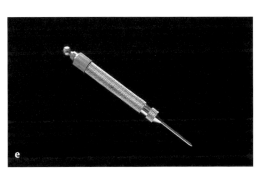

Fig. 6.9 The author's preferred *shonishin* scratching instruments. **(a)** *Chokishin*, **(b)** *kakibari*, **(c)** rollers, **(d)** needle brush, **(e)** rough edge of large *yukoshin*.

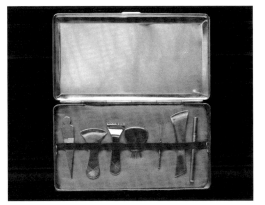

Fig. 6.10 Typical boxed set of *shonishin* instruments.

Most Recommended Tools

Fig. 6.11 shows those tools that are usually easier to obtain and should form the foundation for one's *shonishin* treatment tool kit. These tools usually have more than one application, as summarized here:

Tapping: *herabari/heragata, yoneyama, chokishin*
Stroking: *yoneyama, chokishin*, round end spring-loaded *teishin, enshin*/small Korean *enshin*
Pressing: spring-loaded *teishin/tsumo-shin*, small Korean *enshin*, point of *enshin*
Scratching: *chokishin*, edge spring-loaded *teishin*

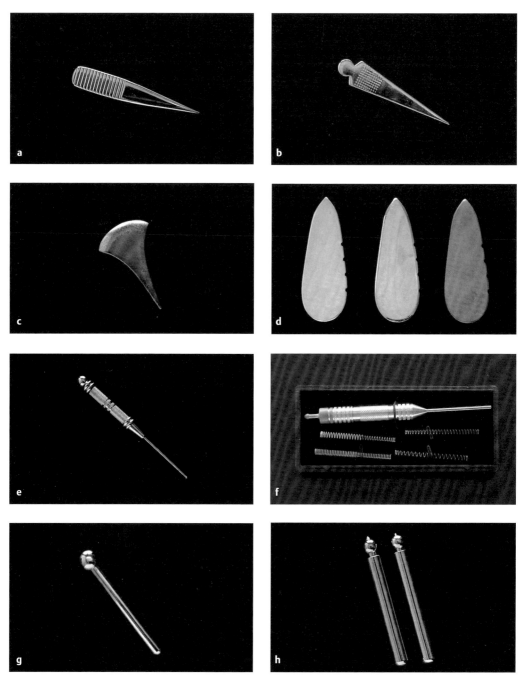

Fig. 6.11 A set of basic *shonishin* treatment tools. **(a)** *Herabari*, **(b)** *heragata*, **(c)** *yoneyama*, **(d)** *chokishin*, **(e)** spring-loaded *teishin*, **(f)** *tsumo-shin*, **(g)** *enshin*, **(h)** *enrishin*.

Thus, with only a few tools one can start applying all of the treatment. Through practice you will develop your personal preferences for which tools and which techniques to use.

Care of the Tools

None of the instruments pierce the skin and thus they do not need to be sterilized before use. However, they do need to be kept clean. They can be cleaned with rubbing alcohol before and after use. Sometimes a small child will get hold of one of the instruments and place it in his or her mouth before you or the parent can intervene. If this happens it is good to wash the instrument with soap and water, and when dry, clean it by rubbing with alcohol. Obviously some of the instruments are dangerous for children to place in their mouth because they are a little sharp, or they are small and could be swallowed, so when using one of these instruments, such as the *herabari*, always make sure that it is placed out of the child's reach when not in use.

Disposable Tools

In the 1980s after pioneering the disposable needle, the company Seirin started manufacturing disposable *shonishin* tools. **Fig. 6.12** shows the two tools that were available. There appear to have been several purposes for these tools. They come presterilized in a sealed container and were intended to allay fears of cross-infection. Each instrument has all four treatment techniques built into it: a flat edge for stroking, a bumpy edge for scratching, a rounded end for pressing, and either a blunt-needled end or a pointed end for tapping.

When these instruments first appeared in the United States in the 1980s I found them especially useful to give to parents for home therapy. They were not very expensive and were easy to replace, whereas the regular *shonishin* tools not only cost more but are often hard to replace when lost. The instruments were also unused and sterile when first given to the parents, which they seemed to appreciate. I will discuss tools used for home therapy in Chapter 8. Unfortunately, these disposable

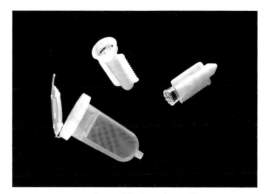

Fig. 6.12   Seirin's disposable *shonishin* tools.

instruments are now unavailable. I have not seen them in the United States or Europe for a long time and they are no longer available in Japan. It seems that the public fears that were triggered with the rise of AIDS and HIV infection in the 1980s, which triggered the development of the disposable single-use needles, is no longer carried to noninserted instruments like the *shonishin* tools. In the 1980s, in that climate, it was thought to be a good idea for public relations to present disposable single-use *shonishin* tools. But time has passed, and with it the accumulated experience and greater knowledge of the risks involved.

Treatment Applications

The instruments that are described in this chapter are used for both root and symptomatic treatment. Chapter 7 describes the use of stroking/rubbing and tapping tools for the "non-pattern-based root treatment." Chapter 10 describes the use of the spring-loaded *teishin* or *tsumo-shin* and the *enshin* for Meridian Therapy "pattern-based root treatments." Section 5 describes the use of the various tools, especially tapping and pressing tools for targeting symptoms.

Monitoring and Assessing Treatment Effects

As mentioned in the previous chapter, when you apply the tapping technique, if your other hand is free, you can regularly touch the area you are working on to monitor for changes in the condition of the skin. This can be done continuously while you are tapping or stroking. When stroking, your free hand can follow the treating hand alternately. When tapping, you can move your free hand over the area you are working on as you tap other regions within that area.

Often when working on a leg or arm area, you need to secure the limb with one hand while you apply the treatment techniques with the other. If tapping, you can apply several taps, then quickly touch with the same hand to see how things feel, apply more taps, then recheck again, and so on. While doing this, you keep hold continuously of the limb to keep it extended, unless the child starts to become very resistant and shows an emotional reaction to what you are doing. If this happens you need to let go and move on to another area, coming back to finish working on the first area later. This "dance" of the treatment is discussed again in Chapter 7, The Core Treatment Model. If you are holding the limb with one hand while applying the stroking method, you can hold the instrument carefully in such a way as to be able to use the finger of that hand to monitor changes as the instrument and hand pass over the treatment areas. Content available on MediaCenter. thieme.com shows how to hold the round and flat-edged instruments so that the finger and edge of the hand are free to stroke behind and monitor changes.

The techniques discussed here are illustrated at MediaCenter.thieme.com, both in the relevant sections and in the clinical examples. It is advisable to watch these portions to make sure you have a good clear sense of how to touch, hold the instruments, apply the instruments, monitor the changes, and so on.

Recommendations of Methods to Practice and Improve Your Tapping and Stroking Techniques

It is a good idea, especially as you are learning and starting to use this core non-pattern-based

shonishin root treatment, to practice and refine your techniques. This can be especially important given how sensitive pediatric patients can be. There are two basic approaches that can be recommended.

■ Practicing on Friends or Colleagues

Organize to meet with a friend or colleague who is willing to let you apply the stroking and tapping techniques. The person should lie or sit on a surface with arms, legs, abdomen, and back exposed so you can palpate and work on them.

Before you start applying the techniques, examine the basic pulse qualities of depth, strength, and speed. Pay attention to whether the pulse seems a bit floating or sinking, whether it feels hard or soft, and whether it is a bit rapid or slow. It is good to do this because as you apply the techniques these basic pulse qualities can change to give you some feedback about what you are doing. For example, if the pulse is felt to be a little floating, rapid, and hard before you apply the techniques, when you start to apply them you can feel the pulse start to soften, sink, and slow down, which is a clear sign of improvement. Similarly, if the pulse is generally deeper, softer, and rapid, after you apply the techniques effectively it will be less deep, less rapid, and less soft. These changes are relatively easy to feel on most people, but on some it will be less clear, but regardless of how easy it is to feel the changes on your friend, it is worth examining to see if these changes have occurred. These same pulse changes can be felt as you apply the pattern-based Meridian Therapy root treatment (see Chapters 9 and 10). On babies and small children these are difficult to feel, but on older children they are much easier to feel, so this can also help for practicing pulse monitoring with that root treatment method as well.

You should also lightly palpate the skin over the yang channel surfaces of the arms, legs, back, and abdomen, where you will be applying the stroking and tapping. Pay attention to the sense of thickness of the skin, the sense of firmness of the subcutaneous tissues, the sense of tension/looseness of the skin, the sense of dryness/moisture of the skin, and the relative temperature. All of this can be felt with very light touch (not pressure) and by light touch or stroking of the hand over the area. When you touch you can touch with only the pads of your fingers, but better to touch with more of or the whole of the palmar surface of the hands and fingers. As you apply the tapping, and especially the stroking, over these areas these often quite subtle feelings of skin texture and other factors can change. On a child these changes are generally easier to feel, but by starting to practice on your friends, you can train yourself to start feeling these subtle changes more readily.

Application of the Tapping Technique

Apply this to a few areas or acupoints to see what the reactions are. Around GV-12 and CV-12 is good, as is LI-4. Check the skin texture over and around the area where you tapped and then see if the basic pulse qualities have changed. It is also good to instruct your friend to give feedback. You can vary the extent to which the tip of the instrument contacts the skin, so that it should not be felt, it should be felt very slightly, or it should be felt more obviously, but not painfully and too sharp. You can ask how well the person's feelings of what you did matched what you were trying to do. This is good to practice with a variety of different tapping instruments so that you can get used to using the different instruments.

Application of the Stroking Technique

As you apply this technique, make sure that you apply the stroking on the same areas and in the same directions that are indicated in Chapter 7 in the non-pattern-based root treatment. You can vary the number of strokes on each region and the relative weight or pressure of contact of the stroke, and you can do it with or without your other hand following up behind to monitor the changes as you apply each stroke. With the stroking it is generally easier to feel skin changes and pulse changes. You can deliberately apply the technique more firmly to see how that feels and how the skin responds. You can also apply the stroking many times over the same area and see how the moisture of the skin may change (overtreatment can lead to slow opening of the skin pores, which slowly increases moistening of the skin).

When you practice like this on friends you train not only the application of the techniques of treatment but also the ability to observe how the tissues and body respond to what you are doing. The following additional practice methods were developed by my colleague Manuel Rodriguez to give other forms of feedback for your training of *shonishin* treatment.

■ Practicing on an Inert Surface

Buy some soft plasticine or modeling clay. The clay usually comes in a block. Keeping the clay in a block place it on a hard flat surface like a wooden board. With your fingers and then with a metal instrument like a spatula, smooth the surface so that it has no depressions or bumps on it. When you apply light pressure to this surface it should show a slight depression where the pressure was applied. Once flat and smooth this surface can now be used for practice of both tapping and stroking.

Using typical kitchen aluminum foil, cover the surface of the clay block, carefully smoothing the foil so that it lies smoothly over the surface of the clay (**Fig. 6.13**). The foil acts like a fine skin over the clay that allows you to perceive the differences between lighter and slightly heavier contact with both stroking and tapping.

Tapping

With the tapping, your contact should be very light and comfortable, so that the tips of the finger and thumb make very light contact; the other fingers of the tapping hand may also make a light and springy contact. To test this apply tapping without holding an instrument on the surface and do not cause any depression in the surface. Then repeat with slightly more contact so as to cause a very slight depression, and so on. **Fig. 6.14** shows the slight depression that might occur with this light tapping. Repeat the same tapping on yourself to see what it feels like.

Now repeat this holding an instrument like the *herabari* and apply the tapping. Always first apply the tapping on yourself to check what dose of tapping you are applying.

- With very low dose tapping, the instrument contacts the skin with no feeling at all of sharpness, and usually you hardly feel anything

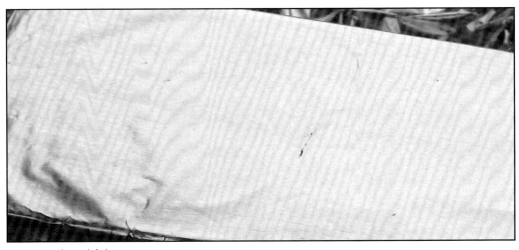

Fig. 6.13 Clay with foil.

except the finger tips. When you tap on the foil/clay surface, your tapping leaves tiny, low depressions in the foil, but when you look at the clay underneath, there are no obvious depressions in the clay (**Fig. 6.14a**).

- For slightly more dose tapping you allow the tip of the *herabari* to protrude slightly more, with tapping on the skin; you may be very slightly more aware of the instrument, but it is still not sharp. When you tap on the foil/clay it will cause a slightly deeper depression in the foil and there will appear very slight depressions in the clay (**Fig. 6.14b**).

- With slightly more dose tapping, you feel the instrument more clearly but it is still not felt as sharply. The tip of the instrument can be seen very slightly beyond the end of the tips of the finger and thumb. When tapping on the foil/clay it will cause not a small depression but a small hole in the foil, more obvious depressions will appear in the clay.

If the instrument protrudes too much from the fingers, the tool is felt to be sharp on the skin. There will be obvious holes in the foil and clear holes in the clay. This is how *not* to apply the tapping (**Fig. 6.14c**).

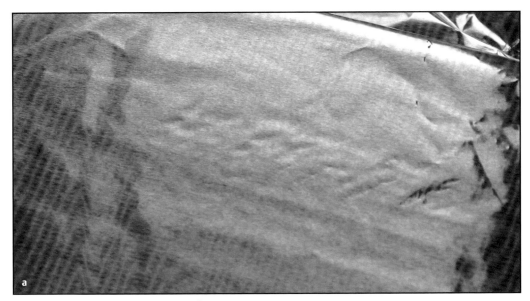

Fig. 6.14 (a-c) Doses of tapping. (*Continued*)

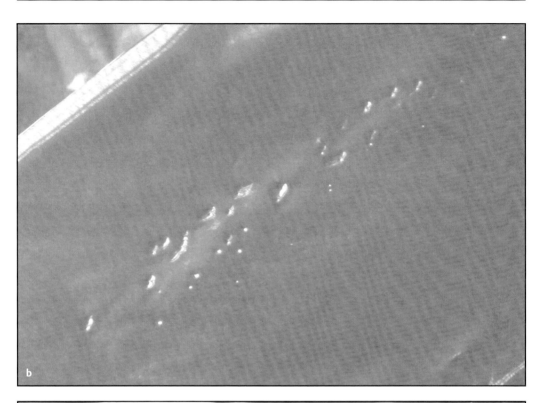

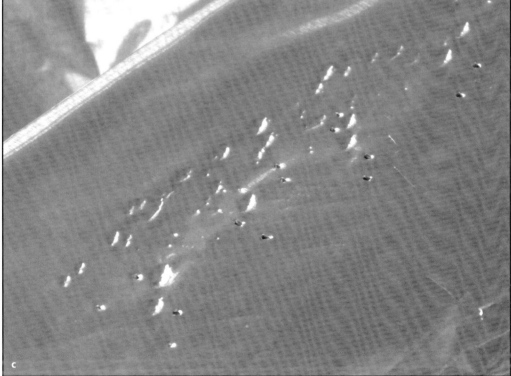

Fig. 6.14 (*continued*) **(b,c)**   Doses of tapping.

As you repeat this exercise, always make sure to tap on yourself to see what it feels like. For each type of tapping what does it feel like in your tapping hand? How do you best position the instrument?

Stroking

Smooth the surface of the clay and cover with fresh foil, making sure it is flat and fully contacting the surface of the clay.

Before you use any instruments for stroking, practice the stroking with only your hand to understand the force of contact for different doses. With each force of contact always make sure to apply the same on yourself to see what it feels like. Using only the fingers of your stroking hand, very lightly stroke along the clay/foil. With very low dose contact virtually no depressions are visible in the foil and clay. As you increase the dose of the contact, first very slight depressions appear in the foil but not the clay. Then as you slightly increase the dose of the contact, the depressions in the foil become more obvious and depressions start to appear in the clay.

Can you apply light stroking that leaves no obvious depression in the foil or clay? When you apply this on yourself, what does it feel like? For different pressures what does this feel like?

Now repeat this using an instrument like a small *enshin* or the *yoneyama* instrument. Always first apply the stroking on yourself to check what dose of stroking you are applying.

With very low dose stroking, the instrument contacts the skin but almost no force of contact is felt. When you stroke on the foil/clay surface, your stroking leaves tiny low depressions in the foil, but when you look at the clay underneath, there are no obvious depressions in the clay (**Fig. 6.15a**).

- For slightly more dose stroking with stroking on the skin, you may be very slightly more aware of the instrument, but it is still very light. When you stroke on the foil/clay it will cause a slightly deeper depression in the foil, and very slight depressions will appear in the clay (**Fig. 6.15b**).
- With slightly more dose stroking, as you stroke on the skin you feel the instrument more clearly but it is still not as heavy. When stroking on the foil/clay it will cause a slightly deeper depression in the foil and more obvious depressions will appear in the clay.

On older children stroking can be applied a little like a gentle massage, so that clearer pressure is applied. When you apply this on yourself, it will feel like a gentle stroking massage. On the clay/foil you will see more obvious depressions in both the foil and the clay.

As with the tapping exercise, as you repeat this exercise, always apply the stroking on yourself to see what it feels like both on the skin stroked and in the hand holding the instrument.

These home practice methods can help you more rapidly develop your sense of touch and

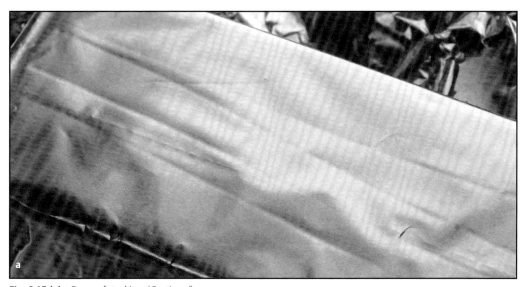

Fig. 6.15 (a)   Doses of stroking. (*Continued*)

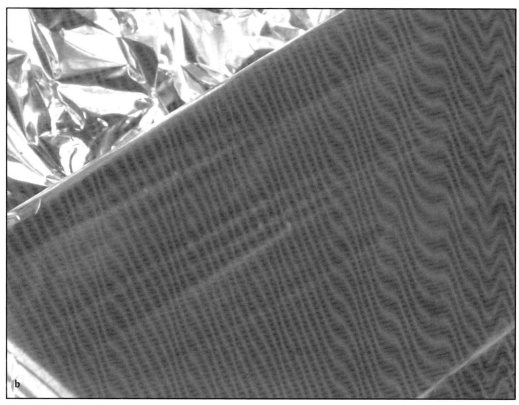

Fig. 6.15 (*continued*) **(b)** Doses of stroking.

ability to observe subtle change, the feelings of how best to hold the instruments, and how to vary the ways of applying the instruments that can be important for dose control on the patient. As the teacher always says: practice makes perfect, so practice, practice, practice.

Section III Root Treatment Approaches and Techniques

- Down the bladder channel on the legs
- Down the lateral (*yang*) aspects of the arms
- Down the stomach channel on the abdomen

To this is added light tapping around GV-12. Additional light tapping can be added to target specific symptoms, such as around GV-3/GV-4 for lower abdominal, lower body symptoms; the occipital region for symptoms of the head, eye, ear, nose throat, and face; or behavioral problems.

When teaching this simplified non-pattern-based treatment to parents, I always give them a drawing that shows the body areas, directions of stroking, number of strokes, and number of taps in each area. Parents might tend to do too much if you don't specify clearly in writing what you want them to do. To help with this, I keep printed copies of the basic treatment of stroking and tapping copied in black ink. I then draw with a red pen the arrows for stroking and mark with shaded areas for tapping and write the numbers of actions next to each.

Most parents, in our experience, will apply treatments at home as best they can, similar to what you ask of them. You need to monitor the child to make sure he or she is not being over-stimulated. If the parent applies the technique too strongly or does too much, you might start seeing some signs of overtreatment. In this case, have the parents explain and demonstrate to you how they are doing the treatment. On a later visit you can correct any misunderstanding and improve their techniques.

An additional component of the home therapy often involves having the parent change the press-spheres or Pyonex press-tack needles (Seirin-America) regularly at home to help reduce or prevent irritation, and to prolong treatment effectiveness. This should be an automatic part of treatment when you leave press-spheres on the child as part of treatment. You can choose in some cases to have the press-tack needles changed as well. These can be left throughout the time between that visit and the next, provided they are regularly changed according to the instructions in Chapter 12.

Other aspects of home treatment might involve care in relation to other treatments, such as retaining press-tack or intradermal needles (see Chapter 12), and, of course, any dietary recommendations you make. On some rare occasions you may need to have *moxa* applied daily at home. For example, in cases of atopic dermatitis or severe chronic eczema, one of the best symptomatic treatments is to apply *okyu* (direct *moxa*—see Chapter 13) to LI-4, LI-10, LI-11, or LI-15 (choose by palpation) and sometimes to *uranaitei* (extra point) (see Chapter 16, p. 105, and Chapter 19). On a younger child this can be difficult to do, and it is only feasible when done by you in the clinic at each visit. However, on older children it is possible to have the child receive regular home *moxa*. Sometimes the parent does this; sometimes the child prefers to do it. An example of this can be found in Chapter 19 (p. 144), where the 12-year-old boy Han decided to do the *moxa* himself since his mother's technique was too hot. In severe cases such as this, daily home treatment with the *moxa* is what helps keep the symptoms quieter and the child more functional.

9 Pattern-Based Root Treatment: Meridian Therapy Applied to Adults

In the previous chapters I described the basic *shonishin* approaches of the non-pattern-based root treatment. This root treatment does not require identification of specific problems couched in the language and framework of traditional ideas and methods. Instead, it applies a general treatment that helps influence the healing process, regardless of the specific diagnosis of the child. To do this, the treatment uses modified forms of a very mild stimulation, typically with rubbing and/or tapping. This method takes advantage of the sensitivity of pediatric patients and the easily accessed homeodynamic mechanisms of the pediatric patient.

This chapter describes a simplified approach to pattern-based root treatment.[1] The term *pattern-based* refers to the identification of a specific pattern of disturbances, and treatment of it to help correct the healing process. In Meridian Therapy, the pattern-based approach involves identifying and correcting disturbances among the 12 channels (or meridians), so that after treatment, the channel system is in a more balanced state, thereby aiding the healing process.

The two treatment approaches combine easily and naturally, so that it is often helpful to add at least some simple aspect of this pattern-based approach to *shonishin's* non-pattern-based approach. This additional simple treatment usually increases the overall effectiveness of the treatment and will be applied to many pediatric patients.

There are, however, some patients where the only form of root treatment that is available is the pattern-based root treatment. This occurs, for example, in children with fevers or skin lesions over all or much of the body, such as in atopic dermatitis. In such cases, it is difficult or contraindicated to apply any of the techniques used in the non-pattern-based treatment. The Meridian Therapy root treatment approach is then used as the primary root treatment for those patients. It is thus important to fully grasp this basic treatment approach to maximize treatment for all pediatric patients.

The history, nature, and theories of Meridian Therapy are described in detail elsewhere. It can be helpful to read those articles and books for such details. (For the history and an overview of the system see Birch 1999; Birch and Felt 1999; Birch and Ida 2004. For an explanation of the whole system and details of its practice methods, see Shudo 1990.) In Chapter 10 I summarize the essential features of Meridian Therapy as they relate to treatment of children:

- The diagnostic patterns
- How to choose the patterns based on age and willingness of the child
- How to treat the patterns and evaluate what you have done
- The point locations

Before discussing pediatric modifications and applications of the Meridian Therapy system, we need to briefly explain the nature of the thinking processes, diagnostic methods, pattern identification, and treatment techniques used in normal clinical practice on adults. Most readers will be coming from a traditional Chinese medicine (TCM) background and will thus expect that with needling the patient should feel the usual sensations of *deqi*. It will also often be assumed that the complex theoretical descriptions of physiology and pathophysiology that are the focus of TCM treatment are needed. Neither of these assumptions will bear out in what follows. *Deqi* in TCM is an interpretation of modern China, and is even now under dispute within China itself. I have written on this at length in my book *Understanding Acupuncture* (Birch and Felt 1999), and more recently in greater depth (Birch 2015). For the purposes of what is described in this chapter, I

---

[1] For the development of this simplified approach see Birch (2010). A number of textbooks were also used, such as Fukushima (1991); Ono (1988); Shudo (1990).

avoid discussion of *deqi* during needling. The techniques covered in Chapter 10 can work regardless of someone feeling *deqi* or not. Although knowledge of basic ideas from historical texts in early China forms the backbone of how many modern practitioners practice traditional acupuncture in Japan, the specific TCM interpretations and patterns of those ideas are usually not used in Japan outside of the practice of herbal medicine. When the TCM models were crystallized in the 1950s they developed under very specific historical and cultural influences in China. Instead, as the reader will see in the following discussion, in Japan different patterns have been described following different interpretations of some of the same traditional ideas and texts, developed to suit the different historical and cultural backgrounds of those practitioners in Japan in the 20th century. It is therefore probably helpful to suspend judgment about the basic approaches and patterns of diagnosis until you have learned and tried them. Like the TCM patterns of diagnosis and treatment, the patterns of diagnosis and treatment in Japanese Meridian Therapy represent practical systems that have been made to work (Birch 2014; Birch and Felt 1999). Try them first before judging whether they make sense and are effective.

Basic Theories of Meridian Therapy

The core treatment approach of Meridian Therapy can be summarized in the following figures (Birch 2009):

Fig. 9.1 represents an idealized state where the channels (level 2—middle circle) are balanced and the internal organ-functional system that they regulate (level 1—inner circle) is operating at optimum, shown by the arrows, and the vitality or overall energy state of the patient (level 3—outer circle) is very good (shown by the arrows and solid line of this circle).

Fig. 9.2 represents the state in which a patient presents for treatment. The channel system (level 2—middle line) is distorted by depressions (vacuity) and bumps (repletion). The organ-functional system (level 1—inner line) that the channel system helps regulate has been disturbed so that it no longer operates well, triggering symptoms, and the vitality (level 3—outer line) is smaller,

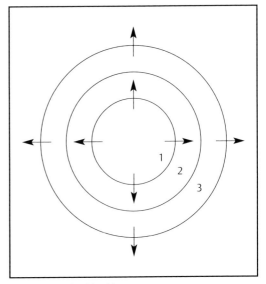

Fig. 9.1   Idealized healthy state:
Level 1—functional systems (*zangfu*, etc.)
Level 2—channel systems
Level 3—vitality: global *qi* of the body

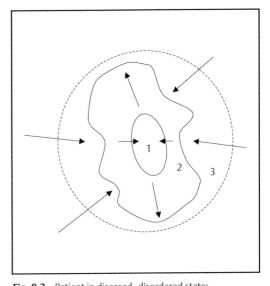

Fig. 9.2   Patient in diseased–disordered state:
Level 1—weakening, dysfunctional
Level 2—imbalanced
Level 3—weakened

less solid, with arrows no longer directed outward.

Fig. 9.3 represents the effect of treatment, applying supplementation and draining to the appropriate channels so that they return to a state

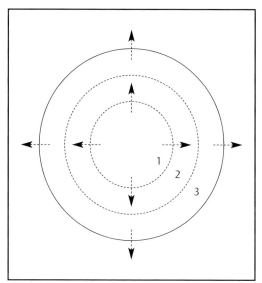

Fig. 9.3   Patient after treatment in a more balanced state:
Level 1—functions improving
Level 2—more balanced
Level 3—stronger

of balance (level 2—middle circle), which in turn helps regulate the organ-functional system (level 1—inner circle) so that it returns to a state of higher functioning (indicated by outward directions of all arrows) leading to improvement of symptoms, and improvement in vitality (level 3—outer circle more solid and outward-directed arrows).

The basic approach of Meridian Therapy is to correct disturbances of the channel system (seen as the bumps and depressions of the middle line in **Fig. 9.2**), using the supplementation method for the vacuous channels (shown as depressions) and, as needed, the draining method for the replete channels (shown as bumps). The tried and tested rules of Meridian Therapy instruct us to choose an underlying pattern of vacuity and treat that, followed by correction of repletion disturbances if they are found, or additional vacuity if found.

A well-performed Meridian Therapy root treatment (Chinese *zhibenfa*, Japanese *honchiho*) results in a rebalancing of the channel system (level 2), which in turn helps reregulate the internal functional systems (level 1). This, in turn, increases overall vitality (level 3). With the more experienced practitioner and a practitioner with the right training, the root treatment also directly increases and improves the overall vitality, which

in turn also helps regulate the channel system and thus the internal functional systems (Birch 2009; Birch 2014).

Meridian Therapy Treatment Principles

After researching the diagnosis and treatment methods outlined in the *Nan Jing (Classic of Difficulties)*, the original Meridian Therapy study group (founded in the 1920s by Sorei Yanagiya) chose to focus on the treatment principles described in *Nan Jing*, Chapter 69:

First, "always supplement before draining" (meaning focus on that which is weak or vacuous as the first target of treatment, and then apply the supplementation technique).

Second, "for vacuity supplement the mother." Here the language of the five-phase engendering cycle is used. To supplement a weak lung we should supplement its mother, the spleen. Since the time of the well-known acupuncturist Sa A'm of Korea in the late 1500s this has been interpreted to mean supplement both lung and spleen channels for vacuity of the lungs (Birch and Felt 1999, p. 311). Practically speaking this makes no sense unless the spleen is also weak alongside the lung. Thus Yanagiya's study group examined patients to see if they showed these patterns of weakness. The study group found that these patterns exist and that they form the basis of diagnosis and treatment.

Meridian Therapy Diagnostic Methods and Patterns

These underlying or primary patterns of vacuity are called the *sho*. There were found to be four of these:
- Lung vacuity—involving vacuity of spleen and lung
- Spleen vacuity—involving vacuity of spleen and heart
- Liver vacuity—involving vacuity of liver and kidney
- Kidney vacuity—involving vacuity of kidney and lung

In the case of adults, the process of selecting the pattern on which to focus treatment involves the integration of different clinical data in an orderly manner. Current and past symptoms and health issues are classified in terms of which channels they are more likely associated with. The channels are palpated, the abdomen is palpated (**Fig. 9.4**), and then the pulse is examined, looking for a pattern of differences in the six positions (**Table 9.1**). The pattern is most commonly confirmed by finding congruence between the pulse and abdominal findings, and the other clinical data often support this conclusion, but it is not a problem if they do not match. Experienced clinicians such as Toshio Yanagishita or Denmei Shudo can gather and integrate these data very quickly.

Fig. 9.5 shows a simple diagrammatic way of summarizing the findings of an examination of the *six yin* channel (deeper) pulses. A circle is a relatively normal-strength pulse; a dot is

a relatively weak pulse. Thus, finding stiffness, discomfort on the right side of the abdomen (ST-25 to ST-27 area) with relative weakness in the right *can* and *guan* pulses (lung and spleen channel pulses) is a sign of the lung vacuity pattern being present. **Figs. 9.6–9.9** show the core palpation findings that help one select each pattern.

Meridian Therapy Treatment and Techniques

■ Step one

Once the pattern is selected, treatment usually follows. The same principles that helped guide selection of the pattern (from *Nan Jing*, Chapter 69) also guide selection of the typical treatment points for each pattern. The following points are usually selected for treatment:

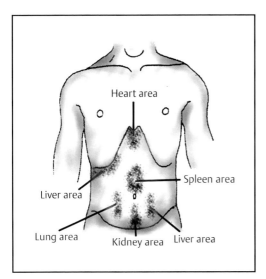

Fig. 9.4   Typical five-phase channel correspondences.

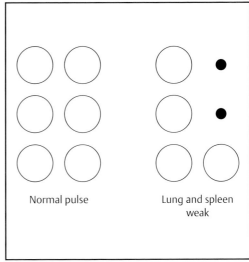

Fig. 9.5   Diagrammatic representations of the six *yin* channel (deeper) pulses—all "normal" and spleen and lung weak. A circle is a relatively normal-strength pulse; a dot is a relatively weak pulse.

Table 9.1   Radial pulse—channel correspondences

Left wrist	Channels	Right wrist	Channels
Left *cun*	Arm *tai yang*/SI and arm *shao yin*/HT	Right *cun*	Arm *yang ming*/LI and arm *tai yin*/LU
Left *guan*	Leg *shao yang*/GB and leg *jue yin*/LV	Right *guan*	Leg *yang ming*/ST and leg *tai yin*/SP
Left *chi*	Leg *tai yang*/BL and leg *shao yin*/KI	Right *chi*	Arm *shao yang*/TB and arm *jue yin*/PC

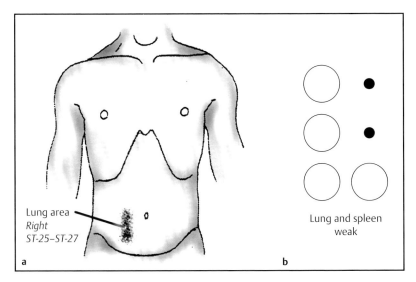

Fig. 9.6 **(a)** Abdominal and **(b)** pulse pictures for the lung vacuity pattern.

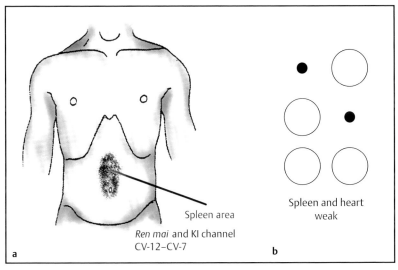

Fig. 9.7 **(a)** Abdominal and **(b)** pulse pictures for the spleen vacuity pattern.

Lung vacuity pattern:	LU-9 + SP-3
Spleen vacuity pattern:	SP-3 + PC-7
Liver vacuity pattern:	LR-8 + KI-10
Kidney vacuity pattern:	KI-7 + LU-8

Experience found that it is usually better to needle the pair of points on one side of the body only. Simple guidelines have been developed to help with deciding which side to treat:

- If there is a symptom or symptoms on only one side of the body, supplement the other side.[2]

For example, painful right shoulder and neck: treat the points on the left side.
- If there are symptoms on both sides or internal symptoms, for males treat the left and females treat the right.

Typically in Meridian Therapy very thin needles are used. Shudo (1990) uses mostly 0.12 mm gauge needles; others may use slightly wider gauge, but no more than 0.16 mm gauge. Needles are to be inserted painlessly and shallowly (0.5–2 mm) in the direction of the flow of the channel. The needles are retained for a few minutes, but this amount varies by practitioner and patient—usually around 10 minutes can be good. But within the field of Meridian Therapy there

---

[2] Traditional justification for this one-sided treatment can also be found; see my publications on this (Birch 2013, 2014).

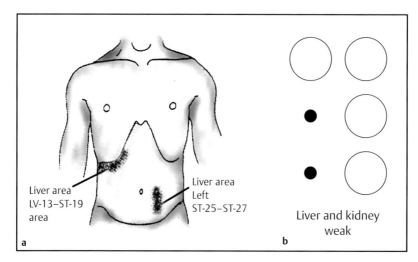

Fig. 9.8 (a) Abdominal and **(b)** pulse pictures for the liver vacuity pattern.

Liver area
LV-13–ST-19 area

Liver area
Left
ST-25–ST-27

Liver and kidney weak

a

b

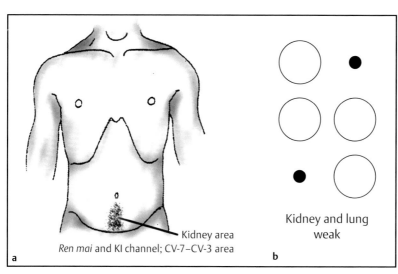

Fig. 9.9 (a) Abdominal and **(b)** pulse pictures for the kidney vacuity pattern.

Kidney area
Ren mai and KI channel; CV-7–CV-3 area

Kidney and lung weak

a

b

are also many practitioners who use noninserted needling methods, such as those we find in the Toyohari (East Asian needle therapy) style of Meridian Therapy. This kind of needling technique requires a lot of structured study to be safely and effectively used on patients—see the discussions in Chapter 11.

The core component of the Meridian Therapy root treatment is the treatment of the first two acupoints. Since the 1930s this has characterized the Meridian Therapy treatment. Over time some Meridian Therapists added additional components to the root treatment to increase the effectiveness of the channel balancing achieved.

For example, in the Toyohari it has become routine to examine the condition of the two *yin* channels that are in controlling cycle relationship to the primary channel that the pattern is named after, and to apply supplementation or draining according to what is found. Thus, for example, for a lung vacuity pattern, after supplementing LU-9 and SP-3, the liver and heart pulses are checked for any disturbances (metal controls wood and fire controls metal). Additionally after performing this second step of treatment, the *yang* channels are then also examined and draining or supplementation applied according to what is found (Birch 2010) as the third step of treatment.

This systematic approach is both theoretically more complete and relatively easy to use, provided one can read the radial pulses. Judgments of what to do for the second and third steps are based almost exclusively on pulse findings.

▪ Step Two

This step of treatment is applied on the other side of the body from which the first step is applied. Source points are commonly used.

After treating a lung pattern (LU-9 and SP-3) examine the liver and heart pulses and treat according to what is found—drain or supplement LV-3 or PC-7 as needed.

After treating a spleen pattern (SP-3 and PC-7) examine the liver and kidney pulses and treat according to what is found—supplement KI-3 or drain or supplement LV-3 as needed.

After treating a liver pattern (LV-8 and KI-10) examine the lung and spleen pulses and treat according to what is found—drain or supplement LU-9 or SP-3 as needed.

After treating a kidney pattern (KI-10 and LU-8) examine the spleen and heart pulses and treat according to what is found—drain or supplement SP-3 or PC-7 as needed.

▪ Step Three

This step of treatment is usually applied to the corresponding *yang* channel luo point, most commonly using a draining technique on the replete channel(s). Hence, if the bladder pulse is replete with pathological disturbance, drain BL-58.

A typical treatment on an adult identified as a lung vacuity pattern might involve the following:

Supplement LU-9 and SP-3 on the left side, then drain LV-3 on the right side, then drain ST-40 on one side and TB-5 on one side. With each step of treatment the pulse quality improves further and the relative balance of what is felt among the six positions becomes increasingly equal.

Conclusion

This brief introduction to Meridian Therapy describes the essentials of the treatment system. However, to use it effectively on adults, it is necessary not only to read the more detailed texts that are available but also to study with a qualified teacher(s) in appropriate courses and programs (see Appendix, p. 332). With practice, the diagnosis and treatment of adults becomes easy and routine. The treatment of children is another matter altogether. Although the basic system remains simple, several practical issues in the treatment of babies and small children require that we modify the approach considerably. For older children on whom we can make the observations related to pulse and abdominal findings and judge the pattern of diagnosis and treatment, a simple form of the preceding treatment can be used. The next chapter describes how to use this system on babies and smaller children and then on older children. In general, steps two and three are more difficult to apply, especially on younger children, due to the difficulties of needing to use pulse diagnosis to determine what to treat.

10 Pattern-Based Root Treatment : Meridian Therapy Applied to Children

Diagnosis to Select the Primary Pattern in Babies and Small Children

We have to select the primary pattern in babies and small children differently than on adults or older children. Abdominal diagnosis on the baby and small child can be difficult to do and yield unclear findings. On babies and toddlers the whole abdomen often feels full, rounded, and springy with unclear or no regional differences; on children aged 2 to 5 or 6 the abdomen is often ticklish. Either of these can make abdominal diagnosis difficult for the inexperienced practitioner. Pulse diagnosis can also be difficult to do, or may yield unclear findings. Babies and small children will not remain still; furthermore, the positional and depth differences are hard to discriminate because the region where you palpate the arteries is very small. Taken together these factors make pulse diagnosis on babies and small children difficult.

Even when you are able to palpate the pulses, you generally cannot spend much time palpating the pulses on children; many young children are not very patient and will not remain still for longer periods of time. A simpler and easier approach is needed. My teacher, Toshio Yanagishita, whose experience in over 60 years of practice extended to the delivery of well over a million treatments, taught a very simple approach that works very well. We take advantage of the fact that babies and young children will tend to manifest symptoms that arise out of their constitutional tendencies. As people age, lifestyle issues start triggering problems in addition to those associated with their constitutional tendency, so that the clinical patterns become more complex. In babies and young children this is not usually the case and we can take the symptoms as a reasonable indicator of the pattern to focus on.

■ Typical Symptoms Associated with Each of the Four Patterns

Lung vacuity pattern: breathing problems; skin problems; easily catching cold, and so on; allergic or atopic constitution

Spleen vacuity pattern: digestive problems; nourishment problems (the child that is underdeveloped, "failure to thrive")

Liver vacuity pattern: behavioral problems; sleep problems; muscle spasm or spasticity problems

Kidney vacuity pattern: birth defects; physical or mental development problems; slow development; cold feet; urinary problems such as bed wetting

As children become older (age 6 or older) we are usually able to apply the other diagnostic methods and follow and identify the changing conditions. Thus, although this simple rule for making a diagnosis based on symptoms can still be followed, sometimes one finds through palpation diagnosis an evolved pattern due to lifestyle and other factors (see later for details).

Typical Examples of the Four Patterns

- The 10-week-old baby who will not settle or sleep well and cries a lot is typically a liver *sho*-type pattern (see Case 1, Chapter 21). In this case some basic pulse information was accessible; the left deep pulses felt weaker than the right deep pulses, supporting the selection of the liver pattern. No clear signs were apparent on the abdomen.
- The 4½-year-old child who repeatedly catches cold, has chronic nasal congestion/infection, and tends to develop cough easily is a typical lung vacuity pattern patient (see Case 2, Chapter 27). The pulse of the right wrist at a deeper level will generally appear weaker than the same depth pulse on the left wrist.

Obviously, things are not always this simple. There are, of course, patients with more complex conditions, due to having more complex constitutional tendencies, complex diseases, early influence of lifestyle issues, influence of medications, or other medical interventions like surgery. The symptom and medical history pictures are more complex, and one has to think through the possible pattern and eventually choose one for treatment.

Example of More Complex Patterns

- The 5-year-old hospitalized patient with very severe and serious digestive disturbance due to an improperly developed gastrointestinal system (see Case 1, Chapter 28). This patient had both spleen (digestive problems) and kidney (developmental disorder) patterns, and both patterns needed to be treated. Although the pulse diagnostic information was accessible, it was not possible to palpate the abdomen and complete a normal (adult) assessment. The pulse findings helped differentiate how to focus the treatment as a primary spleen pattern (spleen and heart pulses weak) with kidney secondary pattern (kidney pulse weak).

Diagnosis to Select the Primary Pattern as Children Become Older

Provided the child will stay still for you and will lie on their back on the table for you, it is usually possible to start getting clearer pictures of the abdominal and pulse findings so that you can make more refined judgments about the primary pattern that needs treating. If this is the case, the basic diagnostic information for selecting the primary pattern is described in the previous chapter. Although it can still be somewhat difficult on a 6- or 7-year-old, it can also be quite easy. The pattern more commonly follows the symptoms that the child presents with. As the child becomes older the ability to identify the primary pattern from abdominal and pulse findings increases and becomes easier. This naturally allows for the possibility that the pattern might have changed due to the various factors identified earlier. As the possibility of change gradually increases, the possibility of selecting the pattern from the abdominal and pulse findings also increases; they almost follow hand in hand.

Typical Example on an Older Patient

- An 8-year-old boy had a bedwetting problem (see Case 4, Chapter 22, p. 217). The pulse and abdominal findings clearly showed the kidney vacuity pattern, and the pulse also showed that the spleen was weak and needed supplementation.

Of course there are some patients where the findings and/or the medical history are more complex, and one does not choose the right pattern immediately. The result of this is usually that the treatment is not as effective. Often, once one has reevaluated one's choice at a later treatment and started to treat the more appropriate pattern, distinct improvements are seen in the treatment outcome. If we are honest and open, this is not unlike what happens in the treatment of adult patients.

Example of More Complex Patterns

- A 12-year-old boy had a long history of severe atopic dermatitis. Although the child may have started out constitutionally as a lung-vacuity-type patient, the extensive use of steroid creams eventually triggered signs and manifestation of the kidney vacuity pattern (see Case 1, Chapter 19, p. 144). Because the boy was more mature it was possible to obtain other diagnostic information to make this decision. The pulse, abdominal, and other palpation findings pointed primarily toward the lung vacuity pattern but also suggested the possibility of the kidney pattern. At first he was treated as a lung pattern, but later and under the advice of my teacher, Akihiro Takai, it became clear that the kidney pattern was better for him. The results of treatment clearly matched this correction of best pattern.
- A 10-year-old boy had bedwetting problems (see Case 1, Chapter 22, p. 204). The initial impression was of the lung vacuity pattern, supported also by a history of asthma, skin

problems, and the abdominal and pulse findings. The lung pattern was treated on this first visit. On the second visit the pulse and abdominal findings were more suggestive of the kidney pattern. This was treated from that visit onward.

Diagnosis to Select Additional Steps of Root Treatment

The foregoing description covers basic details of selecting the primary pattern, but, depending on the child (age, maturity, condition) and your skills, it may be useful to also use steps two and three by treating the secondary *yin* pattern and even the *yang* channels. As already described, in an adult, after supplementing, for example, LU-9 and SP-3 to address the primary pattern of lung vacuity pattern, LR-3 may also be drained as well as TB-5 and BL-58. The decision to drain each point is based on finding relative strength with hardness in the pulse position depths corresponding to each channel (left deeper *guan* pulse, right surface *chi* pulse, and left surface *chi* pulse). The decision in each case is not based on location or nature of the symptoms, but instead only on the pulse findings. As one can imagine, in children where pulse diagnosis can be very difficult because of the factors already discussed, these judgments can be very difficult to make. It is enough to apply treatment to the two main points for the primary pattern and stop there. This, when well performed, is enough.

Those with experience using the Meridian Therapy system of acupuncture in normal clinical practice, may find that the additional judgments of which *yin* channel is involved as a secondary pattern and which *yang* channels show disturbance are easier to make. Then treatment can be applied to appropriate additional points.

But for those who have no prior experience with these methods and judgments, it is better to stay away from trying to do this until you have completed a course of training in Meridian Therapy and developed an understanding of what the pulse changes feel like that indicate application of draining techniques. As described in Chapter 4, it is better to apply less treatment to regulate

the dose of treatment. Unless one is really clear about such steps of treatment, do not do them; stick with the simplified treatment of the primary pattern.

Once you start to incorporate these additional steps of the root treatment, you will find you do this much more on older children and only occasionally on toddlers and not very often on babies.

Children with Two-Pattern Diagnoses

Some children do not exhibit a clear single pattern but instead manifest two patterns to an almost equal degree. A child might show clear signs and symptoms of a lung vacuity pattern as well as clear signs and symptoms of a liver vacuity pattern. Where does one start? In such cases it can be difficult to decide which pattern should be designated as the primary treatment pattern. This can make one hesitant to begin treatment, but it is better to avoid hesitation and uncertainty. There are two basic approaches to decision making in this scenario. You can see if the weight of symptoms leans more in favor of one pattern compared with the other; this usually places more emphasis on the complaints that the parents consider to be more important for the child. Another approach is to start treatment with the core non-pattern-based treatment and then recheck the pulse and abdomen to see if a clearer picture emerges as to which pattern should receive the primary focus. Sometimes neither of these two approaches seems to help you decide. In this case use your judgment. It may be that your intuition tells you to start with the one pattern or it may be that you mentally throw the dice to decide. Either way, it is better to start and monitor the patient to see how things unfold. The important thing to remember is that probably *both* patterns *are* present, and that there is no one right way to start, just your best strategic guess. You will most likely be supplementing a point for each pattern by applying treatment to the primary and then secondary pattern. The following case from my colleague Bhavito Jansch in Switzerland is a good example of this. With the initial decision and its treatments one set of symptoms can be seen to start improving. Then as the other pattern becomes the primary focus, the other problems start to improve further.

Case 1
Nic, Boy Age 5 Years

Main complaints: Nic catches colds easily and has been having accompanying middle ear infections twice a year. For each ear infection he is usually prescribed antibiotics.

He has some skin eruptions that are very itchy, and he scratches a lot, especially in the fall. He also has a problem with itchiness on the back. Additionally he has some shortness of breath. Finally he has been having problems of sleep disturbance with some nightmares over the last 2 months.

Observations: The mother does not mention it, but he shows signs of hyperactivity. In the clinic he cannot be quiet for a second, constantly running around while constantly talking. He is big for his age and a little bit overweight with a slightly red face and cool feet.

Diagnosis: I judged him as a "jitsu" or repletion type of person. From the symptoms I thought to judge him as the lung vacuity pattern with liver vacuity as the secondary pattern. But his feet where slightly cool and his red face showed some counterflow signs. The kidney area on the belly was slightly depressed and somehow cooler. The pulse was not easy to compare because he wouldn't stay still. But given the clear lung vacuity pattern signs and the additional signs of kidney involvement I decided on the diagnosis of kidney vacuity pattern and spleen vacuity pattern, which seemed to account for the majority of his symptoms.

Treatment: Using a teishin, supplementation was applied to left KI-7, LU-5, and right SP-9.

Using the teishin, light stroking was applied down the large intestine and triple burner channels.

Using a Yoneyama instrument, light stroking was applied down the yang channels on the abdomen, back, and legs to descend his qi. Additionally, tap-

ping was applied around the ears.

A cone of chinetsukyu moxa[1] was burned on the lower abdomen around CV-4.

Second visit—21 days later

He had gotten anear infection around Christmas, but antibiotics were not needed. The other symptoms had not changed. I decided to repeat the treatment from the first visit.

Treatment: Using a teishin, supplementation was applied to left KI-7, LU-5, and right SP-9.

Using the teishin, light stroking was applied down the large intestine and triple burner channels.

Using a Yoneyama instrument, light stroking was applied down the yang channels on the abdomen, back, and legs to descend his qi. Additionally tapping was applied around the ears.

A cone of chinetsukyu moxa was burned on the lower abdomen around CV-4.

Third visit—7 days later

His behavior was slightly calmer. His mother also confirmed this. He had no colds or ear problems.

Treatment: Using a teishin, supplementation was applied to left KI-7, LU-5, and right SP-9.

Using the teishin, light stroking was applied down the large intestine and triple burner channels.

Using a Yoneyama instrument, light stroking was applied down the yang channels on the abdomen, back, and legs to descend his qi. Additionally tapping was applied around the ears.

A cone of chinetsukyu moxa was burned on the lower abdomen around CV-4.

The next three treatments were similar with not much to report. Shortly after the sixth treatment he caught a cold again but without an ear infection. After 1 week recovering from the cold he was very tired, and for the first time my clinic was safe from his hands and his exploration. In this seventh treatment, because he was calmer and I was better able to read signs, such as the

---

[1]   The chinetsukyu moxa technique is described briefly at the end of Chapter 13.

pulse, I was able to confirm that the primary pattern was now liver vacuity with secondary lung vacuity. Thus using the *teishin* I supplemented LV-8, KI-10 on the left, with LU-9 on the right. I treated only this that day.

Eighth visit—14 days later

Was this the same child? Except for talking a lot he behaved very quietly and acted like other calmer children in my clinic.

Treatment: Using a *teishin*, I supplemented LV-8, KI-10 on the left, and LU-9 on the right.

I could have stopped here since he was asleep. I finished by doing a little stroking and tapping here and there (just to earn my salary). I sent home a speechless mother and a happy child.

After this he came every 2 weeks for a couple of months. After that we started to do follow-up visits once a month. He hasn't caught cold or had any ear infections for almost 1 year. He has become much calmer and is a much more socially oriented child. We had a lot of fun together.

Comments: In this case the judgment as to which pattern to start with was very complex. There was an abundance of lung vacuity pattern signs (infections, skin problems, minor breathing issues), with signs of kidney vacuity involvement (cool feet, lower abdominal reaction), and clear liver vacuity signs (restlessness, hyperactivity, recent sleep disturbance). Notice how the focus on kidney (which included treating the lung and spleen channels) improved the general lung and kidney signs and notice how quickly the liver vacuity signs (behavior problems) changed once that became the focus. There was no irritation of symptoms because the "wrong" treatment was done. This is a good example of a patient with a complex picture of signs and symptoms that imply multichannel involvement. He probably would have improved regardless of which of the three possible foci were chosen, but Mr. Jansch chose to focus on the pattern that incorporated the signs and symptoms of more concern to the mother since she did not mention his behavioral problems.

Modifying Point Selection for Treatment of the Primary Patterns

The usual point combinations for the four patterns were listed earlier. These are based on a systematic interpretation of *Nan Jing* (*Classic of Difficulties*), Chapter 69, theory and confirmed through clinical experience. The theory predicts which channels to apply the supplementation technique to and on which points to apply treatment on those channels. In the lung vacuity pattern, lung and spleen channels are vacuous; thus treatment is directed to both of these, and usually LU-9 (the mother/supplementation point). But it may be advantageous to modify the points on the targeted channels using other clinical ideas. There are many theories of point selection, just as there are many schools and styles of acupuncture (Birch and Felt 1999). A simple theory that complements the basic Meridian Therapy model comes from *Nan Jing*, Chapter 68. This chapter talks about the use of the five *shu* points according to certain symptomatic manifestations, which we can extend into modern clinical practice—see **Table 10.1**.

Some of these indications are clear. For the child with fever use the *ying*-spring points instead of the usual points; for example, LU-10 and SP-2 instead of the usual LU-9 and SP-3 for the lung vacuity pattern patient. But clinical experience has shown us that we can extend these indications, partly as extended interpretations of what the *Nan Jing* describes and partly based on their five-phase correspondences. **Table 10.2** lists examples of how we might extend selection of acupoints from **Table 10.1**.

Table 10.1   *Shu*-stream point indications—*Nan Jing*, Chapter 68

Acupoint	Indications
Jing-well	Feeling fullness and discomfort below the sternum
Ying-spring	Fever or feelings of body heat
Shu-stream	Joint pains or heaviness of the body
Jing-river	Cough, alternating fever and chills
He-sea	Counterflow *qi*, leakage of fluids such as diarrhea

Table 10.2   *Shu*-stream point indications—extended uses

Acupoint	Indications
Jing-well (wood)	Epigastric pain, bloated abdomen, especially epigastric region
Ying-spring (fire)	Fevers, overheated child (the very active child)
Shu-stream (earth)	The lethargic child with difficulty raising limbs, problems of the limbs; chronic digestive problems
Jing-river (metal)	Cough, cold-flu symptoms, lung problems in general; alternating fever and chills; skin problems in general, such as eczema
He-sea (water)	Counterflow *qi* with signs of heat above and cold below—this can show in some very kidney vacuous children; it also shows in children with skin disease, such as eczema, atopic dermatitis, with a very reddened appearance around the head, face, neck, more inflamed-looking lesions on the upper part of the body; leakage of fluids, such as diarrhea, urination problems, very runny nose

Examples of Modified Point Selections

- A 1-year-old child with lung vacuity pattern but with fever: LU-10, SP-2 instead of LU-9, SP-3.
- A child with atopic dermatitis with more severe lesions on the upper part of the body who shows the kidney vacuity pattern: KI-10, LU-5 instead of KI-7, LU-8
- The liver vacuity child who comes with early-stage cold symptoms without fever: LR-4, KI-7 instead of LR-8, KI-10
- The spleen vacuity child with symptoms of chronic diarrhea: SP-9, PC-3 instead of SP-3, PC-7

Usually we start treatment with the common point combinations once we have chosen the pattern for that child, and, if after some treatment(s) you feel at a later visit that progress is insufficient, you can try the modified point selections. It is, of course, all right to start treatment on the first visit with a modified point selection provided the condition of the child very clearly matches. On most patients we use the common or typical point combinations for treatment.

Treatment Methods in Meridian Therapy

Following the traditions of Meridian Therapy that emerged during the 1930s, needle techniques either involve the sensationless, or at least painless, very shallow insertion of very thin needles for supplementation techniques, or the use of noninserted needling methods.

Sensationless or painless needling requires the use of the correct type and gauge of needle, and reasonable skills with practice. If needles are inserted, they are retained for a few minutes, for example, up to 10 minutes on adults.

Noninserted needling is completed quickly, once the *qi* reaction has been felt and one has responded appropriately to it. However, the use of fine needles without insertion requires either considerable self-developed experience that has evolved through decades of practice, or a systematic training program with qualified and experienced teachers. Programs such as Toyohari that teach noninserted needling require at least a year of careful repetitive study with qualified teachers.

When treating children, especially babies and very small children, these techniques can be difficult. It has already been discussed how the insertion of needles in the desired manner can be difficult, so it is not a good idea to attempt this on a regular basis. With good insertion technique the retention of needles for a while, especially at key treatment points on the extremities, can also pose considerable challenges. Babies and small children rarely stay still enough for such needles to stay in place. Even with the use of noninserted needling methods there can be difficulty because the children will not stay still and can have a tendency to bump into the needle tip, and then they feel a needle prick, which is usually distressing.

Thus, an alternative approach is needed on babies and small children and even older children who are very afraid of needles. We can take advantage of the high sensitivity and responsiveness of children (see discussions in Chapter 4) and are able to use the blunt-tipped needle, the *teishin* (see Birch and Ida 1998, pp. 50–51) instead of a regular filiform needle (**Fig. 10.1**). Keiri Inoue, one of the fathers of the Meridian Therapy movement, extended the *teishin's* use further by developing the spring-loaded *teishin*, which is ideal for use with babies, or on small and frightened children (**Fig. 10.2a**).

With sufficient training the *teishin* can be used for applying treatment on adults. The high sensitivity of children makes them sufficiently responsive that with minimal training it is possible to treat them effectively with the spring-loaded *teishin*. The techniques for using the spring-loaded instrument for a pattern-based Meridian Therapy root treatment are easy to learn and easy to apply.

The *teishin* that is to be used on babies and children must have a very soft spring inside, so that it gives little pressure to the skin and certainly no discomfort at all. The spring-loaded *teishin* made in Japan is usually good for this. But many available spring-loaded *teishin* have springs that are too stiff to use on children. If you are unsure about how stiff the spring is in the *teishin* you are about to purchase then a good alternative is the *tsumo-shin* (**Fig. 10.2b**), which comes with a variety of springs, the softest of which is good for use with babies and children. The *tsumo-shin* is available from companies in the United States and elsewhere (see Treatment Equipment, p. 335). The *tsumo-shin* guarantees to provide a soft spring suitable for treatment of children and babies.

Treatment Technique with Spring-Loaded *Teishin or Tsumo-shin*

I learned the basic methods for use of the spring-loaded *teishin* for performing supplementation and draining techniques in the mid-1980s from my teacher, Dr. Yoshio Manaka, while I was studying with him in Odawara, Japan. At first I did not use the spring-loaded *teishin* for these techniques because I also started learning Toyohari and the use of the regular *teishin* to perform these techniques. But later, I had the chance to reflect on and then revisit what I had learned from Dr. Manaka and found that, at least

for babies and small children, the spring-loaded *teishin* can produce quite clear supplementation and draining effects when applied as described following here.

After selecting the pattern to be treated one should securely hold the limb and place one's finger and thumb of the left hand together (the *oshide*, or supporting hand position) over the acupoint to be treated—being careful not to be forceful or trigger resistance (see MediaCenter. thieme.com for details). Notice how the other fingers of the hand lightly hold the limb of the child so as to help secure the limb nonforcefully and to stabilize the acupoint. Place the point of the

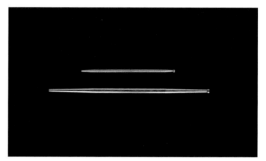

Fig. 10.1   *Teishin.*

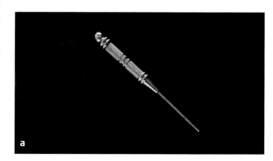

a

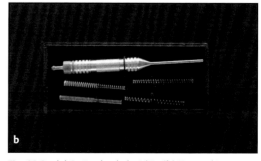

b

Fig. 10.2   (a) Spring-loaded *teishin.* **(b)** *Tsumo-shin.*

teishin/tsumo-shin carefully between the finger and thumb so that it touches the skin at ~ 90° to the acupoint (see MediaCenter.thieme.com).

Without delay, softly and slowly press and release the *teishin/tsumo-shin* handle so that the *teishin/tsumo-shin* bounces slightly on the acupoint. Do this several times and then remove the *teishin/tsumo-shin,* making a very slight pressure between the thumb and finger of the *oshide* as the *teishin/tsumo-shin* is removed slowly away from the skin. There are several important points to pay attention to:

- When you place the *teishin/tsumo-shin* between the finger and thumb over the acupoint, place it so that the round point is virtually level with the tips of the finger and thumb or protrudes very slightly from between the finger and thumb.
- Lightly squeeze the tip of the instrument so as to hold it still within the *oshide* (be careful not to squeeze hard or become tense when you squeeze).
- Make sure that the pressure and bouncing on the skin are very light. The pressure and bouncing are done approximately once per second or second and a half.
- You may press and release/bounce three or more times to get the effect.
- When you do this you should be relaxed and quietly focused on the acupoint you are treating.
- The younger or more ill the child, the less the tip of the instrument presses beyond the tips of the finger and thumb and the fewer presses and releases/bounces are necessary to regulate the dose.
- Remove the *teishin/tsumo-shin* by first pulling it slightly away from the point, allowing the finger and thumb to close over the end of the *teishin/tsumo-shin,* and then slowly remove the instrument completely, leaving the *oshide* on the point for a short time. The different aspects of this technique are covered in detail at MediaCenter.thieme.com.

If you are doing the draining technique with the *teishin/tsumo-shin,* place it to the skin between the finger and thumb in the same manner. The movement is quicker, and the pressure is slightly greater so that it is very slightly stimulating. The *teishin/tsumo-shin* is removed slowly without any increase of pressure between the finger and thumb of the *oshide.* This is covered in detail at MediaCenter.thieme.com.

It is important if you have not taken a *shon-ishin* workshop and studied this technique directly to first study the information at MediaCenter. thieme.com, comparing how the two techniques are applied, and then to try them on yourself before trying them on pediatric patients. You must become comfortable with the techniques so that they feel natural and unrestrained before you try them on a child. Your hesitation may be interpreted differently by the child.

On occasion it is simply too difficult to find the acupoint and place the *oshide* so that you can treat it with the *teishin.* Mostly this occurs because the child is moving around a lot and doesn't want to be touched. If this happens you can use a round-headed instrument, such as an *enshin,* and apply very gentle stroking along the flow of the channel across the acupoint. For example, if treating LU-9, hold the child's wrist so that the lung channel is exposed, then starting around LU-8, gently and relatively slowly stroke the instrument along the lung channel over LU-9, then remove and repeat. Do this some three to four times. Although not ideal, it is better than not applying the treatment.

On children over age 12, and certainly with more emotionally mature children who are not afraid of the needles, one can apply both supplementation and draining techniques with thin (0.12 mm) needles shallowly inserted (0.5–2 mm). Provided your technique is painless it is usually no problem. In the next chapter I describe a few tricks you can use to make the insertion of the needle painless. In that chapter I focus on neutral needling of the acupoint for the purposes of addressing symptoms. Here I discuss needling that is related to either the supplementation or the draining techniques.

The supplementation involves use of 0.12 mm needles. Insert the needle along the flow of the channel at around a 20 to 30° angle. Insert the needle on the exhalation and remove on the inhalation. Close the point as you remove the needle using a cotton ball. Remove the needle relatively quickly. The needles can be retained for around 1 to 2 minutes.

The draining needle technique involves the use of slightly thicker needles (e.g., 0.16 mm). Insert the needle against the flow of the channel at around a 20 to 30° angle. Insert the needle around 2 to 3 mm deep. Insert on the inhalation and remove on the exhalation. Once the needle is inserted, advance it around 1 mm and then pull back around 1 mm, repeat this rhythmically a few times, at a pace of around one up–down movement every 1 to 1.5 seconds. Remove the needle slowly and do not press the acupoint to close it as you remove the needle.

Much more can be said about the traditional needling techniques of supplementation and draining (Birch 2013, 2014; Shudo 1990, 2003), it can be very helpful to read up on these details and variations.

Practicing to Refine Your Technique

■ Practicing on Colleagues or Friends

Learning something new requires a number of steps to be able to use it. First one has to remember the basic details. Next one has to practice the basic techniques until they are done right. Next one has to practice them further until they are done well. And since babies and children are very sensitive, it is better to get to the level of doing the techniques well as soon as possible. Thus after reading and assimilating the information here it can be important and helpful to try it out on yourself, colleagues, or family members. My teacher, Dr. Manaka, strongly suggested this as a good idea before using it on actual patients. For many both the diagnostic techniques and their patterns will be unfamiliar and the treatment methods unfamiliar. It is thus helpful to practice both.

Diagnosis

Examine a colleague, friend, or family member, following the diagnostic procedures described earlier, and choose a pattern to treat (lung, spleen, liver, or kidney vacuity pattern). Be sure to note clearly the basic pulse qualities of depth, strength, and speed as described in Chapter 6. These basic pulse qualities will change as you start to apply treatment techniques; thus it is good to monitor them to see how you are doing. If the pulse is more rapid, hard, and floating it will sink, soften, and/or slow as a sign of improvement. If the pulse is more rapid, soft, and deep it will be less rapid, less deep, and/or stronger/firmer as a sign of improvement.

Treatment

Using the spring-loaded *teishin* or *tsumo-shin,* once you have chosen the pattern for treatment, apply treatment to the appropriate points. Can you make the pulse quality improve? Check the pulse after each point you have tried to supplement with the instrument.

Repeat this using very thin needles very shallowly and painlessly inserted as you might on an older child, such as a teenager. Can you needle painlessly? Can you make the pulse quality improve?

■ Practicing on an Inert Surface

Use a small block of soft modeling clay or plasticine, smoothing the surface and covering the block with aluminum foil as described in Chapter 6.

Placing the *Oshide*

1. Place the finger and thumb on the clay/foil. Hold it still with a constant force of contact. Can you do this and leave no depression in the foil or clay?
2. When treating a small child that will not stay still for you, it is often necessary that you use the other three fingers of your *oshide* hand to stabilize the *oshide.* This is done by grasping the limb of the child between those fingers and the palm of the hand so that the finger and thumb that form the *oshide* can be placed lightly on the skin surface over the point to be treated (**Fig. 10.3a**). Practice this by picking up and holding the clay and placing the *oshide* (**Fig. 10.3b**). When you do this, can you place and hold the *oshide* still for a few seconds so as not to cause a depression in the clay? A slight depression in the foil may be observed. Repeat this moving your hand around slightly, all the while trying to maintain a constant force of contact of the *oshide* to the skin.

Applying the Technique

1. Place your *oshide* on the clay/foil, holding it steady. Place the *teishin/tsumo-shin* so that the rounded tip is level with the tips of your finger and thumb. Gently squeezing the tip in the oshide, apply a light and slow press and release (bounce) of the instrument, repeat a few times, then remove the *teishin/tsumo-shin.* If done

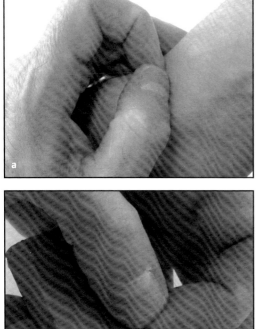

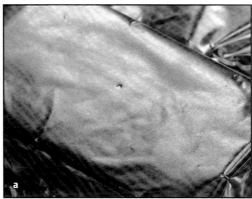

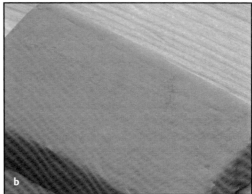

Fig. 10.4 (a, b)   Applying the *teishin*.

Fig. 10.3 (a, b)   *Oshide* placement.

well there will be barely a visible depression in the foil from the instrument and almost nothing in the clay **(Fig. 10.4a)**.

2. Repeat this but with the tip of the *teishin/ tsumo-shin* extended very slightly more. After this a somewhat more obvious depression in both the foil and the clay will be visible **(Fig. 10.4b)**.

3. Repeat step 1, but hold the clay tablet in your *oshide* hand and keep your hand still. With this low-dose treatment, can you produce the same kind of depression as found in step 1? Repeat again, but while moving the *oshide* hand a little. How is the depression in the foil and clay?

4. Repeat step 2, but hold the clay tablet in your *oshide* hand and keep your hand still. With this

slightly increased dose of treatment can you produce the same kind of depression as in 2? Repeat again while moving the *oshide* hand a little. How is the depression in the foil and clay?

These simple practice methods will allow you to more rapidly develop skill at this simple technique. When done well, hardly any depression is visible in the clay, while a slightly more obvious one is visible in the foil. When you do this always try to remain relaxed. Practice this in different postures. When standing straight up with the clay tablet directly in front of your belly. When leaning over at an angle with the clay tablet not quite in front of your belly. How does your posture affect the results? What do you need to do as you have to change your posture to maintain the best results? Being relaxed and calm is a very useful tool for treatment. Staying relaxed and calm can be difficult at times as you respond to the child's activities and cries. There is no better teacher than to practice these techniques both on friends and with the clay exercises and then on actual patients. My colleagues and I have described a series of simple exercises that can help you develop these skills more quickly. It can be helpful to practice some of these simple body-work exercises to help with your skill development.[2]

Point Location of Main Treatment Points

Many textbooks of acupuncture detail the location of the acupuncture points that are to be treated. The trend started as early as 280 CE with Huang-fu Mi's attempt to systematize the knowledge of acupuncture in his *Zhen Jiu Jia Yi Jing (The First Systematic Classic of Acupuncture and Moxibustion)*. However, not only were early descriptions much more vague than those we use today, but the earliest literature on acupoints specified them as not being anatomically based entities, rather as places where *qi* comes in and goes out of the body.[3] These two factors have encouraged many variations in descriptions of the acupoints, which have invariably tried to focus on anatomical landmarks to help the practitioner remember where to apply treatment. These inherent point location variations are self-evident to anyone studying different modern forms of acupuncture. It should thus not be surprising to the reader that the point locations described following here may be different from what you have studied in acupuncture school. Additionally, as explained in Chapter 2, the acupoints are not yet fully matured in babies and small children; they are more like zones rather than discrete points; thus the kind of anatomical precision that is required on adults for treatment to be effective is less of an issue on babies and small children.

Next, we cover the basic location of the major treatment points and the typical reactions that are palpated at those points so as to help make localization more precise.

LU-9 is at the juncture of the edge of the tendon extensor pollicis between the tendon and radial artery, on the wrist crease.

LU-8 is along the same ulnar edge of the tendon extensor pollicis level with the high point of the styloid process.

LU-5 (following historical descriptions) is located on the artery in the elbow crease. The brachial artery is palpable in the elbow crease and on most people is located on the ulnar side of the tendon of the biceps brachial muscle. The point is located on the radial edge of the artery in the elbow crease. First find the tendon with the elbow slightly bent, then straighten the elbow to feel the artery.

PC-7 is between the tendons of the flexor carpi radialis and the palmaris longus on the wrist crease.

To find **KI-10,** place the index finger on the popliteal fossa and pull it medially until it meets the posterior margin of the sartorius muscle. The point is at the juncture of the popliteal fossa and the posterior margin of the muscle.

LR-8 is on the anterior margin of the sartorius muscle and is touched by the thumb as one softly pinches the muscle between finger and thumb. It is on the line between the middle of the patella and **KI-10** as it intersects the anterior margin of the sartorius muscle.

LR-8 and **KI-10** are usually found and treated with the knee straight.

KI-7 is ~2 *cun* above the level of **KI-3** along the anterior margin of the Achilles tendon.

To find **SP-3** wiggle the big toe from side to side. The tendon of the abductor hallucis brevis muscle along the spleen channel can be identified. **SP-3** is on the lower margin of this tendon as it intersects the proximal margin of the distal head of the first metatarsal.

On many children SP-3 can be ticklish, and they have difficulty keeping the foot still, in which case we use the next five-phase point coming up the channel, SP-5. SP-5 is found in front of the medial ankle in a depression roughly at the juncture of a line that runs along the inferior edge of the ankle and another line that runs along the anterior edge of the ankle.

Fig. 10.5 shows the locations of the acupoints.

Because the needling is shallow, to find the treatment points, touch very softly to examine the condition of the skin. The point will show signs of weakness: such as a small depression, softness, weakness, swollen/puffy feeling, sticky feeling.

---

[2]   See *Restoring Order in Health and Chinese Medicine,* Chapters 9 and 10 (Birch, Cabrer, Rodriguez 2014).

[3]   For details of this historical development and the nature of the acupoints see Birch (2014).

To locate the point most precisely and to help place the treatment tool (needle or *teishin*) to the point more precisely, it is advised to softly stroke along the channel flow with the ulnar distal corner of the index finger. Once signs of weakness are found in the vicinity of the point you want to treat, stop moving the finger and place the thumb next to the finger over the point. This process is shown at MediaCenter.thieme.com. But sometimes the best you can do is find the point rapidly and fix it with your *oshide* finger and thumb, while the rest of your fingers grasp the limb to stabilize the *oshide* and then apply the treatment as quickly and precisely as you can. When the child is moving around a lot it is better to apply the treatment even somewhat inelegantly and quickly than not at all.

Five-Phase Correspondences and Clinical Practice

The system of Meridian Therapy, following the models proposed in the *Nan Jing*, uses five-phase theory extensively. Five-phase theory has two main aspects to it. First, the cycles of interaction, such as the engendering (*sheng*) and restraining

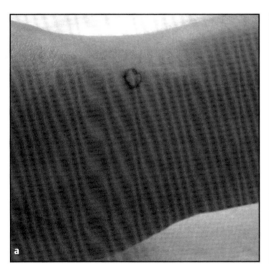
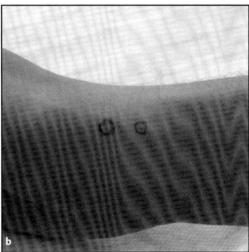
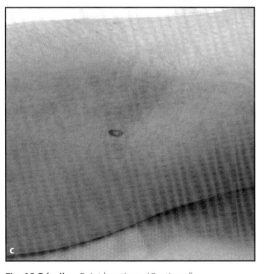
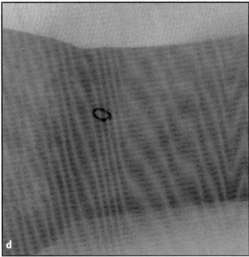

Fig. 10.5 (a–i)   Point locations. (*Continued*)

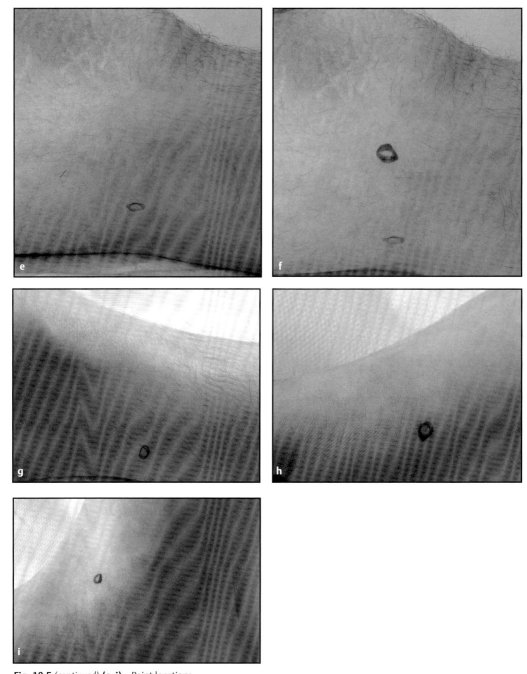

Fig. 10.5 *(continued)* **(a–i)**   Point locations.

(*ke*) cycles. These form, in accordance with *Nan-Jing*, Chapter 69, ideas, the backbone of the diagnosis by patterns in Meridian Therapy. The other main feature of five-phase theory is the "theory of systematic correspondence," including the multiple correspondences that each phase has. Examples of these correspondences are shown in **Table 10.3.**

Table 10.3   Common five-phase correspondences

Correspondence	Wood	Fire	Earth	Metal	Water
Channels	Liver + gallbladder	Heart + small intestine + pericardium + triple burner	Spleen + stomach	Lung + large intestine	Kidney + bladder
Season	Spring	Summer	"Long summer" or 18 days between season periods	Autumn	Winter
Color	Green	Red	Yellow	White	Black
Odor	Rancid	Burned	Sweet	Frowzy	Rotten
Voice	Shouting	Laughing	Singing	Wailing	Groaning
Tastes	Sour	Bitter	Sweet	Spicy	Salty
Orifices	Eyes	Tongue	Mouth	Nose	Ears
Tissues controlled	Muscles/sinews[a]	Blood vessels	Flesh[a]	Skin/hair	Bones
Climate (*Su Wen*)	Wind	Heat	Dampness	Dryness	Cold
Climate (*Nan Jing*) (*external factors*)	Wind	Heat	Overeating/overdrinking/overwork	Cold	Dampness
Emotions	Anger	Joy	Pensiveness	Grief	Fear

[a] Clinically, the difference between the liver controlling the *jin* or sinews and the spleen controlling the *ru* or flesh (including the muscles) is that with liver problems the muscles are usually tight, in spasm; with spleen problems the muscles are usually weakened, the patient feels the limbs are heavy.

We do not use many of these correspondences to form the diagnosis of the patient in Meridian Therapy. Classification of some of the signs in **Table 10.3** can be difficult, such as the precise smell and color. On adults it has become common to use these signs more in terms of overall assessment of the patient's condition rather than choosing a treatment. If something clear shows on a child, it can also be used in this way.

One of the principal issues that comes up for many of those studying Meridian Therapy who have a background in traditional Chinese medicine (TCM) or other Chinese-based models of acupuncture practice lies in the role of external climatic factors and the classification by signs or association. The *Huang Di Nei Jing Su Wen (The Yellow Emperor's Inner Classic—Basic Questions)* and *Nan Jing* clearly describe different correspondences in relation to external factors that mostly relate to climatic influences (Shudo 1990, p. 27). This can be confusing, but in practice, both sets of correspondences seem to be applicable; thus we need to be flexible and not so theoretical in our approach.

If a child shows a lot of phlegm or mucus, the condition is not automatically (as seems to be common in TCM practice) seen as being spleen related. However, if the mucus is disturbing the digestive functions (e.g., causing a blocked nose with anosmia [lack of sense of smell] leading to poor appetite), this could eventually become spleen related. Likewise, the heavily congested lungs with a lot of phlegm and chronic coughing, could be seen as spleen related if, for example, the repetitive coughing triggers problems of regurgitation or vomiting.

For the child whose symptoms are worse when cold, one needs to look at other factors to see if this is lung or kidney related; one cannot automatically assume one or the other. If the feet tend to easily cool, this is kidney related, if the hands easily cool this is lung related. However, if the peripheral circulation in all limbs is diminished and both hands and feet tend to be cool, you need to examine other signs to differentiate.

A final comment on the external (including climatic factors) is also necessary. In TCM and other styles of acupuncture, great care is paid to differentiating the presence or effects of these different factors. However, in Meridian Therapy, it makes little difference in practical terms which is present or creating problems.[4] We apply the draining needle technique regardless of whether the affliction was cold, damp, heat, wind related, and so on. The draining needle technique is varied more in relation to the relative strength of the hardness felt in the pulse position of the channel that is being drained, rather than the more abstract classification system. Similarly, by and large, we do not vary the acupoints that we treat on the basis of these factors. Rather, if we vary choice of acupoints, we tend to use the ideas above from *Nan Jing*, Chapter 68.

Assessing Treatment Effectiveness

With the core non-pattern-based root treatment we see a range of changes on the body surface in the skin condition and texture, and changes of tonus of the underlying tissues. These changes can also occur with the pattern-based root treatment, but they can be less obvious than with the core non-pattern-based treatment. It is useful to continue monitoring the condition of the skin and underlying tissues to see if that also changes further with your pattern-based root treatment. But these are not the most common things we pay attention to in the pattern-based root treatment.

When we use Meridian Therapy on adult patients we can see quite specific changes in the pulse and other findings that can be used as feedback for how well you have done the treatment (Birch 2009). The pulse quality will move toward a more healthy state. How is this understood and defined? If we note the basic pulse qualities of depth, strength, and rate, you will notice that these tend to move toward their healthier state. A healthy pulse is one that is not too fast, not too slow, not too strong, not too weak. In babies the

pulse rate is always rapid; this generally won't respond much, just as the slow pulse on an athlete will tend not to change much with treatment. Thus, in babies and small children the rate of the pulse is not usually very sensitive to treatment. In older children (over age 3) you can feel the pulse rate change more easily.

Thus, in a baby, if the pulse had been weak and more superficial, it will be less weak and less superficial after the root treatment. For a child whose pulse was weak, a little deep, and a little rapid, the pulse changes following successful needling will be that the pulse becomes less weak, less deep, and slows down. Likewise for the pulse that is strong, rapid, and more floating; it will sink, soften, and slow down. It is thus a good idea to get a quick sense of the pulse quality before you start treatment and monitor the pulse quality periodically during and after the treatment. This can give you further information about how well you have applied treatment and/or the extent to which the child responds to treatment. In adults, a good treatment also triggers changes in breathing: the breath often becomes slower and more rhythmic. We often see the patient become more relaxed. These are also good signs to look for in the child.

But regarding all of these signs it can be difficult to obtain the information clearly when the child is upset, moving a lot, being resistant, playing too much. You have to practice making your observations very quickly and without hesitation. The touching of the body surface can be done quickly and unobtrusively, but palpating the pulses can be tricky. Often the child is a bit calmer as you apply treatment and he or she will let you feel the pulses. But just as often the child will have had enough, and will want to stop the treatment, so he or she becomes more resistant. The only way to improve on this aspect of treatment is to practice.

---

[4]   This is not the case in all styles of Meridian Therapy, but for what is described in this chapter it is so.

Section IV Symptomatic Treatment Approaches and Techniques

11 Needling

Introduction

Once the root treatment has been administered, in most cases one then adds some light stimulation to target relief of the child's symptoms. What is done, where, and with what level of dose varies considerably depending on age, sensitivity, symptoms, and overall health of the child. Some of the *shonishin* tools and treatment techniques can be applied to start addressing symptoms. The most common technique is the use of tapping at specific acupoints or over specific regions of the body; the next being the application of gentle pressure to specific acupoints. Most regular adult acupuncture methods can also be used on children, provided they are modified and made suitable for the child. This includes the use of needling, moxa, cupping, bleeding, retention of press-spheres, intradermal needles, or press-tack needles. This section covers the tools and methods of applying them on babies and children. The book *Japanese Acupuncture: A Clinical Guide* (Birch and Ida 1998) covers each of these techniques in detail in individual chapters. What is described here should be complemented by reading the relevant chapters of that book. The content available on MediaCenter.thieme.com also describes the techniques of needling, moxa, and the use of the press-sphere, press-tack needle, and intradermal needle. Please watch the relevant sections at MediaCenter.thieme.com for further details of these techniques.

In general when inserting needles into a baby or child we have two simple approaches:

- The "in and out" method: the needle is inserted, manipulated slightly for a short while, and then withdrawn.
- The "retained needle" method: the needle is inserted and retained for a while, a technique called *chishin* in Japanese.

For the in and out method, after insertion the needles are usually manipulated slightly with an up-and-down movement of the needle for a few seconds and then withdrawn. For the retained needle method, after insertion the needles are left for as long as 2 minutes or more, the time depending on the child's condition and sensitivity and whether he or she stays still or not. The techniques of insertion are illustrated at MediaCenter.thieme.com. To understand how to use these techniques on babies and children it is necessary to consider several important issues. The insertion of needles and the fearful reactions of the child have made many acupuncture practitioners avoid the use of acupuncture on babies and children.

In Chapter 2, I discussed the development of *shonishin* and the likely influences that gave rise to it. One of these is that inserting needles can be difficult on babies and children because they find it painful or distressing. This is not only stressful for children and their parents but also for the practitioner. Further, one of our primary goals in treatment is not to trigger unnecessary emotional expressions and outbursts since we are, as practitioners of traditionally based acupuncture, interested in helping regulate the *qi* of the patient, not cause it further disturbance. Therefore, we have to think about how we are to needle a child, where the reactions can be quite unpredictable. Before discussing the actual techniques of treatment in detail, I first discuss the handling of the child and parents and the choice of needles and other instruments.

Needle Types

To needle a child and minimize emotional reactions to what you do, you must use the right kind of needle. It is desirable that the child does not feel your needle or at least does not feel it as a threatening, uncomfortable, or painful thing. Thus we use only high-quality, thin needles. The moved up and down on an amplitude of around 1 mm a few times and then removed. Following my teachers' recommendations I feel it is better not to tell you to focus on feeling the *qi* arrival (which you probably will not be able to do for a while); rather, it is better to focus on whether you can feel the resistance at the tip of the needle as it is lightly moved up and down. If you do, and if, as the needle is moved you feel a change in that feeling of resistance, then this is the time to remove the needle. Even this feeling of resistance at the tip of the needle is very subtle, and something you will not immediately get a sense for. Thus the simplest approach is to move the needle up and down a few times according to the idea of dosage needs you have for the child. For example, for a lower dose move the needle up and down four or five times over 2 to 3 seconds, and for a greater dose maybe six or seven up and down movements over 3 to 4 seconds, whether you feel anything or not. The important thing to remember is the issue of dosage. If you try to take time to feel these things and you are not yet able to do this reliably and quickly, you will take more time than you have for the technique, and you will run the risk of overtreating the child. Do not do this.

For the *retained* needle method the issue of timing is also important. The fact that the needle has been inserted will provoke *qi* reactions. But you have applied the technique on a point where you want the stiffness in the underlying tissues to change, for example, for the stiff muscles around GB-20 to soften up. Although there will be a *qi* reaction, without additional needle manipulations it takes a short while for the local tissues to respond; hence we leave the needle for 1 to 3 minutes. As well as judging according to the dosage requirements of the child (leave the needle for less time for the more sensitive, more time for the less sensitive), you can watch the reactions and behavior of the child to give you a sense of when to remove the needle. If a child who had been more active starts to become calmer, and if his or her complexion improves, it is enough: remove the needle. If the child starts to show an interest in trying to reach the place where the needle has been inserted, it is enough: remove the needle. If the muscles look less tight around where you have needled, it is enough: remove the needle.

Needle Insertion

It is important that your needling is not uncomfortable. Often (especially with the *retained* needle method) you do not want to draw the child's attention to the inserted needle, and so it is preferable that he or she feels nothing and certainly nothing distressing. How to do this?

On babies and small children you cannot negotiate with them; you simply get permission from the parent. Once you are ready to needle, it depends on where you needle as to how to proceed. Sometimes, you need to needle a point without the child seeing what you have done. For the area around GB-20, have the child sit, put something in front of the child for him or her to focus on, then, hiding the tube and needle in your hand, reach behind the child, find the point (stiff muscles) place the tube and needle, press it slightly into the skin and tap it so that the needle inserts as much as the tube will allow with one tap. Then continue tapping on the tube—this gives the child the impression that you are simply applying the tapping technique (with which he or she is already familiar) over the area. Since the needle was not felt, the child cannot tell that you have inserted a needle. If you are applying the *in and out* technique, then remove the tube, apply the up and down movements of the needle quickly, and then remove the needle. If applying the *retained* needle method, simply remove the tube, leaving the needle inserted into the point. Remove the needle when enough has been achieved.

If the acupoint you want to needle is, for example, on the hand, such as LI-4, you will normally be using the in and out method. Have the child lie down, have the parent distract the child or give the child something to hold with the other hand. Take the hand you want to needle and place yourself between the child and his or her hand (in the space between the side of the body and the arm), so that your body blocks what you are doing from the view of the child. Insert the needle as described, with additional tapping; remove the tube; give the few up and down movements; remove the needle; then give the hand back. If the child did not feel the insertion he or she has no idea that you just inserted a needle. With this method it is important to hold the arm/hand of the child so that the child cannot pull it back while you are performing the needle technique. Don't grasp the limb tightly, hold it softly but firmly. Here, using your *oshide* or supporting hand (see Chapter 10) can be important and useful. As you start to look for the LI-4 acupoint securely hold the wrist/arm of the child between your third to fifth fingers and the palm/base of the hand. Your index finger and thumb are free to find the point and secure it, placing the tube with needle in the space between the thumb and index finger (the *oshide*). While the needle and tube are held between the thumb and index finger securely and without moving over the point, your other three fingers are securing the arm/wrist of the child in a grip between the finger and palm of the hand. You keep this grip at all times while you insert and manipulate the needle. This not only helps prevent the child from pulling the limb back but it allows you to move with the moving limb *without moving* the needle and tube placement at the acupoint.

If the acupoint you want to needle is on the back, such as BL-20, you can apply the *retained* needle method. But this area can be very sensitive for needling. Thus, with the child lying on his or her abdomen, find the point, place the needle and tube at the point, press the tube firmly into the skin so that it gives a clear sensation of pressure, tap the needle quickly into the point, applying more taps to give further distraction from the needling.

On a younger child it can be easier to insert a needle, for example into LI-4, in front of the child. The 2-year-old does not know that you are holding a needle. He or she will watch you needle the point and move the needle, but because it is quick and painless, the child only feels the tapping of the tube, and does not become frightened or upset.

Generally you will want to use the *in and out* needling method on acupoints where the child will not stay still, on points on the limbs where the child can move the limb to look at what he or she may be feeling, and on children who are in the oral phase and you want to make sure they do not grab the needle and try to place it in their mouth. The *retained* needle method is easy to use

on the back of the body and on older children who will stay still for you. Needling techniques are described at MediaCenter.thieme.com and in the book *Japanese Acupuncture: A Clinical Guide* (Birch and Ida 1998, pp. 60–77).

Key Points to Remember

When you place the needle and tube to the point to be treated, immediately apply a gentle but firm pressure. The pressure gives distracting sensations thus making pain on insertion less likely. It also stretches the skin within the space of the tube so that the force of the tap is met by less resistance of the soft, flexible skin, and the needle inserts more easily.

Immediately tap the needle so that it inserts as far as the tube will allow, then continue tapping the tube. After the needle is inserted the child then only feels a continuous tapping, which, while different in quality than tapping with, for example, the *herabari*, appears to be a form of tapping and not as frightening as inserting a needle.

Practice Methods to Improve Your Needle Insertion Skills

1. Needle yourself. You can do this on points or areas on relatively neutral areas of your leg, such as on your thigh between the spleen and stomach channels, or on more sensitive points or areas on the feet or abdomen. Can you *routinely* insert the needle painlessly? What pressure of tube is optimal for less sensitive regions and for more sensitive regions?
2. As you apply the needle insertion technique, vary how you do this to see which is more likely to give painless, and the even better sensationless, insertion.
3. After the needle has been inserted apply tapping to the tube. What does that feel like and what force of tapping is comfortable?

press-spheres or the 0.3 mm press-tack needles on these points after the root treatment. If after a couple of treatments we notice no change in the asthma symptoms and no signs of overtreatment, we then leave 0.6 mm press-tack needles for a day and a half, to be replaced by press-spheres. If there is still no change in the symptoms and there are no signs of overtreatment, we start leaving intradermal needles to give a stronger treatment effect.

Precautions

There are certain important precautions to be observed with the use of these three instruments.

Press-spheres and press-tack needles should not be used on areas that receive a lot of pressure, such as the buttocks. Neither should they be given any further stimulation by parent or patient. They should not be touched until removed.

Generally do not leave needles or press-spheres of different metals, for example, a stainless steel press-tack needle on one point and a gold plated press-sphere on another. The metals should always be the same. Thus, if you want to leave only press-spheres, they can all be stainless steel or gold plated. If you want to leave, for example, a press-sphere on GV-12 and press-tack needles on the asthma *shu* points, since the press-tack needles are stainless steel, the press-sphere should also be of stainless steel.

If the child plays sports, such as football, it is a good idea to have the needles removed before the game begins, and you should recommend this to the parents.

There are additional important rules for the use of intradermal needles:
- Always follow skin folds, and if no skin folds are apparent, insert the needle along with the flow of the channel that the acupoint lies on.
- Insert the needle almost flat to the skin.
- Don't insert the intradermal needle more than half the actual length of the shaft of the needle (for the 3 mm needle this means insert the needle ~ 1 mm).
- After inserting the intradermal needle always make sure it is not too deeply inserted, so if you press on the handle you should see the point of the needle raise the skin.

- Leave the intradermal needle for several hours and never more than 3 days. If the child is older and plays sports, it is better to recommend that the parent remove the needle before the activity starts.
- Tape the needle with two pieces of tape, a small piece under the handle of the needle and a larger piece over the top of the needle. Make sure that the larger piece is longer than the length of the needle and covers the needle completely. As you tape the needle, stretch the skin slightly—this will help counter the normal movements of the skin, which could tend to loosen the tape.
- The parent should be given instructions about when and how to remove the needle. If the intradermal needle causes discomfort it should be removed.
- Instruct the parent in the safe care of the needle: that is, do not rub the area where the needle is placed too vigorously. When drying after a shower or bath, be careful drying that region. If the tape starts peeling up at the edge, place a new piece of tape over the edge to protect it, or remove the needle.
- Do not place more than one needle (intradermal or press-tack) along the path of a channel. For example, do not leave needles at both right BL-18 and right BL-23. Occasionally this can be too much stimulation and can be too much for the patient.

The press-sphere provides continuous pressure to the point on which it is placed. Over time, this can irritate the skin. To prevent unnecessary skin irritation Hyodo (1986) recommended changing them regularly. After 1 or 2 days[2] have the parent remove the press-sphere. When it is removed a small depression will be visible where it had been placed. Place another press-sphere right next to the point, but not in the depression. Repeat this every 1 or 2 days, moving around the original spot you placed the first press-sphere. This reduces the risk of irritation and keeps the acupoint continuously stimulated. Give the parents a strip of press-spheres so that they can replace them regularly at home. If the skin does

---

[2] For the more sensitive child with thin sensitive skin, change daily. For other children, change every other day.

become irritated, which happens in a small number of cases, or through prolonged stimulation of the same point, stop applying the press-spheres until the skin has healed, and you may start to use the 0.3 mm press-tack needles instead.

Application of Press-Spheres, Press-Tack Needles, and Intradermal Needles

To place the press-sphere you need to be careful not to touch the tape with your fingers because this will reduce the stickiness of the tape. Always use tweezers. Peel the tape with the press-sphere above the strip it comes on, holding the tape by only a small portion. Find the point to be treated, lightly stretch the skin, and quickly press the tape and sphere onto the point, making sure with the pad of your finger that the tape sticks all the way around its edges.

To place the new Pyonex press-tack needle, tear open the packaging of the needle to expose it. The needle is on a piece of tape, placed onto a paper surface. Fold down the plastic base of the container the needle comes in. This exposes the edge of the tape, which adheres to a small piece of white nonsticky paper. Pick up the needle holding it by the piece of paper. As you do this, the tape and needle are peeled off the rest of the surface they were originally placed on. Now the needle is ready to be inserted. Making sure not to touch the tape at all with your fingers, find the point to be treated. Stretch the skin slightly, then quickly place the tape and needle on the point, pressing with the pad of the finger to make sure that the tape sticks all along its edges smoothly. The child should not feel the insertion of this needle.

To place the intradermal needle, carefully open the top of the packaging that the needle comes in, making sure not to drop the needle. I recommend holding the needle firmly between the middle fingers pressed together on the outside of the packaging. Then slowly peel back the packaging to expose the handle of the needle. Then using tweezers, carefully grab the needle by the handle. The tweezers need to have a good grip on the handle so that the needle does not move. When you find the point to be treated, decide the angle and direction of insertion of the needle. For example, if inserting a needle at the asthma *shu* point, angle down the back; for BL-23, angle toward the spine. Place the tip of the needle at the point to be treated, in the correct angle for insertion, then slowly, while pressing the needle tip gently into the skin, pull the skin from behind so that the skin is made to slide up over the needle. By this method the needle is inserted without pushing the needle and is much more likely to be painless and sensationless. Once the needle is inserted, check visually how much of the needle appears to be inserted (it should be about one-third to half the length of the needle shaft), adjust as necessary by pulling the needle out a bit or inserting a bit more, then press on the handle of the needle to make sure that the tip raises the skin. Tape by placing a piece of tape on the skin under the handle, and then a larger piece over the needle and smaller tape. As you place the tape, slightly stretch the skin to ensure better adhesion.

These three methods are described at Media-Center.thieme.com and each method is described in the book *Japanese Acupuncture: A Clinical Guide* (Birch and Ida 1998, pp. 139–158,[3] 165–171, 175–180).

In recent years the new Pyonex press-tack needles from Seirin have become more commonly used than the press-spheres, even on babies and small children. The intradermal needles are also less commonly used, tending to be used in certain conditions, such as asthma or bedwetting, and more likely on older children.

---

[3] The book describes the use of the older press-tack needles; although different it is useful to read this for additional information. The new Pyonex press-tack needles are much easier and safer to use than the older press-tack needles.

15 *Shiraku*—Bloodletting (*Jing* Points and Vascular Spiders)

Bloodletting can be a commonly used technique, depending, of course, on the preferences of the practitioner. However, on children we tend not to use it very often because of the difficulties of applying the technique and such issues as parental approval and upsetting the child. The most common uses are to bleed *jing* points or stab and remove some blood from small blood vessels, such as vascular spiders. The techniques and details of these methods are covered in *Japanese Acupuncture: A Clinical Guide* (Birch and Ida 1998, pp. 209–242).

For bloodletting we no longer use the three-edged bloodletting needle that has been used historically in Asia. It is much easier using the lancets that diabetic patients use. They are finer, sterile, inexpensive, and disposable. They have been manufactured and improved for use by diabetic patients who routinely check their blood sugar levels by taking blood from the fingertips—a very sensitive area.

Of course, when you are to come in contact with the body fluids of a patient you must protect yourself and be careful about contamination. The following basic rules need to be followed:

- Always wear latex or rubber gloves.
- Prepare the lancet needles, alcohol-soaked cotton balls, and dry cotton balls in advance. Place these on a nonporous surface that can either be sterilized afterward (e.g., a metal tray) or disposed of (e.g., a plastic surface).
- Wipe the skin to be punctured with alcohol. Let the alcohol dry.
- Apply the lancet needle (yet to be described), remove the small amount of blood desired, being careful not to touch anything with your contaminated hands, and place the needle and contaminated cotton balls only on the nonporous surface.

More details of this are given in *Japanese Acupuncture* (Birch and Ida 1998, pp. 216–217).

In the following section I list indications that have been edited from Maruyama and Kudo (1982) and describe the techniques in each style of bloodletting (*jing* points and vascular spiders).

Jing Point Bloodletting

Bloodletting can be used if one modifies the manner of needle use and blood removal to modify and control the dose of treatment and make the technique completely painless. Bloodletting *jing* points can be very helpful for certain pediatric conditions as indicated in the following edited list from Maruyama and Kudo (1982). But it is also good to remember that any symptom in the related channel can also be targeted. The primary findings that indicate the use of *jing* point bloodletting are location of symptom, channel affected, signs of blood stasis, and reactions at the *jing* point, such as redness, swelling, puffiness, or pressure pain. For details of the methods of *jing* point bloodletting, its precautions, and doses see *Japanese Acupuncture* (Birch and Ida 1998, pp. 233–241) and Shimada (2005).

■ Indications for the Nail Corners of the Fingers

Thumb: mainly applied at the radial corner (LU-11), but can be applied at both corners
 Good for: tonsillitis, pharyngeal catarrh, mumps, bronchial asthma, teething fevers of infants
Index finger: mainly applied at the radial corner (LI-1)
 Good for: lymphadenitis of the neck region, bronchial asthma, toothache of the lower jaw
Middle finger: radial corner (PC-9)
 Good for: diseases with high fever
Fourth finger: mainly the ulnar corner (TB-1)
 Good for: headache, congestion of the eye, pharyngeal pain
Little finger: ulnar corner (SI-1)
 Good for: dyspnea, pharyngeal pain, convulsive disorders

■ **Indications for the Nail Corners of the Toes**

These areas are not as frequently used as the fingernail corners, but they do have wide application and distinctive effects for the indicated symptoms. These are interesting areas for the application of bloodletting techniques. Their indications are as follows:

Big toe: medial corner (SP-1)
Good for: indigestion, acute gastroenteritis, infantile seizures

Lateral corner (LR-1)
Good for: eye problems (especially if with severe pain), convulsive disorders

Second toe: mainly the lateral corner (ST-45)
Good for: toothache of the upper jaw, gastroenteric disorders

Fourth toe: usually the lateral corner (GB-44), but sometimes the medial corner is very effective
Good for: headache, eye pain, ear pain

Selection of points should be based on the finding of appropriate signs at the *jing* point, such as redness, swelling, pressure pain, as well as associated symptoms.

To bleed the point, hold the digit firmly with the fingers and thumb of the nondominant hand (most commonly left). Hold the lancet between the index finger and thumb of your dominant hand (most commonly right) so that the tip of the lancet lies *just behind the level of the tips of the finger and thumb*, which should be level. Carefully place the tip of the lancet directed toward the point, almost touching the point. Make sure that either the tip of the index finger or the tip of the thumb lightly touches the finger near the point. With a smooth *rapid rolling* motion, roll from the fingertip touching the skin over to the other fingertip, pulling away from the child's digit as soon as the other fingertip touches the skin. As you do this the tip of the needle very rapidly presses the skin at the point to be bled, making a tiny cut. When done correctly, the needling is painless and the drops of blood can be squeezed out one at a time. You are not stabbing the point, rather the motion you make presses the tip of the needle into the skin, and since the skin is very fine, it makes a very small superficial cut. Remove the number of desired drops of blood using the wet cotton ball; to stop, press the point with the dry cotton ball—when done correctly the blood stops when you want it to. The amount of blood removed relates to the desired dose for the child and the point. Sometimes a single drop is enough, but you may want to take up to five drops.

This technique needs to be thoroughly practiced before you try it on a child. The action of rolling over the point quickly is very important. If you get this wrong you will cause a deeper stab than you intend (making dose regulation more difficult) and cause unnecessary pain (making treatment management more difficult). Do not do this on a child until you have been able to routinely apply it painlessly on adults.

Vascular Spider Bloodletting

The bleeding of vascular spiders can also be a very useful therapy to treat blood stasis and relieve symptoms associated with it. The two most common areas where vascular spiders occur are in the lower cervical and upper thoracic region (C6 to T4) and in the lumbar-sacral region. The upper spine region is indicated for any symptom in the upper half of the body, and the lower spine region is indicated for any symptom in the lower half of the body. Maruyama and Kudo (1982) list certain symptoms associated with each area, an edited version of which follows. For details of the methods, precautions, and doses of vascular spider bloodletting see *Japanese Acupuncture* (Birch and Ida 1998, pp. 213–229).

■ **C6-T4 Region Indications**

Look for vascular spiders on the back of the shoulders in patients whose main complaints are accompanied by stiff shoulders and can include difficulty breathing, expectoration, problems such as bronchial asthma, chronic bronchitis, and so on; and patients whose main complaints are problems of the eyes, ears, nose, face, neck, and throat. We can add to this symptoms of the cervical or thoracic spine and any symptoms of the upper limbs.

■ **Lumbosacral Region Indications**

The lumbosacral region extends from L4 to the sacrum and is effective for problems of the lower half of the body, especially chronic problems of the urogenital system, bowels, locomotor system. In some cases, with repeated bloodletting, we can obtain unexpected improvements. In this region, when we cannot find vascular spiders, we look for small superficial venules. They seem to function the same as the vascular spiders.

Bloodletting in this region can be good for problems in the lower half of the body including urinary disturbances, or skin problems of the lower body.

To bleed the vascular spider we use the same kind of lancet needle as for the *jing* points. The technique is very different. For the *jing* point, the needle is held so that its tip lies just behind the level of the finger and thumb; the lancet needle is rolled over the point quickly. For the vascular spider the lancet is held so that the tip extends very slightly beyond the level of the tips of the finger and thumb. The lancet is placed almost perpendicular to the vascular spider and inserted with a rapid down and up motion of the needle. To do this, first make sure that the tip of the needle is lined up with the vascular spider so that, as you press the needle down, it stabs into the middle of the vascular spider. One way of making sure you have lined up the needle tip correctly is to lightly press the skin with the needle tip. When lined up correctly you will see blood pressed back inside the vascular spider either side of where the needle tip is pressing. To apply the technique *do not* let the needle move up from the skin before applying the downward stabbing (this usually causes the stab to miss the vascular spider). The stabbing is done with a quick downward pressure followed immediately by withdrawal (like a bounce). Essentially you are trying to cut the upper edge of the vascular spider

so that a small amount of blood can be removed through the small cut on the upper surface of the vascular spider.

On children we don't use cupping with this method; it is enough to squeeze the blood out. To squeeze, place your fingers around the stabbed vascular spider; press the fingers gently into the body and then toward each other. These actions force blood into the vascular spider and out through the small cut you have made.

Practice

This is probably a technique you will not use often on children, but if you need to use it you must first learn how to do it effectively and painlessly.

You can practice on your own *jing* points, either of your toes or of your nondominant hand.

Can you apply the technique in such a way that it is painless, hardly any sensation is felt? It can be helpful to press the skin next to the point with a finger nail as a distraction just before applying the needle. What is the optimal position of the needle tip relative to your finger tips for a painless application? What is the best movement of your hand to roll the needle tip over the point painlessly? Can you do this so that blood only comes out one drop at a time as you squeeze the digit? Does the blood stop exactly when you want it to stop?

You can learn very quickly what are the best ways to apply the technique painlessly, but on the other hand some of you may give up trying if you are unable to do it painlessly. Like a concert pianist, you can only play the piece properly if you practice it a lot.

16 Point Location—Location of Extra Points for Symptomatic Treatment

Josen

This point is located at the juncture of L5 and S1. In the Chinese books it is the one "below the 17th vertebra point." Palpate for pressure pain at the exact location on the midline of the spine and in a slowly widening circle spreading out from that epicenter. The most reactive point may not be on the exact midline of the spine. Akabane (1986) recommends leaving an intradermal needle at the reactive *josen* for problems such as back pain, gynecological problems, labor pain, or hemorrhoids. We have found it can show reaction with and help conditions such as sciatica, intestinal problems, and urogenital problems. The point can also be treated with moxa instead of an intradermal needle. In general this point is used more on older children than on younger children. It could, for example, be used if clearly reactive for bedwetting or low back pain.

Uranaitei

Uranaitei or "below *nei ting*" or "below ST-44" is located on the sole of the foot proximal to the second toe. Two methods are used to find this point. The first involves placing a dot of ink in the center of the pad of the second toe then folding the toe over until it touches the sole of the foot. Where the dot of ink touches the sole of the foot is the point. But many people don't have flexible enough toes to do this so a second method is used. Measure the distance of the crease on the plantar surface of the foot where the digit intersects the foot. Make an equilateral triangle with that distance. The point is at the tip of that triangle when the line along the crease is the base of the triangle. This point is measured and not palpated. It is good for acute gastrointestinal problems, including food poison-

ing (hence one of its names the "food poisoning point"), acute gastric or intestinal distress (e.g., vomiting, diarrhea, acute gastroenteritis), and food allergies (although allergies are a chronic problem, they have acute manifestations when the wrong foods are eaten).

The point is treated only with moxibustion. To treat, apply equal shape and size (half a rice grain) moxa on both the left and right sides. Usually, with acute symptoms, one foot does not feel the heat, whereas the other does. Treatment is directed to the point that does not feel the heat, and treatment is repeated until heat is felt at the point at least three times. This may require many moxa cones. If both feet feel the heat, apply moxa until both feet feel the heat three times. For food allergies one usually applies moxa to feel the heat three times to both sides because there is not usually a difference of heat sensitivity as there is in, for example, acute gastrointestinal irritation. Also note that the skin here is thicker than on other parts of the body, and the child may not feel much heat until the moxa is burned closer to the skin.

Shitsumin

This point is located in the center of the heel of the foot. It is treated with moxibustion only and has been described by various moxa therapists (Fukaya 1982; Katsuyoshi 2006). It is especially indicated for problems of urinary disturbance with oliguria (infrequent urination), and frequent urination. It helps reduce edema subsequent to diminished urinary output and when moxead is able to increase urinary output. It is also indicated for sleep problems such as insomnia. On adults its uses may be more extensive, including pain in the feet, pain and swelling of the knees, psychological problems, tension in the lumbar and upper back areas, and so on

(Katsuyoshi 2006). The skin is quite thick here and will turn brownish or blackish with repeated moxa. It generally does not blister with moxa. It is a good point for parents to treat at home for chronic urinary problems that cause, for example, decreased urinary output. Usually it takes time for the patient to feel the heat and many more than three moxa cones are needed if the patient is to feel the heat at least three times.

Asthma *Shu* Point

This point is described in the moxibustion literature by authors such as Fukaya and Shiroda. The point is located slightly lateral to BL-17 and slightly superior to the level of BL-17. It is found as a hard, jumpy, painful knot in the area defined by this method. It can be reactive on either left or right sides or more commonly on both sides. In my experience anyone with asthma shows reaction at these locations. Although the point is first described in the moxibustion literature we found that patients with reactive asthma cannot tolerate treatment of the points with moxibustion because the smoke of the moxa can trigger an asthma attack. Consequently, I started leaving intradermal needles at the point(s) instead, with good effects. It is possible to lessen the frequency, intensity, and duration of asthma attacks by simply leaving intradermal needles or the new short press-tack needles at these points. The point also shows reaction quite frequently in patients with chronic congestion of the lungs as in recurrent bronchitis. It might be better on the particularly young or sensitive child to use press-spheres instead. If the press-spheres are well tolerated but show insufficient treatment effects, then try using the new press-tack or intradermal needles, but for a shorter period of time than usual (a few hours to 1.5 days only).

"Stop Coughing" Point

This point is ~ 0.5 *cun* distal to the traditional Chinese medicine (TCM) location of LU-5 (on the radial side of the tendon biceps brachii) and usually slightly lateral to the line of the lung channel. It is found as a hard, very painful point on palpation. To find the point, bend the elbow to locate the tendon, then, placing your finger at the modern Chinese LU-5 location, straighten the elbow and move your finger slightly distal and lateral, then squeeze. You will find a hard, painful point. This point can be used to help contain the symptom of coughing in both acute and chronic cases and can be used in, for example, asthma patients when the asthma manifests with a cough. It is treated with moxibustion, intradermal needles, press-tack needles, or press-spheres. On children I recommend using press-spheres or the short (0.3 mm) press-tack needles; press-spheres are easier.

Lateral *Pigen* Point

Historically, there were said to be three *pigen* points, which, when used together with moxa, are good for abdominal masses. On the back there are two *pigen* points, one more lateral than the other. Although there have been two different descriptions for this more lateral point, one 0.5 *cun* lateral to BL-51 and the other 0.5 *cun* lateral to BL-52, I recommend a more flexible location. The point is found in a depression below the margin of the 12th rib, not quite as far as the end of the 12th rib (where GB-25 is located). To find the point, locate the lower margin of the 12th rib at the spine and run your fingers lightly along the inferior margin. If the point needs to be supplemented, your finger will naturally move into and stop in a depression. This point is treated with *chinetsukyu* (warm moxa) (see Chapter 13), supplementation technique, and can also be treated with the *ryu* or press-sphere (see Chapter 12).

Moving LR-1

This is an extra point on the liver channel between LR-1 and LR-2. It is treated with moxa if a reaction is found. Although it is difficult to needle here, it is good to treat with moxa for night urination problems. To find the point, use your fingertips to find pressure pain. Once you have found some pressure, examine with a probe, such as the rounded end of the *teishin*, to define the precise location for treatment. It can be possible to apply the pressing *shonishin* technique to treat the point.

Section V   Treatment of Specific Problems/Diseases

of increased ordering of the levels below. The application of the core non-pattern-based root treatment primarily works on the vitality level, level 3, helping trigger increased regulation of the levels below it. The pattern-based root treatment primarily regulates the channels at level 2, helping regulate the level below it. The various symptomatic treatments help further change the functional structural, physical systems to relieve symptoms; that is, they work mostly at level 1. Thus the whole treatment when taken together can access and work at all four levels.

Of course, treatment can be applied only by doing the core non-pattern-based root treatment or pattern-based treatment with simple procedures to target symptom relief. We will see that this alone can be a very successful treatment approach. In fact, it is what has given *shonishin* the reputation that it has in Japan. It is also possible in some cases that you only have a chance to apply root treatments (either the non-pattern and/or the pattern-based) with no targeting of symptoms (see treatment Chapter 28, Improving Vitality). However, by applying all the various methods described in this book in an integrated, simple, properly balanced treatment, one is able to create a big change that can have profound long-lasting effects for the child.

When one adds the home treatment (see Chapter 8), where the parent applies some regular simple form of therapy at home, modifies diet, and so on, we find that this can contribute to changes and improvements in the tensions in relationships between parent(s) and child. This can contribute to changes in the psychosocial context where the child lives. This is represented by level 5, the space surrounding the four levels contained within the box (**Fig. 17.3**).

Although we have avoided extensive discussion and application of traditional East Asian medicine (TEAM) theory and Western medical knowledge in the discussions of how to diagnose and treat children, one can see in this five-level model that the whole system can be complete in itself. A well-performed treatment can help regulate the psychological, regulatory, and functional states of the child. With the addition of simple home therapy this is further enhanced through influencing the psychosocial context. It is not my purpose to expand here on these theoretical considerations, only to point out that your treatments using the methods recom-

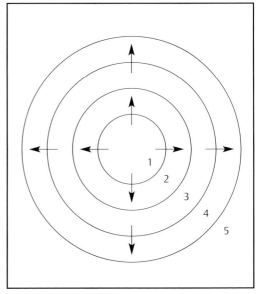

Fig. 17.3   Five-level model:
Level 1—functional systems (e.g., *zang fu*)
Level 2—channel systems
Level 3—vitality: global *qi* of the body (e.g., *zheng qi, sheng qi, yuan qi*)
Level 4—mind: heart/mind (e.g., *yi:* intention/attention/awareness; *zhi:* will)
Level 5—environmental systems (e.g., ecological/social systems, including "earth"; cosmological systems, including "heaven")

mended in this book can have quite broad and often surprisingly strong treatment effects.[1]

In this and the following chapters I shall describe the basic approach to treating a variety of common and uncommon health problems. The chapters contain examples and recommendations for the treatment of a variety of more commonly seen health problems or circumstances that may present when children come for treatment. Chapter 29 lists recommendations of treatment for some less commonly seen health problems.

Many books on acupuncture tend to be prescriptive; that is, they list points and associated

---

[1]   I have elaborated on this model in several places. The simple three-level model was published in 2009. A more elaborate seven-level model is in process (Birch , in preparation [a]) and explorations of how these might be understood and seen to work in the chapter on acupuncture in the recent book on *qi* and the *jingmai* (Birch 2014, pp. 218–226).

techniques for each symptom, and this is the main manner of describing treatment for the different conditions the book addresses. Not only do I not like or find the typical prescriptive treatment books on acupuncture to be very helpful, I also feel clinically one needs to be armed with a variety of treatment tools and ideas and be flexible enough so as to be able to apply them routinely and in modified form as needed. This is especially so in the treatment of children. When you put the whole treatment together you often find that you are adapting your approach and methods around the child to carry out the treatment as efficiently and easily as possible. I call this the "dance" of treatment (see Chapter 7). To help capture this approach so that the following treatment chapters are useful, I have given each the same order:

1. Clinical case example(s) of the treatment of that symptom
2. Basic ideas and recommendations for the use of the core non-pattern-based root treatment
3. Basic ideas for the use of the pattern-based root treatment
4. Basic ideas of which techniques used on which points or areas have been shown to be helpful
5. Additional clinical information pertaining to that health problem, as needed
6. Further case(s) to illustrate how the various methods have been selected from, combined, and when they worked and sometimes when not

The goal is to present a spectrum of treatment ideas and recommendations and show their use through case histories. I have collected cases from colleagues around the world who have had success treating children with these treatment methods, and I have, of course, included many of my own.

Treatment Chapters 18 through 28 will thus cover the following:
• The most likely pattern-based root diagnosis
• Core non-pattern-based root treatment and its modifications
• *Ryu* or press-spheres
• *Empishin* or press-tack needles
• *Hinaishin* or intradermal needles
• Needling (typically a modified form of *chishin*, retained needling or simple in–out needling)
• *Okyu*—direct moxa
• *Kyukaku* or cupping
• *Shiraku* or bloodletting

• Other considerations
• Dietary recommendations
• Home treatments

The final Chapter 29 lists recommendations for the treatment of several less commonly seen conditions and thus does not have case histories, and Chapter 30 contains examples of how skilled TCM and Japanese acupuncture practitioners integrated *shonishin* treatment methods into their overall treatment for some very ill little girls.

How to Use These Treatment Chapters

For each condition I have presented cases. In some cases it is self-explanatory what was done and why. In some cases I have added explanations to help the reader follow the logic and thinking. In other cases I have not given explanations. This is not because I am lazy or have forgotten what I did and why. I have done this to encourage you to think about what was done. It has been my experience teaching for over 20 years, and following Asian models of education and thoughts about the nature of knowledge and understanding, that we have to figure things out for ourselves if we are to really internalize an understanding of things. Sometimes, simply being told something only makes one forget and not understand. But when we do it for ourselves, we tend not to forget, and can also develop a greater ability to reason things through, which shows a greater understanding.

Putting aside my personal biases about the nature of learning and studying, there are a few things that I think it is helpful to explain in terms of how to construct the patterns of diagnosis and treatment, integrating as needed the different methods covered in this book.

Putting Your Treatment Together into a System

After evaluating the patient you should proceed quickly into treatment. In general it is better not to have the child (especially small children)

It is, for example, good for the overactive child to avoid sugar or have minimal exposure to sugar. I have had parents who thought it fine to let their hyperactive child drink lots of caffeinated, sugared soda every day. The constipated child may resist eating vegetables or foods with fiber, and the parents may not have a good understanding of what is needed in the diet. In such cases, you can give some straightforward recommendations. Probably the most common dietary factor that I pay attention to is cow's milk and cow's milk products.

Cow's Milk Products

In serious cases allergies to cow's milk can cause severe colitis, with bleeding, leading to severe gastrointestinal disturbance, hemorrhaging, and anemia. We tend not to see children in such severe states because they are usually being treated at the hospital, and appropriate dietary measures are being followed. Most commonly, we see children who are allergic to cow's milk products, or who are sensitive to consumption of such products, lactose intolerance, with a different set of symptoms. The baby can be colicky or have problems with vomiting and/or diarrhea. Other symptoms of sensitivity to cow's milk products include eczema, urticaria, asthma, rhinitis, behavioral problems, and migraine. Experience shows us that, whenever the child has a problem with congestion of the nose or sinuses (rhinitis, sinusitis), congestion of the lungs (catches cold easily, croup, asthma), recurrent ear infections after catching cold and always being congested, we should look to consumption of cow's milk products. The products themselves may not be a cause of the symptoms, but they are an irritant that obstructs recovery, tending to make the problems become more chronic. It seems that cow's milk in many people stimulates production of mucus or phlegm to the extent that this causes further congestion when congestion is already present, obstructing the ability to recover. The symptoms associated with sensitivity to cow's milk represent a large percentage of children who come for treatment with us. Thus it is worthwhile to further examine this issue.

Some parents will have already figured out, either by themselves or with their doctor's help, that there is an allergy or sensitivity to cow's milk products. Others may have no idea, and in some countries where milk and cheese products are consumed in large quantities, this can be quite common. It is necessary to establish a relationship between the child's symptoms and the consumption of cow's milk products. The following is a simple and quite reliable method of testing[2]:
- Have the child go completely without cow's milk products for a week (including milk, cheese, cream, butter, yogurt, ice cream).[3]
- If after 1 week the symptoms seem a bit better, have the child restrain from consumption for another month.
- At the end of the month challenge the child by letting them eat a bit of cheese, drink some milk, and so on.
- If there is a problem, the symptom will show an acute flare-up.

This process of testing is important because many parents are not convinced by words alone, and many are concerned that some important nutritional ingredients will be missing in the child's diet.[4] After this test shows the clear association, it becomes easy to get the parents to help the child stay away from the cow's milk products.[5] Older children also come to understand the need to avoid these products. This process of testing is

---

2   The following recommendations come from a professor in pediatrics who specialized in cow's milk allergy and lactose intolerance and who lectured on this subject when I was a PhD student at Exeter University.

3   You often need to be very explicit about which products this includes. Many parents, for example, do not realize that the yogurt their child consumes is cow's milk based.

4   I have even had one parent who had been told that it was tantamount to child abuse to withhold vital nutritional content that could only be found in cow's milk products!

5   Sometimes the association between milk products and the child's condition is more difficult to see. One of the factors that makes the testing harder to interpret is that we are also applying the *shonishin* and associated acupuncture treatments during the time that they are testing for the sensitivity to cow's milk products. Thus the initial improvement after a week free of milk products can be hard to interpret. In this case skipping this initial 1-week step and going straight into the month-long milk-free test can help make the association clearer. It can also happen that the child reacts to the replacement milk products in the same way, so that no clear change is perceived. You need to question the parent about whether there are any new symptoms or clear worsening associated with the consumption of the replacement milk product. If so, stop the use of that product and have them try a different replacement product and run the test again.

not always clear; sometimes the child has accidental exposure to the products during the time of avoiding them, and the results of the test are not as convincing.

It is important to help the parents find an alternative. An easy alternative is fortified soy milk. However, recent work suggests that soy milk consumption may be a problem for babies. Therefore, we need to have several alternatives to offer. Goat's milk and goat's milk products are usually acceptable to children, but some either don't like them or they react to them as well. Fortified soy milk products can show the same reactions. There are also fortified rice milk and oat milk products available in grocery stores and especially health food stores. In some countries, the apothecaries or chemists carry special processed milk products where the cow's milk has been treated so as to break the offending protein chains down to peptide chains. This can be a good alternative for drinking milk; however, these products can be expensive. In Holland some parents have objected to using them without a doctor's prescription (so that the insurance company pays for them).

For the child that likes drinking or eating cow's milk products, it is usually necessary for the whole family to help. Keeping milk, cheese, cream, and yogurt in the refrigerator exposes the child to them. Many will not have the understanding or discipline to stay away from them. Thus, sometimes the whole family has to stop consuming these products, at least until the child has improved.

In the chapters that follow, many cases arise where it was necessary to test for and avoid cow's milk products.

■ Environmental Sensitivities

Some children have environmental allergies or sensitivities, such as airborne allergens, contact allergens, or chemical sensitivities. The atopic child can show several different allergies and/or sensitivities, triggering a variety of symptoms. Often the specific factors that the child reacts to are unknown. Consequently, it is difficult to reduce exposure to the factors the child is reacting to. The allergic child may not yet have had a full battery of allergy tests or parents may not have been able to figure out everything to which the child is reacting. Sometimes we find cases where the parents are unwilling to part with their favorite family pet that may be a contributing factor to the environmental reactions. Some parents may be making a great effort to control the environment at home (twice daily cleaning and vacuuming, etc.) but cannot eliminate the environmental factors that the child is reacting to. It can be difficult to help the parent navigate this maze of issues to gain some measure of control, but we must pay attention to those children with such environmental sensitivities.

A simple model is to have the parents start using high-powered air-filtering systems at home and leave them running all the time. The air filters should have three different filter levels, including the high efficiency particulate air (HEPA) filter. These remove particles, dust, and chemicals from the air. Leaving them running all the time does not stop the introduction of the reactive factors into the home environment, but it does reduce the level of exposure by keeping the amount in the air at any one time down to a minimum. For some children, this is enough to help stop the reactions. For some it helps reduce the pressure on the body that triggers the symptoms, allowing your root treatments to be more effective in terms of changing the overall condition of the child so as to be less sensitive in the future. Case 1 in Chapter 26, Weak Constitution, is a good example of the use of this strategy. It is best if the air filter is set up in the place where the child spends most of his or her time (e.g., the bedroom), or if the house or apartment is larger, have two air filters set up to cover the larger area. You can find appropriate filters through the Internet and provide the parents with model names and contact details for purchasing them.

Sources Used in the Treatment Chapters of This Book

The compilations below cover three main areas of treatment: pattern-based root treatment, core non-pattern-based root treatment, and symptomatic recommendations.

For the pattern-based root treatment, the main source of materials has been my teachers, especially my Toyohari teachers. Books such as *Meridian Therapy* by Fukushima (1991) and *Japanese*

Stroking with an *enshin* was applied down the arms, legs, and abdomen.

Using a *teishin*, supplementation was applied to left LU-9 and SP-5, draining to right LR-5 and TB-5.

Press-spheres were left on right BL-13 and the "stop coughing" points on the elbows.

Third visit—5 days later

He woke on this day with a cold at 5.30 a.m. with symptoms of coughing. He was still coughing, but with signs of improvement. He had diarrhea over the weekend as well.

Treatment: Tapping with a *herabari* was applied to GV-20, ST-12 region, neck region, LU-1, GV-12, and LI-4.

Stroking with an *enshin* was applied down the arms, legs, back, and abdomen.

Using a *teishin*, supplementation was applied to left LU-9 and SP-3, draining to right LR-3.

Press-spheres were left bilaterally on the asthma *shu* points and GV-12.

Fourth visit—2 weeks later

His cough was much better, but he was still coughing a little in the early morning.

Treatment: Tapping with the *herabari* was applied to GV-20, ST-12 region, GV-12, and LI-4.

Stroking with an *enshin* was applied down the arms, legs, back, and abdomen.

Using a *teishin*, supplementation was applied to right LU-9 and SP-3, draining to left LR-3.

Press-spheres were left on bilateral asthma *shu* points and behind *shen men* on the back of the left ear.

Fifth visit—1 week later

The cough was much better again, but he had started coughing a little more 2 days before this visit.

Treatment: Tapping with the *herabari* was applied to the head, ST-12 region, occipital region, LU-1.

Stroking with an *enshin* was applied down the arms, legs, back, and abdomen.

Using a *teishin*, supplementation was applied to left LU-9 and SP-3, draining to right LR-3.

Press-spheres were left bilaterally on the asthma *shu* points and behind *shen men* on the back of the left ear.

Sixth visit—13 days later

The cough had again improved, but he had started coughing a little more in the early morning with a cold that started 1 day before this visit.

Treatment: Tapping with the *herabari* was applied to GV-20, ST-12 region, LU-1, GV-12, LI-4, and LI-11.

Stroking with an *enshin* was applied down the arms, legs, back, and abdomen.

Using a *teishin*, supplementation was applied to left LU-9 and SP-3, draining to right LR-3.

Press-spheres were left bilateral on BL-13 and behind *shen men* on the back of the left ear.

Seventh visit—2 weeks later

No symptoms of coughing and his condition was overall much improved. There were no sleep disturbances.

Treatment: Tapping with the *herabari* was applied to GV-20, ST-12 region, GV-12, LI-4, and LI-11.

Stroking with an *enshin* was applied down the arms, legs, back, and abdomen.

Using a *teishin*, supplementation was applied to left LU-9 and SP-3, draining to right LR-3 and left SI-7.

Press-spheres were left on GV-12 and behind *shen men* on the back of the left ear.

Eighth visit—22 days later

On holiday he started with a lung infection and was prescribed antibiotics. He fully recovered and had had no coughing before or since then. This was a significant milestone because any time he had gotten sick like this before his cough had severely worsened. This time, he had no coughing!

Treatment: Tapping with the *herabari* was applied to GV-20, the neck region, GV-12, and LI-4.

Stroking with an *enshin* was applied down the arms, legs, back, and abdomen.

Using a *teishin*, supplementation was applied to left LU-9 and SP-3, draining to right LR-3.

Press-spheres were left on GV-12 and behind *shen men* on the back of the left ear.

Treatment finished because the family moved away. In the final discussions with his mother she revealed that she had not talked to the doctor who had prescribed the inhaler. She had always kept it with her, but since the first visit Gilbert never needed the inhaler. She was very happy with treatment and promised to contact me for a referral should the need arise in the future.

Reflection: In a case like this, one cannot determine the degree to which improvement is possible. It is possible his lungs were weakened due to having been born premature. It was also possible that he was sensitive to cow's milk products, and that eliminating them after the first visit had contributed to his improvements. It is also possible that he actually had an asthmalike condition, such as croup, rather than asthma per se. Also, I did not prescribe the mother to do daily home treatment since he was responding so well to treatments. I prefer to use this additional therapy when the condition of the child is not changing or the changes are slow in coming. In Gilbert's case, this was not necessary. Although he caught a few colds during the time he was receiving treatment, none progressed to a major worsening of his symptoms, which I took to be a good sign of the change of his condition. Also, I felt that as well as having a trend toward weak lung constitution he also had a strong tendency toward liver repletion. Hence, even after his sleep problems had improved I continued treating points that would be helpful for this tendency, such as the point behind *shen men* on the back of the ear, GV-12, and so on.

■ General Approach for Patients with Asthma

Generally when we treat patients who have asthma, we are using treatment to augment or complement the existing therapy that they usually receive—the daily inhaled medications. Asthma is a serious condition that can kill the patient. Since we have no evidence that acupuncture can save

the life of an asthmatic patient who is having an asthma attack, we do not use acupuncture in place of the usual drug therapy. These drug therapies do not generally cure the illness, but they help reduce the asthma attacks. Although in the past acupuncturists have had to try using acupuncture to stop asthma attacks when such medications did not exist, we do not usually do this. The principle goal of acupuncture treatment of an asthmatic child is to slowly change the overall condition of the child so that he or she is less prone to having asthma attacks in the future. In other words, most of our work is preventive. This does not mean that we cannot use specific techniques or acupoints to try to keep the asthma symptoms quieter, reducing the frequency or severity of attacks, but our primary goal is to use the root treatments, both pattern-based and core non-pattern-based, to change the overall condition of the patient. Thus, if the patient has an asthma attack in your clinic, it is advisable to wait for the parent to administer the inhalant medication to the child. Once the attack has calmed down you can start to apply your treatment on the child.

■ Most Likely Pattern-based Root Diagnosis

In a baby or young child, where full diagnostic examination can be more difficult, it is advisable to focus on the symptom as the constitutional type of the patient and thus treat the lung vacuity pattern. If the child is a little older and has a longer history of taking medications for the condition, it is possible that the pattern has changed. If you are able to get more detailed information from the pulses and other methods, you can follow the pattern that emerges. In my experience kidney or liver vacuity patterns seem to emerge. One of my teachers, Akihiro Takai, suggested that with extended use of steroid medications the patient can start to show the kidney vacuity pattern. Check for softer or cooler lower abdomen and cool feet, as well as the specific pulse findings. Sometimes the liver seems to become reactive to the extensive use of medications and the liver vacuity pattern emerges. To check for this as well as the usual liver pulse findings, check to see if the right subcostal area has started to become stiffer than the left or is more sensitive or jumpy than the left.

For the lung vacuity pattern we usually treat LU-9 and SP-3, but following the ideas of

History: Like her brother (Gilbert, in Case 1), this was diagnosed as asthma, and she was prescribed an inhaler to be used daily, which she had been using. She had a tendency to catch cold easily, the cold triggering worsening of the asthmatic cough.

Diagnosis: From the symptoms and the fact that the right pulse was weaker than the left, I diagnosed lung vacuity pattern.

Treatment: I discussed with her mother the need to test for sensitivity to cow's milk products.
  Tapping with the *herabari* was applied to GV-20, GV-12 area, ST-12 area, and LU-1.
  Stroking with an *enshin* was applied down the arms, legs, abdomen, back, and neck.
  Using a *teishin*, supplementation was applied to LU-9 and SP-5, draining to right LR-3.
  Press-spheres were left on GV-12 and bilaterally on the "stop coughing" points on the elbows.

Second visit—7 days later

No symptoms of cough this week. These changes came immediately after treatment. Also her mother discontinued use of the inhaler this week.

Treatment: Tapping with the *herabari* was applied to GV-20, GV-12, ST-12 area, and on the abdomen.
  Stroking with an *enshin* was applied down the arms, legs, abdomen, back, and neck.
  Using a *teishin*, supplementation was applied to left LU-9 and SP-5, draining to right LR-3.
  Press-spheres were left on GV-12 and bilaterally on the "stop coughing" points on the elbows.

Third visit—5 days later

She had a cold over the last few days. She had more vomiting than usual and a problem with diarrhea on this weekend as well.

Treatment: Tapping with the *herabari* was applied to GV-20, ST-12 region, abdomen, LU-1, GV-12, and LI-4.
  Stroking with an *enshin* was applied down the arms, legs, back, abdomen, and neck.
  Using a *teishin*, supplementation was applied to left LU-9, SP-5, and left GB-37.
  Press-spheres were left bilaterally on the asthma *shu* points.

Fourth visit—8 days later

The cough was much better, but she was still coughing a little in the early morning. The problem of vomiting was unchanged.

Treatment: Stroking with an *enshin* was applied down the arms, legs, back, chest, abdomen, and neck.
  Using a *teishin*, supplementation was applied to right KI-7 and LU-5, draining to left SP-9.
  Press-spheres were left on left BL-20, GV-9, and CV-12.[4]

Fifth visit—7 days later

The cough was much better; she had almost no symptoms at all. But the problem of vomiting persisted. As the mother described this, Claire threw up on my treatment room floor.

Treatment: Tapping with the *herabari* was applied to PC-6, CV-12, GV-12.
  Stroking with an *enshin* was applied down the arms, legs, back, abdomen, chest, and neck.
  Using a *teishin*, supplementation was applied to right LU-9 and SP-5, draining to left LR-3.
  Press-spheres were left on bilateral PC-6 and left BL-20.[5]

Sixth visit—13 days later

The cough was still better, but had worsened slightly with a cold that started the previous day. The vomiting was a little less frequent.

---

[4] She did not show the lung pattern, probably because the respiratory symptoms were better. Instead it was clear that the spleen was replete; thus to accommodate this I chose kidney vacuity pattern with spleen repletion. I also applied only stroking downward on the body as the core non-pattern-based treatment, thinking this might help with the counterflow symptoms of the vomiting. The acupoints chosen for treatment with the press-spheres each showed some reaction and are indicated with these kinds of symptoms.

[5] The pattern had returned to what I had found before on Claire, perhaps because it had not changed as I had thought on the previous visit. Judging changes of pattern in adults can be difficult at times; on children even more so as the findings we use to judge this, the pulses and abdominal reactions, are more difficult to read. PC-6 was added because of its effects on vomiting.

Treatment: Tapping with the *herabari* was applied on GV-20, GV-12, LI-4, and PC-6.

Stroking with an *enshin* was applied down the arms, legs, back, and abdomen.

Using a *teishin*, supplementation was applied to right LU-9 and SP-3, draining to left LR-3.

Press-spheres were left on bilateral PC-6 and GV-12.

Seventh visit—2 weeks later

No problem with coughing at all, and her problem with vomiting had also improved significantly—very few episodes during this time.

Treatment: Tapping with the *herabari* was applied to GV-20, GV-12, LI-4, and PC-6.

Stroking with an *enshin* was applied down the arms, legs, back, and abdomen.

Using a *teishin*, supplementation was applied to right LU-9 and SP-3, draining to left LR-3.

Press-spheres were left on GV-12 and bilateral PC-6.

Eighth visit—22 days later

The coughing remained better and the vomiting had stopped completely.

Treatment: Tapping with the *herabari* was applied to GV-20, GV-12, LI-4, and ST-12 region.

Stroking with an *enshin* was applied down the arms, legs, back, and abdomen.

Using a *teishin*, supplementation was applied to right LU-9 and SP-3, draining to left LR-3.

A press-sphere was left on GV-12.

Treatment finished as the family moved away. Claire exhibited the same improvements in asthma symptoms as her brother Gilbert from Case 1. The problem she had with regurgitation and vomiting took a little more time but responded well to treatment. Once the asthma symptoms had clearly improved, treatment focused on this secondary problem. Treatment of PC-6 was helpful for the vomiting. If she had not responded with the press-spheres I had thought to replace them with press-tack or intradermal needles but was hesitant because they would be easily within her grasp, which could be dangerous. I did not teach her mother any home treatment because Claire's condition clearly improved from the first visit.

Case 3
Miguel, Boy Age 7 Years

Main complaints: Since age 3 he had suffered with asthma.

History: The bouts of asthma would typically be triggered by catching cold, rapidly turning into an asthmatic cough, then to severe wheezing attacks. They were very bad in the fall and winter and into the spring, and less frequent and not as severe during the 3 or 4 hotter months of the year, although humidity could trigger the symptoms. He had some form of the cough for almost the whole year. He had been taking steroids, albuterol (Ventolin, GlaxoSmithKline), and other inhalants almost continuously since the asthma started 4 years earlier, typically not taking the steroids much during the warmer months while taking the Ventolin daily. Pulmonary tests a few months previously had shown that he had borderline pulmonary obstructive disease. The asthma had resulted in several emergency room visits, averaging about two per year. In addition he had many allergies, especially airborne allergies, which could irritate the asthma condition. The asthma made it difficult for him to participate in many activities, especially sports and other outdoor activities. He naturally disliked this as he was unable to keep up with his friends. He came for his first treatment at the end of the summer. He had not had much problem with the asthma during the summer, and his parents were seeking preventive treatments to see if he could have a better fall and winter and to reduce or eliminate his use of the medications.

Additional medical history: He had a tendency toward constipation, which would cause a lot of irritability. He had his tonsils and adenoids removed at age 4. There was a history of rheumatoid arthritis in the family. Everything else was unremarkable.

Assessment: He was a normal-looking boy, his skin looked relatively normal and supple, and his complexion was generally with luster. He was nervous at his first visit. His parents were both therapists. During the initial interview, he did little talking. His parents also made it clear that no needles were to be inserted, and that this

19 Skin Disease

Eczema

Case 1
Julie, Girl Age 5 Years

Main complaints: Since the age of 10 months, she had had eczema—skin problems on the chest and back of shoulders, but especially on the genitals.

History: Born 10 weeks premature. At the age of 2 she had double pneumonia, and at age 3, minor pneumonia—since then her lungs had generally been fine. Her father had a significant history of eczema. All other systems were normal.

Diagnosis: Based on the symptoms, abdomen, and pulse, I diagnosed her as having lung vacuity pattern.

Treatment: Tapping was applied with a *herabari* to LI-4, LI-10, LI-11, ST-36, BL-40, abdomen, chest, neck region, GV-20, GV-12, and on the back.

Using a *teishin*, very light stroking was applied down the back and on the bladder channel on the legs, then supplementation was applied to right LU-5, SP-9, draining to left LR-8.

A press-sphere was applied to bilateral BL-25.

Second visit—1 week later

She had a problem with itching on the buttocks and upper thighs, but the vaginal itching was much better, and the shoulders and chest were better.

Treatment: Tapping was applied with a *herabari* to LI-4, LI-10, LI-11, ST-36, BL-40, abdomen, occiput, neck region, GV-20, GV-12, and on the back.

Using a *teishin*, very light stroking was applied down the back and on the bladder channel on the legs, then supplementation was applied to right LU-9, SP-3, with draining to left LR-3 and BL-58.

A press-sphere was applied to bilateral BL-25.

Third visit—1 week later

Overall improvement in her skin problems; some small spots remained on the buttocks, the vaginal region was much better, but she was slightly more irritable.

Treatment: Tapping was applied with a *herabari* to LI-4, LI-11, LI-15, ST-36, BL-40, abdomen, occiput, neck region, GV-20, GV-12, and on the back.

Using a *teishin*, supplementation was applied to right LU-9, SP-3, draining to left LR-4 and BL-58.

Press-spheres were applied to right BL-18 and left BL-25.

Fourth visit—15 days later

She had some minor skin problems on the buttocks (small patches), but overall the eczema was much better.

Treatment: Tapping was applied with a *herabari* to LI-4, LI-10, LI-11, ST-36, BL-40, abdomen, occiput, neck region, GV-20, GV-12, and on the back.

Using a *teishin*, very light stroking was applied down the back and on the bladder channel on the legs, then supplementation was applied to right LU-9, SP-5, draining to left LR-3.

Press-spheres were left on left BL-18 and right BL-25.

The mother said she wanted to take a break from treatment because Julie was much better, and it was difficult making the trip to the clinic on a regular basis due to scheduling difficulties and the long travel distances. She agreed to call for further treatment if the problem started worsening.

Case 2
David, Boy Age 9 Months

Main complaints: He had eczema over the whole body. He was sleeping poorly, and he had a congested nose with some coughing.

History: Soon after birth he started developing red skin blotches, which soon gave rise to eczema over the whole body. The dermatologist immediately prescribed a cortisone cream, saying that it was a constitutional type of eczema. The parents used the cream, which helped, but the symptoms came back as soon as they stopped. They did not want to continue with the cortisone cream. The itching was very bad, causing him to wake five to seven times a night, so everyone became sleep deprived and tired. He had stopped breast feeding 1 month before and was eating relatively widely without a worsening of the symptoms. He became a bit phlegmy with a regularly congested nose and occasional mild cough. He had Vaseline applied regularly to keep the skin more moist and was bathed daily.

Examination: The parents had not been advised by the dermatologist to examine whether there was a dietary problem that might be contributing to the eczema. He was a healthy-looking, largish child. His abdomen looked full and rounded. The skin over the abdomen was rough and a bit dry. The right deeper pulses were weaker than the left deeper pulses.

Diagnosis: Lung vacuity pattern was confirmed by the symptoms, abdominal findings, and pulse.

Treatment: Using a *teishin*, a light stroking above the skin was applied quickly down the large intestine channels on the arms, the stomach channels on the abdomen and legs, down the bladder channel on the back, and down the neck and shoulders.
Light stroking was applied using a silver *enshin* down the backs of the legs.
Using the *teishin*, supplementation was applied to right LU-9, SP-3, left LR-3, *yin tang*, and GV-12.
A gold-plated press-sphere was placed and retained on CV-12.
The parents were counseled about testing the effect of cow's milk on the eczema. They were advised to try stopping the milk and milk products to see if there was any change in symptoms.

Second treatment—7 days later

He continued to be itchy and sprouted two teeth during the week. The stuffiness of the nose was better.

Treatment: Using a *teishin*, a light stroking was applied quickly down the large intestine channels on the arms, the stomach channels on the abdomen and legs, down the bladder channel on the back, and down the neck and shoulders.
Using a silver *enshin*, light stroking was applied down the backs of the legs.
Using the *teishin*, supplementation was applied to right LU-9, SP-3, draining to left LR-3 and GB-37.
Gold-plated press-spheres were placed and retained on CV-12 and GV-12.

Third treatment—7 days later

Over the week his condition had improved, but the day before treatment it was not so good. The itchiness was less and the sleep was better. The skin looked clearer. It was discussed that the avoidance of milk products seemed to be helping and that the parents should continue having him avoid milk products.

Treatment: Using the *teishin*, a light stroking was applied quickly down the large intestine channels on the arms, the stomach channels on the abdomen and legs, down the bladder channel on the back, and down the neck and shoulders.
Stroking with a silver *enshin* was applied down the backs of the legs.
Using the *teishin*, supplementation was applied to right LU-9, SP-3, draining to left LR-3 and right ST-40.
Gold-plated press-spheres were placed and retained on CV-12 and GV-12.

Fourth treatment—7 days later

He had sprouted two more new teeth, which disturbed his sleep again and left him with more nasal congestion. The skin was still itchy but had improved and looked better.

Treatment: Using a *teishin*, a light stroking was applied quickly down the large intestine channels on the arms, the stomach channels on the abdomen and legs, down the bladder channel on the back, and down the neck and shoulders.

Stroking with a silver *enshin* was applied down the backs of the legs.

Using the *teishin*, supplementation was applied to right LU-9, SP-3, and left LR-3.

Gold-plated press-spheres were placed and retained on CV-12 and GV-12.

It was recommended for the parents to briefly apply light stroking with a rounded silver instrument down the large intestine channels on the arms, the stomach channels on the abdomen and legs, the bladder channels on the back and the backs of the legs, and on the forehead around the nose. They were instructed to do this daily.

Fifth treatment—7 days later

He had had the best week in months. The skin was much less itchy, with an improved appearance, and his sleep was much better. It was discussed that this would be the last treatment until further intervention was needed. The parents could continue on a diet free of cow's milk and continue the daily treatments, which they had been able to do every day over the last week. The parents agreed to call up and reschedule if the symptoms started recurring.

Treatment: Using a *teishin*, a light stroking was applied quickly down the large intestine channels on the arms, the stomach channels on the abdomen and legs, down the bladder channel on the back, and down the neck and shoulders.

Stroking with a silver *enshin* was applied down the backs of the legs.

Using the *teishin*, supplementation was applied to right LU-9, SP-3, left LR-3, and right ST-36.

Gold-plated press-spheres were placed and retained on CV-12 and GV-12.

■ General Approach for Patients with Eczema

Skin problems usually take time to improve and sometimes cannot be changed much with treatment. Most children show some degree of responsiveness, but it can be a complicated problem to treat. In general, the pattern-based treatment is very important because it will allow you to start changing the underlying constitutional tendency of the child. The non-pattern-based treatment is more limited for eczema and skin problems in general, and tends to be applied only around the affected regions, which means it is not usually a "root" treatment per se. It is also more difficult deciding what or if home treatment can be applied. Sometimes you are unable to have the parents apply any home treatment, due to the nature and extensiveness of the symptoms. Thus we need to place more emphasis on the pattern-based root treatment. There are a few symptomatic treatments for eczema (e.g., direct moxa), but they can be difficult to do on small children. Because of these typical complications, I recommend not making predictions about how many treatments before the problem is better, rather to suggest trying a certain number of treatments to see if what you do helps, then to continue or not as needed and based on response.

■ Most Likely Pattern-based Root Diagnosis

The lung vacuity pattern is by far the most common, especially if the eczema problems began as an infant. If the eczema is associated with lung symptoms—as the skin improves the lungs worsen, as the lungs improve the skin worsens—this is also a clear sign of lung vacuity pattern. But extensive use of steroid creams can gradually shift the patient from a lung to a kidney vacuity pattern. To identify this, check the feet. If they are cold or tend to become cold, this is a sign of the kidney involvement. While on small children the pulse may remain difficult to read, the additional sign of cold feet can be taken as an indication to try the kidney pattern.

Sometimes the skin problems show in relation to food allergies. The food allergies themselves can be a sign of spleen or liver involvement. It can depend on the manifestation of associated symptoms. If there is a history of food allergy reactions since infancy, with skin problems showing up as part of that pattern, the child may need to be treated as a spleen vacuity pattern. But this is not always very clear. The spleen signs can be included within the lung vacuity pattern, and if you are unsure, because the pulse and abdominal reaction findings are unclear, it is better to approach the patient as a lung pattern until other symptoms and signs become clearer. If the skin problems show along with food allergies, remember to add moxa treatment of the extra point *uranaitei* as part of the symptomatic treatment.

Generally with the pattern-based root treatment we use the treatment combinations outlined in Chapter 10; for lung pattern supplement LU-9 and SP-3 or SP-5, for kidney pattern supplement KI-7 and LU-8. But if the skin is very red and irritated and especially affects the upper parts of the body, such as around the neck and face, then it could be useful to try using the *he*-sea points instead. One of my teachers, Akihiro Takai, recommended the use of the *he*-sea points in such cases because they are indicated in *Nan Jing* (*Classic of Difficulties*), Chapter 68, as being good for counterflow *qi*, and one can see the heat in the upper parts and generally in the skin as a sign of counterflow. Sometimes such a simple shift of point selection can improve treatment outcome. Thus, for the lung pattern, use LU-5 and SP-9, for the kidney pattern KI-10 and LU-5.

■ Typical Non-pattern-based Root Treatment

Overall, this can be difficult to apply on children with eczema. The general recommendation is to use tapping around the lesions and no stroking or rubbing methods. This is not usually thought to be a root treatment because it targets only the symptom areas themselves. If you are using this approach it is a very good idea to make sure to include treatment by the pattern-based approach.

A method that can be used to perform a non-pattern-based root treatment comes from my teacher, Toshio Yanagishita. He described a modified way of applying the *teishin*, using it with a very light stroking method. Here, the *teishin* is held between the finger and thumb and just touching the skin very lightly. The *teishin* is then moved, almost in a gliding movement rather than a stroking movement, along the body surface relatively quickly. A simple pattern is to stroke down the large intestine channels on the arms, stomach channels on the abdomen and legs, and bladder channel on the back and legs (**Fig. 19.1a**). I have found it often helpful as a light technique for applying the non-pattern-based root treatment when the usual methods of performing that treatment are not possible. Normally for eczema, rubbing cannot be used; however, this technique has such light contact to the skin

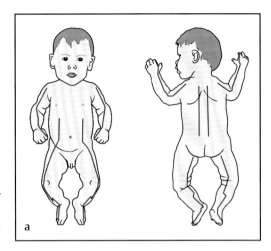

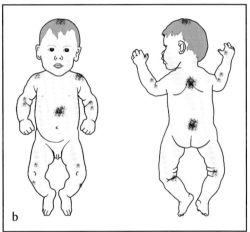

Fig. 19.1 **(a)** Gliding action with *teishin*:
- Down the large intestine channel on the arms
- Down stomach channel on the abdomen and legs
- Down the bladder channel on back and legs

(b) Tap around:
- LI-4, LI-10, LI-11, LI-15
- GV-12, GV-3 (for affected lower limbs)
- GV-20
- BL-40 or SP-10 + ST-36
- CV-12
- And if possible around affected areas

that it does not cause the problems associated with rubbing. This is illustrated in the case histories in this chapter. The limitation of this method is that it is not so easy to teach to parents as home therapy. At least it offers you the possibility of using a *shonishin*-like root treatment approach.

Sometimes the latter technique is also not sufficient when treating skin problems like eczema, or atopic dermatitis, in which cases I recommend the use of the tapping only method, directed neither to the body surfaces nor to the areas around the lesions, but instead to several specific acupoints that are good for skin problems. You can apply tapping to a selection of the following points: LI-4, LI-10, LI-11, LI-15, BL-40, SP-10, ST-36, CV-12, GV-12, GV-3 area. Some of these points are usually treated with moxa for skin problems and some are needled. Applying direct moxa regularly on older children can be possible, and even applying moxa at home, but in general and especially on babies and small children, this is not really an option. Thus we can apply tapping to a selection of the points (**Fig. 19.1b**). Often, there are lesions on the backs of the knees so that we cannot treat BL-40, in which case use SP-10, ST-36 instead. Often there are lesions in the elbows, in which case you may not be able to include LI-11. GV-12 can affect the upper body manifestations, GV-3 the lower body manifestations.

■ Recommendations for Symptomatic Treatment

Okyu—Direct Moxa

It is generally recommended to use acupoints on the large intestine channel with moxa for eczema. Shiroda (1986), following Takeshi Sawada's style of treatment (see Chapter 13 on moxa), recommends the following moxa treatment for allergic skin problems, eczema, sweat rash: moxa BL-12, GV-12, LI-15, LI-11, LI-10. My Toyohari instructors following this kind of idea recommend the following: palpate and select the most reactive points from among LI-4, LI-10, LI-11, and LI-15, and apply direct moxa to them. This can be done regularly in the clinical treatment and additionally as a form of home treatment, having the patient (if older) or parents do the moxa regularly at home. However, this is not an easy treatment to do. If there are food allergies associated with the problem, apply moxa *uranaitei* on the foot.

Needling

Needling can be applied to some of the main treatment points that are usually treated with moxa when it is very difficult to apply the moxa. Thus needling, for example, LI-4 or LI-11,

can be helpful. Choose the more reactive points for treatment. On some children the itching is very distressing and can disturb sleep, and so on such children it may be necessary to needle acupoints such as GV-20 (palpate for a reaction) and around GB-20 (palpate to see if the region is stiff).

Press-Spheres (*Ryu*), Press-Tack Needles (*Empishin*), and Intradermal Needles (*Hinaishin*)

It can be helpful leaving some kind of treatment tool on acupoints, but it can also be very difficult. First, the skin overall can be very dry on some children, in which case the tape generally does not stick well. Second, parents are often using some kind of moisturizing or other cream or salve on the skin, in which case it can be difficult to get things to stick well or at all. Third, the skin of some children with eczema is overall more sensitive, they sometimes react to the tape and sometimes to the metal of the press-sphere or press-tack. If there are any signs of reaction, you usually have to stop using these treatment tools. In general, if you are able to leave something like the press-sphere or press-tack needle, have them left for less time and changed more often so as to reduce the risk of skin irritation. On children who show the lung vacuity pattern, acupoints like BL-13, BL-17, and BL-20 can be palpated and treated. GV-12 is usually helpful to treat as well. For children who show more the kidney vacuity pattern, BL-23 can be treated. If the child has accompanying lung problems like croup or asthma, you will need to stimulate acupoints specifically for that problem and thus choose which acupoint combination is best for the child (e.g., the asthma *shu* points with press-tack needles for the asthma and GV-12 with press-sphere). If the child has concurrent digestive problems, such as food allergies contributing to the eczema, it can be useful to treat acupoints like BL-20, CV-12. If the problem is one of concurrent constipation, it can be helpful to treat acupoints like BL-25 or ST-25, to try to get the bowels moving better.[1]

---

[1]   In herbal medicine, one of the strategies for helping with skin problems is to get the bowels to move better.

Cupping

Cupping can be applied around the navel if there are any food allergies related to the eczema. Be careful to match the dose to the child and make sure it is not uncomfortable.

Bloodletting

Bloodletting can be helpful for some children. If you find vascular spiders on the upper torso, it can be worthwhile trying to bleed these. Use the stab and squeeze method rather than the cupping method, to ensure a lower dose.

■ Other Considerations

Dietary

Dietary issues need to be attended to. Eczema can be a reaction due to sensitivity or allergy to cow's milk products, thus it can be important to test for this. If other allergies are found, it is not uncommon that the parent has figured this out already, either by trying and testing different foods or asking the child's physician to test for different allergies.

Home Treatment

In some cases home treatment can be difficult due to the complexity and extent of the manifestations and various restrictions involved in treating patients with eczema. The basic techniques of stroking are prohibited or need to be significantly modified. It is difficult for parents to do this. Tapping can be applied, but then it is done more as part of the symptomatic treatment rather than root treatment. Often root treatment is only possible in the clinic. When having the parent apply some tapping treatment at home, it is usually over specific acupoints, the selection of which depends on the manifestations of the eczema. Tapping is not applied over a lesion, only on healthy skin regions. Thus it can be applied around lesions on the backs of the knees or in the elbows. If patches occur, tapping can be applied around each. But when there are extensive lesions of eczema covering large parts of the body surface, such tapping is difficult to do. Instead and sometimes as well, apply tapping to a selection of the following acupoints: LI-4, LI-10, LI-11, LI-15, BL-40, SP-10, ST-36, GV-12, GV-3 area. If there are lesions on the backs of the knees, use SP-10, ST-

36 instead. If there are lesions in the elbows, you may not be able to include LI-11.

Egg—Vinegar Folk Remedy

I have learned a simple folk remedy that sometimes is helpful for treatment of eczema. It uses raw eggs and brown rice vinegar. Place a clean raw egg in its shell in a bowl then put enough brown rice vinegar in the bowl to cover the egg. Leave the egg in the vinegar in the bowl for several days. Since the vinegar is acidic and the shell alkaline, the shell will slowly dissolve. After around 8 to 10 days, the shell will have dissolved so that one has a membranous egg in the vinegar. When the shell has dissolved, carefully spoon the whole egg out of the vinegar, being careful not to break the membrane and spill its contents. Place the membranous egg in another bowl, without any additional vinegar. Break the membrane and empty the contents into the bowl. Remove the membranous part. Mix the contents. There will have been a chemical exchange across the membrane of the egg so that the egg becomes slightly "pickled."

For treatment smear some of the vinegared-egg mix over the affected skin regions. Leave the mix on the regions for ~20 minutes, then with warm soapy water wash the mix off. Repeat up to three times daily.

The mix can sting when it is first applied, then after a while the stinging stops and it reduces the itching of the area. On some patients this can be a very effective simple treatment to help the eczema lesions. *Do not use this on children with egg allergy. Do not use this on skin lesions where the skin has been scratched open or has cracked open.* You may find that the stinging is too much for some children and they become upset or increasingly resistant to continued use.

This method is simple and inexpensive; parents can try it at home. A few observations and comments are helpful. The egg in vinegar should be kept in a cooler cupboard, it should be covered, and not allowed to become warm or hot. Make sure that the egg is clean first. I have tried other vinegars when the brown rice vinegar is unavailable; it seems not to work as well. It is best to store the vinegared-egg mix in a covered bowl in the refrigerator with instructions that it is not to be eaten. It usually takes 8 to 10 days for the shell to dissolve, but it can take more time. The vinegar does not need to be thrown away, it can be used several times, thus as soon as one egg is ready, the next can be placed in the vinegar so as to keep a steady supply of vinegared-egg mix going. This technique is much easier to use on adults than children, but it can be worthwhile trying it.

■ Further Case Histories

The following cases illustrate further modifications in the treatment of children with eczema.

Case 3
Paul, Boy Age 5 Years

Main complaints: He has had eczema since birth—itchy skin, especially on the medial thighs, upper arms, and around the eyes. His parents used Vaseline and occasionally hormone cream for the eczema.

History: He was born 10 weeks premature and was hospitalized for several weeks after birth. He had recurrent problems with bronchitis and some episodes of pneumonia. He caught cold easily. His lungs were an ongoing issue for him, a weak spot. He tended to get a stuffy nose very easily. His father had a significant history of eczema. All other systems were normal.

Diagnosis: Based on his symptoms, abdomen, and pulse, I diagnosed him as having lung vacuity pattern.

Treatment: Tapping was applied with a *herabari* to LI-4, LI-10, LI-11, ST-36, BL-40, neck region, GV-20, GV-12, and on the back.
　　Using a *teishin*, very light stroking was applied down the back and on the bladder channel on the legs, then supplementation was applied to left LU-5, SP-9, and right GB-37.
　　A press-sphere was applied and retained to GV-12.

Second visit—1 week later

He was tired after the treatment. He had had a cold with fever on the weekend with coughing, but had recovered quite quickly. The skin appeared to be a little better.

Treatment: Tapping was applied with a *herabari* to LI-4, LI-10, LI-11, ST-36, BL-40, abdomen, neck region, GV-20, GV-12, and on the back.

　　Using a *teishin*, very light stroking was applied down the back and on the bladder channel on the legs, then supplementation was applied to left LU-9, SP-3, draining to right LR-3 and TB-5.
　　A press-sphere was left on GV-12.

Third visit—6 days later

Skin itchiness was better overall—but there were still visible skin signs. He was more moody and irritable.

Treatment: Tapping was applied with a *herabari* to LI-4, LI-11, LI-15, ST-36, BL-40, abdomen, neck, neck region, GV-20, GV-12, and on the back.
　　Using a *teishin*, supplementation was applied to left LU-9, SP-3, right LR-3, draining to right ST-40.
　　Press-spheres were left on right BL-18 and GV-12.

Fourth visit—15 days later

There was some itchiness of the upper arms and legs but overall he was much better.

Treatment: Tapping was applied with a *herabari* to LI-4, LI-10, LI-11, ST-36, BL-40, abdomen, neck area, GV-20, GV-12, and on the back.
　　Using a *teishin*, supplementation was applied to left LU-8, KI-7, draining to right SP-9, then supplementation to right TB-4.
　　Press-spheres were left on GV-3 and GV-12.
　　The next visit was canceled since Paul's condition had significantly improved and he had no more itchiness or skin lesions. They also had to travel more than an hour each way to get to the clinic. His mother promised to call if the symptoms worsened.

Case 4
John, Boy Age 3½ Months

Main complaints: He had had allergic eczema since age 2 weeks.

History: At age 2 weeks, he broke out with facial skin reactions. Two weeks later the skin over most of his body became dry and rough. This was diagnosed as a cow's milk intolerance. His diet was changed to alternating breast feeding with a special powder drink in water. Both he and his mother stopped consuming cow's milk products but the skin was still rough. It was worst over the abdomen, in the joints, especially knees and elbows, and recently was starting to get worse on the back. The face was virtually clear. There was a history of allergies in the family, raising the suspicion of additional allergies beyond the cow's milk intolerance. His skin looked rough and slightly irritated over large parts of his body. Overall, his skin color was off-white. Otherwise he looked like a healthy, largish baby.

Diagnosis: The abdomen and pulse findings indicated a lung vacuity pattern.

Treatment: Using a *teishin*, left LU-9 and SP-5 were supplemented.

Using a *herabari*, light tapping was applied around the most affected areas on the abdomen and back, and around GV-12 and ST-36 on both legs.

A press-sphere was placed at GV-12, with instructions to replace it every 2 days.

Second visit—1 week later

The symptoms were pretty much the same. The abdomen was slightly better, the back slightly worse, the feet slightly worse. His mother announced that she was stopping breast-feeding that day.

Treatment: Using a *teishin*, left LU-9 and SP-3 were supplemented. Draining was applied to right LR-3.

Using a *herabari*, very light tapping was applied around LU-1 on both sides, on the head, and around TB-17 on both sides.

Press-spheres were placed and retained at GV-12 and LU-1 on both sides.

Third visit—2 weeks later

The rash was slightly worse on the arms, legs, and face, but the general nature was unchanged.

Treatment: Using a needle, supplementation was carefully applied to left LU-9, SP-3, GV-12, and GV-4.

Very light stroking was applied over the abdomen, chest, arms, legs, and back. This technique involved holding the needle tip between the finger and thumb of the right hand and moving it over the skin, not along the surface of the skin, so that the fingers made some contact but the needle tip was slightly above the skin at all times.

GV-12 and GV-4 were supplemented.

Press-spheres were placed and retained on GV-12 and LU-1 on both sides.

Fourth visit—3 weeks later

The rash had been slightly worse at times.

Treatment: Using a needle, left LU-9 and SP-3 were carefully supplemented.

Very light stroking needling was applied over the abdomen, chest, arms, legs, back, and head.

Using a *herabari*, tapping was applied around GV-12.

A press-sphere was placed at GV-12.

The parents were instructed in the use of the egg-soaked-in-vinegar treatment.

Fifth visit—1 week later

The rash was the same. He was teething but generally seemed to be sleeping better. The egg–vinegar mix was not yet ready to apply.

Treatment: Using a needle, left LU-9, SP-5, and GV-12 were carefully supplemented, right ST-40 was drained.

Very light stroking was applied over the abdomen, chest, arms, legs, and back.

Using a *herabari*, tapping was applied over the head (to help with the teething).

A press-sphere was placed and retained at GV-12.

Sixth visit—1 week later

The eczema appeared to show a slight improvement. The egg–vinegar mix was not yet ready to use.

He had caught a mild cold this week, seemingly associated with teething. He had a mild cough.

Treatment: Using a needle, left LU-9, SP-3, right LR-3, and BL-12 on both sides were carefully supplemented.

Very light stroking was applied over the abdomen, chest, arms, legs, and back.

Using a *herabari*, tapping was applied around GV-12 and in the occipital region.

Press-spheres were applied and retained at GV-12 and the "stop coughing" points close to LU-5.

Seventh visit—1 week later

He still had some symptoms of the cold, with a congested chest. The eczema had shown a clear improvement during the week. The egg–vinegar mix was still not ready.

Treatment: Using a needle, left LU-9, SP-3, and right LR-3 were carefully supplemented.

Very light stroking was applied over the arms, legs, back, and abdomen.

Press-spheres were applied and retained at GV-12 and LU-5 on both sides.

Eighth visit—1 week later

The cold was better, congestion was better, but still with some residue. The skin continued to improve and was much softer. The egg–vinegar mix had developed a fungus and could not be used.

Treatment: Using a needle, left LU9, SP-3, and right LR-3 were carefully supplemented.

Very light stroking was applied over the arms, back, abdomen, chest, and legs.

Using a *herabari*, tapping was applied over the head and occipital region.

Press-spheres were applied and retained at GV-12 and LI-10 on both sides.

Ninth visit—2 weeks later

A week before, he had been diagnosed with bronchitis and treated with penicillin. Today was the last day of the antibiotics. He was still congested. Two days before, the skin was reddened, and then improved. Overall, the skin was still improved.

Treatment: Using a needle, left LU-9 and SP-3 were carefully supplemented, right LR-3 was drained.

CV-12 was supplemented.

Stroking with the silver needle was applied over the arms, abdomen, legs, and back.

Using the *herabari*, tapping was applied on the back of the neck and head.

Press-spheres were applied and retained at the asthma *shu* points and GV-3.

Tenth visit—1 week later

The skin was improved and was less irritated. He had eaten a kiwi a couple of days before, which had caused an immediate reaction around the mouth and on the back.

Treatment: Using a needle, supplementation was carefully applied to left LU-9, SP-3, right LR-3, and CV-12.

Stroking with the silver needle was applied over the arms, abdomen, and legs.

Using a *herabari*, tapping was applied on the head and back of the neck.

Press-spheres were applied and retained at CV-12, GV-12.

Eleventh visit—10 days later

The eczema was still improving, there were still a few small spots of eczema here and there, but it was much improved. He had now fully recovered from the bronchitis.

Treatment: Using a needle, left LU-9 and SP-3 were carefully supplemented, right LR-3 was drained.

Very light stroking was applied over the chest, abdomen, legs, arms, and back.

Using a *herabari*, tapping was applied around GV-12 and GV-4 and on the head.

Press-spheres were applied and retained at GV-12 and CV-12.

Twelfth visit—2 weeks later

The eczema was much improved again. The parents had finally been able to use the egg–vinegar treatment and noticed it seemed to clear up some of the stubborn spots of eczema.

Treatment: Using a needle, left LU-9 and SP-3 were carefully supplemented, right LR-3 was drained.

Very light stroking was applied over the abdomen, arms, chest, legs, and back.

Using a *herabari*, tapping was applied on the head and neck.

A press-sphere was applied and retained at GV-12.

The parents reported that this was to be the last appointment for a while because the insurance would not pay for any more treatments. Their son was much improved and it seemed that the egg–vinegar mix was helpful. They agreed to continue using this mix and to come back for further treatments if the need arose.

At 1-year follow-up, the boy's skin was still much improved. He had a little dry skin occasionally, but the eczema had been virtually eliminated. He was a very big, strong, healthy boy.

Case 5
Albert, Boy Age 17 Months

Main complaints: Eczema on the backs of the knees, the elbows, and the neck (the worst area), with patches on the upper body and sometimes on the face. The problem had started at age 3 months and worsened over the last 3 months. The dermatologist had prescribed a cortisone cream.

History: He had had a cold with fever the week before. Since starting at day care 5 months before he had routinely had nasal congestion problems, catching cold. His sleep, appetite, and bowel movements were good. The mother used the cortisone cream when the symptoms were very disturbing, but preferred not to use it, as it did not stop the problem without regular use, which she wanted to avoid.

Diagnosis: The right deep pulse was a little weaker than the left. The diagnosis was of a lung vacuity pattern.

Treatment: Using a *teishin*, supplementation was applied to left LU-9 and SP-5, and GV-20, GB-20.
Using the *teishin*, a very light, superficial stroking was applied down the large intestine channels on the arms, the stomach and bladder channels on the legs, and down the bladder channel on the back. A light, circular motion was applied on the abdomen in a clockwise direction.
Tapping was applied with a *herabari* on the head.
The importance of testing for cow's milk sensitivity was explained to the mother. I also inquired further into what the doctors had

described about his condition and we discussed the possibility that he had an allergic-type constitution, which means that he may tend to show symptoms of the skin and lungs together or, alternately, as the skin improves the lungs may become symptomatic and vice versa. I explained that this can be a good sign if we progress from skin improvements to lung irritation to improvement in both.

Second treatment—8 days later

It was difficult to see any effects of the treatment. Albert had been free of cow's milk products most of the week.

Treatment: Tapping was applied with the *herabari* to GV-20 and GB-20.
Using the *teishin*, a very light, superficial stroking was applied down the large intestine channels on the arms, the stomach and bladder channels on the legs, and down the bladder channel on the back. A light, circular motion was applied on the abdomen in a clockwise direction.
Using a *teishin*, supplementation was applied and retained at left LU-9 and SP-5, and GV-20 with draining of right LR-3.

Third treatment—8 days later

No clear signs of change of the skin. Albert had caught cold this week and had a stuffy nose, a cough with disturbed sleep, and 2 days of constipation.

Treatment: Tapping was applied with the *herabari* to LI-4, LI-11, GV-20, GV-22, and occipital region. Using the *teishin*, a very light, superficial stroking was applied down the large intestine channels on the arms, down the stomach and bladder channels on the legs, and down the bladder channel on the back. A light, circular motion was applied on the abdomen in a clockwise direction.
Using a *teishin*, supplementation was applied to left LU-9 and SP-5, with draining of right LR-3.
Press-spheres were placed and retained on GV-12 and bilateral ST-25.

Fourth treatment—7 days later

The skin on the abdominal region was better, no clear signs of change elsewhere. The sleep was good. The cough was still present but now mild.

Treatment: Tapping was applied with the *herabari* to LI-4, LI-11, GV-20, GV-22, GV-12.

Using the *teishin*, a very light, superficial stroking was applied down the large intestine channels on the arms, down the stomach and bladder channels on the legs, and down the bladder channel on the back. A light, circular motion was applied on the abdomen in a clockwise direction.

Using a *teishin*, supplementation was applied to left LU-9 and SP-5, with draining of right LR-3, LI-6.

Press-spheres were placed and retained on GV-12 and bilateral ST-25.

The mother was taught to apply this very light, superficial, gliding-like stroking action on the arms, legs, and torso as daily home treatment using a metal object that could be applied like the *teishin*. The mother used a small piece of silver jewelry for this.

Fifth treatment—7 days later

No additional signs of progress with the eczema this week. Otherwise he was fine. His sleep was good, the cough was gone, and the home treatment was going well.

Treatment: Tapping was applied with the *herabari* to LI-4, LI-11, GV-20, GV-22, GV-12.

Using the *teishin*, a very light, superficial stroking was applied down the large intestine channels on the arms, down the stomach and bladder channels on the legs, and down the bladder channel on the back. A light, circular motion was applied on the abdomen in a clockwise direction.

Using a *teishin*, supplementation was applied to left KI-10, LU-5, and ST-36.

Press-spheres were placed and retained on GV-12 and bilateral BL-25.

Sixth treatment—7 days later

He was generally fine, but the skin on his back was more irritated.

Treatment: Tapping was applied with the *herabari* to LI-4, LI-10, LI-11, GV-20, GV-22.

Using the *teishin*, a very light, superficial stroking was applied down the large intestine channels on the arms, down the stomach and bladder channels on the legs, and down the bladder channel on the back. A light, circular motion was

applied on the abdomen in a clockwise direction.

Using a thin needle, the *sanshin* technique was applied over the back.[2]

Using a *teishin*, supplementation was applied to left LU-9, SP-3, and CV-12 with draining of right LR-3, BL-58.

Press-spheres were placed and retained on bilateral ST-25.

Seventh treatment—7 days later

He was generally fine, and the skin on his back was somewhat better. He had some mild coughing and nasal congestion.

Treatment: Tapping was applied with the *herabari* to LI-4, LI-10, LI-11, GV-20, GV-22, BL-40, ST-36, occipital area, arms, legs, and abdomen.

Using a thin needle, the *sanshin* technique was applied over the back.

Using a *teishin*, supplementation was applied to left LU-9, SP-3, with draining of right LR-3.

Press-spheres were placed and retained on CV-12, bilateral ST-25.

The mother was instructed to stop the previous home treatment methods and only apply tapping over the points LI-4, LI-10, LI-11, GV-12, BL-40, ST-36 daily at home (this remained the home treatment).

Eighth treatment—7 days later

He was generally fine. The skin on his back had improved further. On this day he was very irritable.

Treatment: Tapping was applied with the *herabari* to LI-4, LI-10, LI-11, GV-20, GV-22, BL-40, ST-36, occipital area, arms, legs, and abdomen.

Using a thin needle, the *sanshin* technique was applied over the back.

Using a *teishin*, supplementation was applied to left LU-9, SP-3, with draining of right LR-3.

Press-spheres were placed and retained on CV-12, bilateral ST-25.

---

[2]   The term *sanshin* means "contact needling." There are many variations of contact needling found in the practice of acupuncture in Japan. Here the technique was to rapidly draw and flick the needle across the back, only very lightly touching the skin surface. The idea is that this particular technique is to "disperse" the surface of the body. The rate of movement of the needle is about two times per second, and the back area is covered in 5 to 10 seconds.

Ninth treatment—7 days later

Overall his condition was improved, and the skin on his back was better again.

Treatment: Tapping was applied with the *herabari* to LI-4, LI-10, LI-11, GV-20, GV-22, BL-40, ST-36, occipital area, arms, legs, and abdomen.
    Using a thin needle, the *sanshin* technique was applied over the back.
    Using a *teishin*, supplementation was applied to left LU-9, SP-3, with draining of right LR-3.
    Press-spheres were placed and retained on CV-12, bilateral ST-25.

Tenth treatment—3 weeks later

He had had a cold with a high fever the week before, after which his skin improved overall.

Treatment: Tapping was applied with the *herabari* to LI-4, LI-11, GV-20, GV-22, GV-12, BL-40, ST-36, occipital area, arms, legs, and abdomen.
    Using a thin needle, the *sanshin* technique was applied over the back.
    Using a *teishin*, supplementation was applied to left LU-9, SP-3, with draining of right LR-3.
    Press-spheres were placed and retained on CV-12, bilateral ST-25.

Eleventh treatment—7 days later

Overall the skin remained improved, but he had had congestion in the lungs for the last 3 days.

Treatment: Tapping was applied with the *herabari* to LI-4, LI-10, LI-11, GV-20, GV-22, GV-12, BL-40, ST-36, occipital area.
    Using a thin needle, the *sanshin* technique was applied over the back.
    Using a *teishin*, supplementation was applied to left LU-9, SP-3, with draining of right LR-3.
    Cupping was applied lightly and briefly over the interscapular region.
    Press-spheres were placed and retained on CV-12, bilateral LI-15.

Twelfth treatment—12 days later

His skin and lungs were irritated from exposure to a lot of dust from moving to a new house. His eyes were irritated and he had been crying a lot.

Treatment: Tapping was applied with the *herabari* to LI-4, LI-10, LI-11, GV-20, GV-22, GV-12, BL-40, ST-36, occipital area.
    Using a thin needle, the *sanshin* technique was applied over the back, neck, and shoulders.
    Using a *teishin*, supplementation was applied to left LU-9, SP-5, with draining of right LR-3, left BL-58.
    Press-spheres were placed and retained on CV-12, bilateral LI-15.

Thirteenth treatment—16 days later

Overall the skin was much improved, but his lungs were more congested. He was much more settled emotionally as well.

Treatment: Tapping was applied with the *herabari* to LI-4, LI-10, LI-11, GV-20, GV-22, GV-12, BL-40, ST-36, occipital area, neck.
    Using a thin needle, the *sanshin* technique was applied over the back, neck, and shoulders.
    Using a *teishin*, supplementation was applied to left LU-9, SP-3, with draining of right LR-3.
    Press-spheres were placed and retained on CV-12, bilateral BL-13.

Fourteenth treatment—12 days later

His skin was very good, but his lungs were more congested again.

Treatment: Tapping was applied with the *herabari* to LI-4, LI-10, LI-11, LU-1, GV-20, GV-22, GV-12, BL-40, ST-36, occipital area.
    Using a thin needle, the *sanshin* technique was applied over the back and neck.
    Using a *teishin*, supplementation was applied to left LU-9, SP-3.
    Cupping was applied lightly over the upper back and LU-1 regions.
    Press-spheres were placed and retained on CV-12, bilateral asthma *shu* points.

Fifteenth treatment—3 weeks later

He had had a mild fever and the chicken pox the week before. His skin was generally good and his lungs were much better.

He would have been born weak lung constitution type, which triggered the skin problems and multiple allergies, and with the extensive use of corticosteroid creams he would have become kidney vacuity type, hence the very cold feet. It is possible to view the extensive signs of inflammation of the skin as a kind of counterflow-type symptom, especially since the lesions are worst around the neck and face, thus following the logic of *Nan Jing*, Chapter 68, the *he*-sea points would be better to treat (see discussions of this in Chapter 10). He also suggested trying *okyu*/direct moxa by applying it at LI-4, LI-10, LI-11, or LI-15, whichever was most reactive and did not have skin lesions on it. *Okyu* could also be applied to the extra point *uranaitei* for the food allergy components of his condition. The moxa could also be used by family members at home to give the patient some home treatment options. After this advice, I tried applying his ideas and obtained much clearer treatment effects.

Eighth visit—7 weeks after the fourth visit

The skin was not very good; he was scratching, especially at night, with bleeding.

Treatment: *Okyu* was applied to LI-4 (the more reactive of the four points mentioned by Takai) and *uranaitei*.

Using needles, supplementation was applied to CV-12, left KI-10, and LU-5, draining technique was applied to right ST-40, TB-5, and left GB-37.

The *sanshin* contact needling technique was applied over the ST-12 and inguinal regions.[4]

Press-spheres were placed at BL-17.

His mother was taught to apply moxa to the LI-4 and *uranaitei* points daily.

Ninth visit—2 weeks later

His skin was clearly better and less irritated. The severe flare-up from the summer had started improving immediately after the previous treatment. He complained that his mother's moxa techniques were very bad and asked me to explain them again to her.

---

4   *Naso* and *muno* treatments in the Toyohari system (Birch and Ida 2001; Yanagishita 2001a, 2001b).

Treatment: Essentially the same as the last except that right SP-9 was drained instead of ST-40.

Following this, he was able to maintain a more stable improvement in his skin condition over the next eight twice-monthly treatments. He had taken over doing the moxa himself as he could not tolerate his mother's technique. We found that when he was inconsistent at doing his home moxa, generally the skin was not quite as good, and when he was consistent in the use of home moxa, the skin was better. Intradermal needles were used to replace the press-spheres at BL-17 to increase the dose of treatment.

Treatments became less regular due to financial and scheduling issues. He had a flare-up of the skin symptoms with the next summer holidays. He came for treatment more regularly at that point. Moxa was added to LI-10 as well as the usual LI-4. Additionally, he had been swimming in unclean water while he had open skin lesions, which led to some becoming quite irritated and looking like they may be infected. The use of tea tree oil in the bath water was helpful in clearing up these additional surface lesions. He came for treatment on and off over the next 2 years. He was able to maintain an improved skin condition without the use of drugs, which can have unpleasant side effects (the primary reason the mother had stopped using them in the past). The use of the kidney vacuity pattern-based root treatment coupled with the moxa therapy seemed to create the most lasting changes for this patient. He was in an overall improved state during the time he received treatment and had tools at home to help reduce symptoms.

Reflection: Although atopic dermatitis is an increasingly common problem, it can be difficult to treat. Mild cases generally respond better than severe cases. Han's condition was particularly severe. I was unsure what I could do for him and found the advice of my teacher Takai very helpful in constructing a more effective treatment approach. I was not surprised that I could not "cure" his condition. I have heard some claim to be able to cure conditions like this, but that is not so common. He and his mother were happy with the treatment because it helped him manage the symptoms, leaving him more functional and better able to cope.

■ **General Approach for Patients with Atopic Dermatitis**

This is a difficult condition to treat. You may not be able to cure the condition and may only be able to help improve symptoms and quality of life. Often parents have tried many things to treat their atopic child. Thus you need to caution the parents about long-term treatment usually being needed and that you will, as soon as you are clear what to do, have the parents start doing some treatment at home so as to lengthen the time between visits to you and thus reduce the financial and scheduling burdens of treatment. Often the child is distressed by the symptoms and has difficulty sleeping due to the itchiness. This can leave the child feeling moody.

The atopic condition often comes with symptoms of the lung, congestion in the lungs, shortness of breath, wheezing, and, in more severe cases, asthma or a tendency to catch colds easily. These manifestations are part of the overall weak lung constitution, in which case look at the discussion of this in Chapter 26, Weak Constitution. You may find that you are alternating the focus of your symptomatic treatments between dealing with the skin symptoms and the lung symptoms. Overall, your root treatment is the most important part of the treatment, especially the pattern-based root treatment.

■ **Most Likely Pattern-based Root Diagnosis**

In younger children this is most likely a lung vacuity pattern and can be a manifestation of the weak lung constitution (more severe in constitutional lung vacuity pattern). Thus the usual treatment can be LU-9 and SP-3. But it can also be helpful to use the metal points LU-8 and SP-5 instead, and, if the skin is very reddened and there are more lesions on the upper part of the body, especially around the neck and face, the *he*-sea points are better used, LU-5 and SP-9. If the child shows the lung vacuity pattern and also has disturbed sleep, the liver is often replete, in which case after supplementing the lung and spleen points, apply draining technique to, for example, LR-3 on the opposite side of the body.

The condition is often treated by doctors using corticosteroid creams. Over time with extended use this can weaken the kidneys and one starts to see kidney vacuity pattern (look for signs of cold

feet). In this case the treatment uses KI-7, LU-8, or, with more counterflow signs, such as more reddened appearance around the face and neck, KI-10, LU-5 are better. Although the shift to kidney pattern can be seen in younger children, it is more common in the child who is older and has had the problem for longer with more use of the corticosteroid creams.

If you feel that the condition is part of the more severe weak lung constitution, you can apply moxa to GV-12, but this is not so easy for the younger child.

■ **Typical Non-pattern-based Root Treatment**

Do not apply the stroking technique on children with atopic dermatitis. If the lesions are limited and regional, such as around only the elbows and knees, you can apply the tapping technique over the healthy regions of the skin on the torso and only around the lesions of the arms and legs. However, if the skin lesions are more extensive, you cannot apply tapping techniques over the body surface. Instead, focus the tapping to acupoints that are good for such a condition, such as LI-4, LI-10, LI-11, and LI-15. If any of these acupoints have skin lesions over them, do not tap those points. If BL-40 on the back of the knees is free of lesions, you can also apply tapping there. If there are lesions over the knees, try SP-10 and ST-36 instead, provided neither have lesions on them. Additionally, tapping can be applied over GV-12 and BL-17, provided there are no lesions on these areas. Bl-17 can be helpful in the following cases: if there are more symptoms in the upper part of the body, especially around the head and neck, and if the skin itchiness is triggering sleep disturbance. If there are food allergy problems involved, additional tapping can be applied to CV-12. If there is sleep disturbance and there are no skin lesions in the area, apply tapping to the area around GB-20 and GV-20 (**Fig. 19.2**).

■ **Recommendations for Symptomatic Treatment**

Okyu—Direct Moxa

In general, *okyu* is the recommended treatment for this condition. Palpate and compare reactions at LI-4, LI-10, LI-11, and LI-15. Choose the points that are the most sensitive and apply moxa to those.

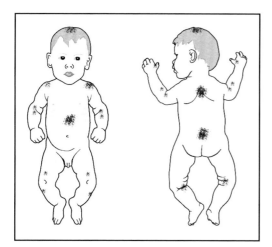

Fig. 19.2   Tap around:
- LI-4, LI-10, LI-11, LI-15
- CV-12, GV-3 (for affected lower limbs)
- GV-20
- GB-20
- BL-40 or SP-10 + ST-36
- CV-12

For example, treatment may be directed to LI-4 bilaterally or LI-10 bilaterally. On small children this can be difficult to do, in which case we apply tapping over the four points (see earlier discussion). Teaching the parents to apply home moxa, or, if the child is older, teaching the child to do the home moxa, can be very helpful. *Uranaitei* is used if there are any food allergy components to the atopic skin complaints. Often in this condition the two *uranaitei* points (on the left and right feet) show the same degree of heat sensitivity, but sometimes one notices that one foot feels the heat much less than the other.[5] If you find this, direct the treatment to only the insensitive point, and make sure that the heat is clearly felt at least three times on that foot.

Press-Spheres (*Ryu*), Press-Tack Needles (*Emp-ishin*), and Intradermal Needles (*Hinaishin*)

Press-spheres can be a useful treatment technique for helping support the pattern-based root treatment. Leaving a press-sphere on GV-12 can be helpful because it is good for all pediatric conditions, and in particular it supports the treatment

of the weak lungs, which are usually involved in this condition. If the child shows the kidney vacuity pattern, press-spheres can be placed at bilateral BL-23 or the more reactive points at the level of BL-23 (often between BL-23 and BL-52 or closer to BL-52). But, because the patient with this skin condition is usually applying creams and lotions to try to keep the skin more moist and reduce the irritation of the skin, you may find that the press-spheres come off easily.

If the condition is worse on the upper part of the body, especially around the head and neck, and a tight band is found around BL-17, this can be a good point on which to place the press-spheres.

Press-tack needles and intradermal needles can be used in place of the press-spheres to increase the dose of treatment when needed. However, it is better not to use these on a child where the press-spheres are difficult to retain because of the daily moisturizing of the skin with creams. On older children, they are easier to use, and you can have the child keep track of them.

Needling

On children where the skin lesions are not responding much with the tapping and pattern-based root treatment, and you are unable to apply moxa because it is too difficult to use on the child, you can try using in-and-out needle insertion to points such as LI-4 and LI-10 or LI-11.

Some children are very disturbed by the itchiness of the skin so that it leaves them distressed and moody, and it disturbs their sleep. In such children if the tight knots around GB-20 do not soften much with tapping, insert needles to these points. Also, the knots at BL-17 can be seen in relation to the sleep disturbance. If the symptoms do not change with other treatment methods, such as tapping or applying press-spheres, you can try needling these knots with the in-and-out needling technique. If GV-20 shows clear reaction when you palpate, this can also be a good point to needle to help reduce the distress caused by the symptoms.

Cupping

It can be difficult to apply cupping on a child with skin lesions, especially if the lesions are open. However, provided the skin will tolerate this, cupping around the navel can be helpful if

---

[5] As occurs with this point when treating adult patients with acute gastrointestinal symptoms, such as food poisoning.

the child has food allergies. Also, many children with atopic dermatitis also have problems of the lungs, which can show as congestion in the lungs and, in more severe cases, asthma or asthmalike symptoms. If the congestion in the lungs is not changing much with overall treatment and the skin condition is good enough to try this, cupping can be applied over the interscapular region to help treat the congestion.

Bloodletting

If vascular spiders are visible in the upper back region, especially around the GV-14 area, it could be helpful in resistant cases in older children to try bleeding these. If the symptoms over the neck and face are bad, LI-1 could be bled; check the point for signs of redness and congestion.

■ Other Considerations

Dietary

Commonly, you will need to discuss diet and help the patient identify food allergies. Cow's milk products are an obvious target, but many different allergies can show, some of which are hard to expect or predict, and there can be difficulty identifying them.

Home Treatment Targets

Usually parents are already busy with things that they do at home for the child with atopic dermatitis. At the very least this involves the application of creams and skin moisturizers. Usually the parents take this extra work in stride, but some find it a bit overwhelming. It is therefore not very helpful if you try to push too many home treatment recommendations. You need to determine what the parents are usually doing, and then figure out strategic approaches to help them start applying additional things, such as home tapping, home moxa, dietary changes, and so on.

Urticaria

With urticaria (or hives) red itchy spots can suddenly appear over various areas of the body, which often become swollen when scratched. The size of the affected areas can vary; they generally have a reddened appearance and can be light or dark. The skin surrounding the urticaria can also redden, and one can also see blisters on the area of urticaria. Generally the itchiness is worse in the evenings and worsens with scratching. In children these outbreaks of urticaria can come and go very rapidly, and in some cases they can become chronic. Generally these problems are caused by food allergies, sometimes as a reaction to medication, and sometimes as a result of internal problems. They are especially caused by metabolic disorders and can result from psychological factors. In some cases urticaria might also be due to a reaction to woolen fabrics, sunlight, coldness, or heat. It is unclear how these reactions can occur, but it is clear that many cases are allergy related.

If, when you start treating the child, you notice the areas you work on become flushed easily, where you stroke leaves a red line, or where you tap becomes reddened, you have to assume that the dose of treatment should be reduced, and you have to be even more careful not to overtreat.

■ Most Likely Pattern-based Root Diagnosis

Urticaria often involves the liver channel. On an older child one can more easily discriminate whether the liver is weak or replete from the pulse; on a baby or smaller child who will not stay still for you, this can be more difficult. One possible pattern is to find a lung vacuity pattern with liver repletion. But, if food allergies are involved, one might find spleen vacuity pattern with liver repletion. You need to check other signs and symptoms to discriminate. In some children you can find liver vacuity pattern as the primary pattern. Thus it is important to first get a sense of whether the liver is replete or weak. Regardless of the child's age or willingness to stay still, try to focus especially on the liver pulse position. Often you have to feel the pulse quickly.

The liver is replete if you feel resistance, and especially an edgy feeling of hardness, while pressing the pulse in the liver position from the level of feeling the artery (between the heartbeats) toward the bone. Once you have identified this feeling of hardness in the liver position of the pulse, then examine the heart and lung pulse positions; does one feel generally weaker than the other? If the lung pulse feels weaker than the

20 Digestive Problems

Constipation

Main complaints: She had had severe problems with constipation since she was a baby. She had very hard stools and passed small quantities at a time because it was painful to pass the stools. She was afraid to go to the toilet because of this pain. Additionally, she had had a lot of intestinal-abdominal pain since birth. She tended to wake every night between 2 and 3 a.m. with this pain.

Additional complaints: She had hernia of the navel, occasional small patches of dry and itchy skin, and a variable appetite. All other systems were unremarkable.

Diagnosis: Based on her symptoms and pulse I diagnosed her as having lung vacuity pattern.

Treatment: Tapping with the *herabari* was applied on the abdomen, chest, back, arms, legs, and especially around GV-12, GV-4, and GV-20.

Using the *teishin*, supplementation was applied to right LU-9 and SP-6 (SP-3 and SP-5 were too ticklish).

Press-spheres were applied and retained on GV-12 and bilateral BL-25 (they were not retained on ST-25 for fear that she might play with or interfere with them).

Second visit—2 weeks later

The stools had been larger and easier over the 2 weeks but were still a bit hard.

Treatment: Tapping with a *herabari* was applied on the abdomen, back, arms, legs, around GV-4 and GV-12.

Using a *teishin,* right LU-9 and SP-5 (SP-3 still too ticklish) were supplemented, left LR-3 drained.

Press-spheres were placed and retained on GV-12 and bilateral BL-25.

The mother was taught to do basic tapping at home daily.

Third visit—3 weeks later

The stools had been much better and were much softer and larger. In the last few days they had become slightly harder again, but there was no more waking at night with pain and no more fear of going to the toilet. Mother and child enjoyed daily home treatments.

Treatment: Using a *herabari,* tapping was applied to the abdomen, back, arms, legs, neck, and GV-12 and GV-4 areas.

Using a *teishin,* right LU-9 and SP-3 were supplemented, left LR-3 drained.

Press-spheres were placed and retained on GV-12 and bilateral BL-25.

Fourth visit—4 weeks later

Bowel movements were normal, with some variation in frequency (not always daily). No more abdominal pain, still no fear of going to the toilet and no constipation.

Treatment: Using a *herabari,* tapping was applied to the abdomen, back, arms, legs, neck, GV-12, and GV4 area.

Using a *teishin,* right LU-9 and SP-3 were supplemented, left LR-3 drained.

Press-spheres were applied and retained at GV-12 and bilateral BL-25.

For financial reasons and because of good progress, treatment was stopped.

■ General Approach for Patients with Constipation

Daily bowel movements may be an ideal concept, but for some people bowel movements at a frequency less than daily can be "normal." It is important to consider what the parent means by "constipation." If the child generally has difficulty passing stools such that the frequency is less than daily and causes some distress to the child, giving pain on evacuation, great strain trying to evacuate, or fear of going to the toilet, this certainly qualifies and should be treated as constipation. But the child who passes stools without effort four to five times a week and with no associated issues may well be "normal."

You may need to pay attention to the secondary symptoms that accompany the constipation. Is the young child afraid to go to the toilet because it has been painful and the child is afraid of that pain on straining to evacuate? Is it that the child usually feels the urge to evacuate after breakfast when he or she is typically at school and afraid of the more public toilets of the school or does not like using them for bowel movements? The first will usually improve once the child starts more easily passing stools. The second may need more attention as you think about how to help the child feel less nervous. Is this second category more related to a *kanmushisho*-type manifestation? How in general is the child's sleep and behavior?

If the bowel movement problem has had a sudden onset and is quite strong, it can also be important to inquire what the parents have done already and whether they have consulted their doctor. A complete stoppage with sudden onset can be a dangerous condition that requires proper medical investigation and attention.

It will, of course, be important to discuss the child's diet with the parents and make some simple recommendations as needed to help improve the diet if there appear to be problems with it. This can include discussing whether there may be sensitivity to certain foods, such as cow's milk products.

■ Most Likely Pattern-based Root Diagnosis

Problems of constipation can occur as a symptom of the spleen or large intestine. If the pattern is spleen vacuity, look also for other signs, such as abdominal bloating (independent of the effects of extended episodes of constipation), general abdominal pain, whether the stools have been passed or not, tendency toward also having periods of loose stools or diarrhea and tiredness. If the large intestine, this steers one toward considering the lung vacuity pattern; look for other problems such as nasal congestion, lung congestion, breathing difficulties, skin problems. Occasionally the problem of constipation arises as a sequela of the *kanmushisho:* look for associated problems with behavior or sleep. If there appear to be such problems, the non-pattern-based root treatment may be enough to deal with this, but it could show a problem of the liver channel. In this case examine the child for the liver vacuity pattern, but be careful to check out also whether the liver is not replete as a secondary problem to the underlying lung or spleen vacuity pattern. Because the problem manifests in the digestive system, it is usually enough to use the earth-source points for treatment. These are normally used for the lung (LU-9, SP-3) and spleen (SP-3, PC-7) vacuity patterns, but if the liver vacuity pattern shows LR-3, KI-3 may be better instead of the usual LR-8, KI-10.

■ Typical Non-pattern-based Root Treatment

For the smaller child apply the stroking and tapping or tapping non-pattern-based root treatment as usual over the limbs, back, and abdomen. Apply targeted tapping to the area around GV-12, GV-3 to GV-4, the navel, LI-4, and on the stomach channel below the shins. Tapping at ST-25 and BL-25 can be helpful. Also apply stroking or pressing in a circular motion (following the colon) over the abdomen around the navel (**Fig. 20.1**). This latter can be ticklish for some children, making it difficult to apply. In such cases use only a pressing technique with a larger instrument, such as the round ball end of the *enshin*.

If the child shows signs of the *kanmushisho*, apply tapping also over the occipital region. If the child is nervous because of the difficulties of going to the toilet (pain, etc.) also apply tapping on the head around GV-20.

■ Recommendations for Symptomatic Treatment

Press-Spheres (*Ryu***), Press-Tack Needles (***Empishin***), and Intradermal Needles (***Hinaishin***)**
In general, for the treatment of constipation we can focus treatment to the main constipation points, such as ST-25, BL-25 (Hyodo 1986). Leaving press-spheres at one or both of these points can be helpful.

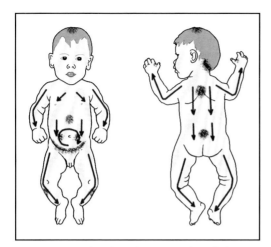

Fig. 20.1   Normal stroking plus extra stroking clockwise around abdomen.

Tapping:
- Around LI-4
- Around CV-12: 5 to 10 times
- ST-25 area: 10 times each
- Around ST-36-ST-37: 5 to 10 each leg
- Sometimes around pubic region: 10 to 20 times
- Around GV-20: 5 to 10 times
- Occipital area: 10 to 15 times
- Around CV-12:10 to 20 times
- Around CV-3:10 to 20 times

On children who are still in the oral phase and tend to place what they lay their hands on in their mouths, it is probably advisable to avoid leaving the press-spheres on ST-25 because the child may see and remove them, and thus potentially swallow them. If on a younger child the press-spheres are not producing a sufficient change one can increase the dose by using press-tack needles. Depending on the child, this is probably better done only to the points on the back (BL-25). For the older child who can handle a larger dose of treatment, one can start by placing press-tack needles on BL-25. If one wants to also stimulate ST-25, apply press-tack needles on BL-25 with press-spheres on ST-25. If there is no change with treatment and one wants to increase the dose again, application of the 3 mm intradermal needles to, for example BL-25, can be very helpful. If you choose to use press-tack or intradermal needles on the abdomen at ST-25, make sure that the parents are aware of this, and do not do this if you think the child might interfere with them.

On the adult we can apply intradermal needles or the short press-tack needles (0.6 mm) to the constipation zone in the ear. This lies along the lower border of the triangular fossa region. On an older child (6–7 years or older) who is not responding to what you have done with enough change, it can be possible to apply the 0.6 or 0.3 mm press-tack needles to this region of the ear on one side with appropriate care instructions to the parents. This is not a good idea to try on the younger child because the child may interfere with the needle.

Needling

On a younger or more frail child, if leaving press-spheres on acupoints such as BL-25 and ST-25 is not producing enough change, one can start applying needling shallowly at acupoints such as ST-25, BL-25, SP-13 (Hyodo 1986). For the older child one can apply needling to these points earlier in the treatment. If the child is older and stays still for you, you can insert the needles to the abdominal points and then begin the pattern-based root treatment. When you finish this root treatment, you can then remove the abdominal needles.

Cupping and Bloodletting

We tend not to use these techniques frequently on children for the problem of constipation, but in more stubborn cases it can be advantageous to try cupping lightly over the lower back and around the navel, using light pressure. If the child's condition is not changing and you notice clear vascular spiders on the lumbar region that are superficial enough to stab, apply the stabbing and squeezing method to these, removing a few drops of blood from each. This last technique can be difficult to apply on very small children because it can be quite uncomfortable on the lower back.

■ Other Considerations

For really stubborn conditions it can be very helpful to have the parents start applying a simplified form of the core non-pattern-based root treatment regularly at home.

■ Further Case Histories

The next case is the sister of the girl in Case 1. One can see that the effects were also quite remarkable.

Case 2
Alexandra, Girl Age 9 Months

Main complaints: She has had severe problems with constipation since birth. The pediatrician had identified problems with cow's milk, which was discontinued and replaced by special milk, but without a change in symptoms. She had very hard, small stools. She usually did not pass them herself, and her mother had to pull them out manually. She would wake some nights with abdominal pain. She had dry skin, and her mother used oils to moisten the skin.

Additional complaints: At 3 months she had had a bad cold; since then she tended to get a stuffy nose and an irritated throat (postnasal drip?) with cough. All other systems were unremarkable.

Diagnosis: Based on her symptoms and pulse I diagnosed her as having lung vacuity pattern.

Treatment: Tapping was applied with a *herabari* on the abdomen, chest, back, arms, legs, and especially around GV-12, GV-23, and GV-20.
Using a *teishin,* right LU-9, SP-3 were supplemented, left LR-3 drained.
Press-spheres were placed and retained on GV-12, bilateral BL-25, and ST-25.

Second visit—2 weeks later

The stools had been much better, almost normal over the 2 weeks, but had become slightly harder again in the last 2 days.

Treatment: Tapping with a *herabari* was applied on the abdomen, back, arms, legs, around GV-4 and GV-12.
Using a *teishin,* right LU-9, SP-3 were supplemented, left LR-3 drained.
Press-spheres were placed and retained on bilateral ST-25 and BL-25.
The mother was taught to do basic tapping at home daily.

Third visit—3 weeks later

The stools remained better, staying soft for the 3 weeks. Mother and child enjoyed the daily home treatments.

Treatment: Using a *herabari,* tapping was applied on the abdomen, back, arms, legs, chest, GV-12.
Using a *teishin,* right LU-9, SP-3 were supplemented, left LR-3 and BL-58 drained.
Press-spheres were placed and retained on bilateral ST-25 and BL-25.

Fourth visit—4 weeks later

Bowel movements were normal; no constipation, no hard stools.
The nose was somewhat less congested and the cough better, but she still had some problems with coughing.

Treatment: Using a *herabari,* tapping was applied to the abdomen, back, arms, legs, chest, GV-12.
Using a *teishin,* right LU-9, SP-3 were supplemented, left LR-3 drained.
Press-spheres were placed and retained on GV-12 and bilaterally on the asthma *shu* point.
Light cupping was applied to the interscapular region.
For financial reasons and because of good progress, treatment was stopped.

Although it is not uncommon for children to come to our clinics with bowel problems like constipation and for the treatments to generally work well, as is evidenced by the first two cases, not all cases of constipation are simply constipation. We have to be alert to complications that require a change in treatment tactic.

Case 3
Gerald, Boy Age 3 Years[1]

Main complaints: Gerald had been struggling with constipation for the previous year and a half. He could go through periods of normal bowel movements, but at least several times a month he would have difficulty passing stools, leading sometimes to abdominal pain and a lot of emotional distress. He could go up to 5 days without stools, but when not having a period of being constipated he usually had some bowel movement at

---

[1]   I treated this child before I had become familiar enough with Meridian Therapy to apply it routinely on children; thus there is no pattern-based diagnosis and treatment.

least every other day. He had no other problems; appetite, sleep, and mood were good. He was a full-bodied, energetic child, with no overt signs of weakness; thus I judged he could handle a slightly larger dose of treatment.

Treatment: Using a *herabari,* light tapping was applied over the abdomen, back, arms, and legs. Extra tapping was focused on the lower abdomen, especially around ST-25 and the lower back—around BL-25 and GV-3—and on the legs around ST-36 to ST-37.

Press-spheres were applied and retained bilaterally to BL-25.

Second visit—1 week later

There was nothing to report. Gerald was a bit relaxed on the day of the treatment. His bowel movements were difficult to assess as yet.

Treatment: The same pattern of light tapping was applied as on the first visit.

Press-spheres were placed and left on bilateral BL-25 and ST-25 (four press-spheres).

I taught the mother to repeat the basic light tapping treatment at home daily.

Third visit—1 week later

Gerald had had slightly more problems with constipation this week, but it was unclear if this was just a normal fluctuation or a worsening of symptoms. I discussed this with the mother and instructed her to apply the home treatment more lightly, with lighter tapping and fewer taps in each area.

Treatment: The same treatment as the second session was applied at a very slightly lower dose (lighter tapping with fewer taps in each area).

Fourth visit—8 days later

The symptoms were similar to those of the previous week; slightly worse than after the first treatment, but not quite as bad as after the second treatment. I decided to try a slightly stronger treatment.

Treatment: The same pattern of tapping was applied as on the first visit.

Needling was quickly applied to BL-25 bilaterally. Needles were inserted 2 to 3 mm, moved up and down very slightly and quickly, and then removed.

Intradermal needles were placed on BL-25 with instructions to remove them by the next morning and replace them with press-spheres.

Press-spheres were also placed and retained on bilateral ST-25.

Fifth visit—12 days later

No change in symptoms; his bowel movements remained erratic and problematic

Treatment: The same as on the fourth visit.

Sixth visit—1 week later

Gerald's bowel movement problems remained unchanged. I was now concerned; it is unusual not to have a clear response of some kind at least after three or so sessions when treating children of this age. I questioned the mother again to see if I had missed or misunderstood anything. Then the problem finally came to the surface. The constipation problems had begun in a period when Gerald was going through the normal growth stage that is associated with the "terrible twos." In his struggle to create more space for himself and learn more about his boundaries he had found a pattern of behavior that usually would get his mother to give him what he wanted. If he could not easily get what he wanted he would turn angry and threaten his mother, saying, "I won't go to the toilet then," following which he would hold his stools, thus creating the episodes of constipation. In other words, he did not have a functional bowel problem, he had the *kanmushisho* pattern, and the constipation was how it manifested in him. I thus changed my treatment accordingly.

Treatment: Light stroking was applied down the arms (three yang channels), legs (stomach and bladder channels), abdomen (stomach channel), and back (bladder channel).

Light tapping was applied around GV-12, GV-20, the occipital margin, and LI-4.

Press-spheres were applied and retained at GV-12 and GV-3.

I instructed the mother to change the home treatment to use the light stroking and tapping of the areas I had worked on.

Seventh visit—1 week later

Gerald was more relaxed. He had had no problems with bowel movements this week, managing to go every day, at least a little bit.

Treatment: The same treatment pattern as on the sixth visit was applied, with the exception that light needling was applied to the area around GB-20 (which felt quite stiff) and LI-4 after the tapping of those points.

Eighth visit—10 days later

He had had normal bowel movements every day, with no distress, and his mood had generally improved. He was no longer using the "no toilet" threat with his mother.

Treatment: Same as on the last visit.

Ninth visit—4 weeks later

Gerald was having normal daily or almost daily bowel movements, and he was generally in a better mood.

Treatment: Same as on the last two visits. I instructed the mother to continue the home treatment for a while longer and come back if there was any recurrence of the constipation problems.

This case was interesting. It shows that simply trying to address the manifestations of the symptom is not always the best approach. As long as I did the usual core non-pattern-based treatment with symptomatic focus to constipation and treatment points specific to constipation, there was no real progress. But as soon as I started treating the underlying problem of the *kanmushisho*, he started changing more and the symptoms started improving. The actual shift in treatment was quite small, but the effects of the small changes were very clear.

Diarrhea

The following case comes from the practice of my colleague Manuel Rodriguez of Barcelona, Spain. It shows the sometimes very surprising and powerful effects of this simple and gentle treatment method. Manuel saw this baby for treatment before he had learned the Meridian Therapy pattern-based treatment system. He only treated the baby with a simple form of *shonishin*. The baby would clearly have fitted the category of "spleen weak constitution" type, but did not need the specific root treatment nor the stronger, more aggressive treatments that can be used for this pattern—see Chapter 26, Weak Constitution.

Case 1
Paul, Boy Age 7 Months

Main complaints: Paul's mother, a nurse, was one of my students. She contacted me when Paul was ~2 to 3 months old because he was showing dermatitis linked with digestive problems. After making an appointment she had to cancel the visit on two separate occasions because she had to take Paul to the emergency room at the hospital, where he was subjected to extensive testing. Finally, at the third attempt to schedule an appointment, she brought Paul to my clinic when he was 7 months old. His medical history was already complex.

History: November 2002: Paul was born by normal birth after a normal pregnancy.

December–January 2003 (while 2–3 months old): He showed dermatitis of the toddler (possibly cradle cap) and a tendency to diarrhea. The analysis by the Western medical doctors concluded that he showed lactose intolerance. They stopped giving him cow's milk derivatives, giving instead rice milk together with cereals. Almost immediately the baby started with major episodes of diarrhea, with frequent passing of semi-liquid feces. The mother started testing different kinds and brands of "milks," including Damira, a hypoallergenic preparation. Paul continued with the diarrhea, which was becoming increasingly strong. Finally his doctor had him admitted to San Juan de Dios, the most famous pediatric hospital in the area.

March 2003 (at age 5½ months): He was still in the hospital. All allergy tests were negative. He was showing hypersensitivity only to egg white (which he had never eaten). Meanwhile the strong symptoms of diarrhea continued. He was referred to the gastroenterology department in the same hospital, where they also were unable to determine the cause of the diarrhea. By this time defecation immediately followed eating anything, and the child was showing deterioration (low weight, failure to thrive). The mother decided to change hospitals and took the baby to Teknon, a private hospital with an outstanding reputation. Once inside this hospital the testing continued. When starch and fat appeared in his stools the pediatrician concluded that Paul had "intolerance to macromolecules" and, after a further round of tests, determined that he had a "deficit of alpha-1-antitrypsin," which is considered congenital and without any possible treatment.

Late May 2003: The hospital made an intestinal biopsy, but could not see anything abnormal. The child was discharged from the hospital. He was still defecating four or five times a day, immediately after eating. His feces were almost liquid, showing scarce or no signs of digestion.

Mid-June 2003: He developed a fever. Within 3 days mucus started appearing in the stools. He was given cefuroxime, an antibiotic. The fever stopped but the diarrhea increased.

Early July 2003: He showed signs of dehydration (apathy, loose skin, etc.). He was taken back to the Teknon Clinic where he received emergency treatment. He was discharged 5 days later.

The next day, his mother brought Paul to see me for treatment. He looked almost normal, he was only a bit small for his age, and his vitality was slightly under par. His skin had a lackluster appearance. He had no dermatitis, and there was nothing else to remark on. At this time he was still defecating four or five times a day, always immediately after eating. His liquid feces contained almost undigested food. The hospital had informed the parents that they had no treatment to offer.

Treatment: I treated him with *shonishin,* the core non-pattern-based root treatment. To do this I applied very light stroking with a silver *enshin* over each of the indicated areas (down the arms, down the legs, down the back, down the abdomen). I added a very soft digital massage or pressure over ST-25.

I instructed the mother to repeat the light stroking treatment daily at home and to call me in 3 days to let me know how he was doing.

Three days later

Paul's mother reported by telephone that starting right after the treatment 3 days earlier, the feces had started to become more consistent. The day after, the child had defecated only three times, with almost normal feces. I instructed her to continue the treatment and report again in 15 days, or to call earlier if something happened.

Two weeks later

His mother reported by phone that Paul was now defecating only twice a day with normally formed feces. He had been gaining weight and increasing in vitality. I instructed her to continue with the treatment as a way to help the child's development.

At later follow-up (3 and 9 months) the mother reported that Paul's problem of diarrhea had never returned. He appeared to have a normal digestive system. I discharged him from treatment as he no longer needed any.

■ General Approach for Patients with Diarrhea

The symptoms of diarrhea (loose watery stools) are not accompanied by other symptoms such as vomiting, fever, or bad disposition. In the infant who is still breast-feeding the stools can range in frequency from several to many times a day. In babies the stools can be greenish and show some mucus. The condition does not usually lead to dehydration or weight gain problems. Yoneyama and Mori state that there is often a psychogenic component (Yoneyama and Mori 1964). In the older child if the tendency to diarrhea or at least relatively frequent loose stools persists, this may result in weight gain or growth problems with a more weakened appearance (i.e., skinny, less active, poorly developed muscles). These are signs of the spleen weak constitution and may be addressed as such (see Chapter 25). Infants may sometimes show signs of a spleen weak constitution, though it is less common. Infants with these problems generally respond much better to treatment than older children. Dietary factors can be a major issue for children with diarrhea, especially the consumption of cow's milk products.

Provided there are no significant medical complications, such as unrecognized allergies or food sensitivities, the infant with the simpler form of diarrhea can respond unexpectedly quickly to treatment using the core non-pattern-based root treatment. The infant with more complicated conditions, such as spleen weak constitution, will respond more slowly and require more focused treatment (see Chapter 25). The older child with this weak constitution will generally have a more weakened condition and will respond even more slowly and require more treatment.

■ Most Likely Pattern-based Root Diagnosis

The most common pattern will be spleen vacuity pattern, usually treated with SP-3 and PC-7. When pulse and abdominal findings are not clear enough to make a judgment of the pattern from them, select the spleen vacuity pattern. When the pulse and abdominal findings are clear, sometimes the lung vacuity pattern will show and the symptoms of the spleen are part of the lung vacuity pattern, in which case supplement LU-9 and SP-3. It is also possible that the kidney vacuity pattern will show, in which case look for signs of cold feet, underdeveloped child, as well as the pulse and abdominal findings. One can treat KI-7 and LU-8 or KI-3 and LU-9. Occasionally with the kidney vacuity pattern, the spleen is replete on the restraining cycle. On a baby or small child this can be difficult to feel in the pulse. There can be slight discomfort when the area above the navel is palpated. If this occurs, on the baby or small child it is better to supplement ST-36 rather than drain the spleen as a counterbalancing treatment for the spleen repletion. If, however, the child is older and you are able to discern the repletion of the spleen pulse clearly, then apply draining technique to SP-9. When applying these secondary treatment strategies for the kidney vacuity–spleen repletion pattern, always remember to apply the treatment points for the kidney vacuity on one side and then the treatment point for the spleen repletion on the other side of the body. Sometimes the liver vacuity pattern will show. In such cases not only will the

pulse and abdomen confirm this, but the child will often show signs of irritability, excessive crying, and sometimes vomiting; supplement LR-8 and KI-10.

It is often helpful to apply the idea from *Nan-Jing (Classic of Difficulties)*, Chapter 68, that the *he*-sea points are good for symptoms of diarrhea, in which case use SP-9 and PC-3 for the spleen vacuity pattern, LU-5 and SP-9 for the lung vacuity pattern, and KI-10 and LU-5 for the kidney vacuity pattern.

■ Typical Non-pattern-based Root Treatment

The core non-pattern-based root treatment can be applied with stroking down the arms, legs, and back, with tapping on the abdomen, LI-4, GV-12, and GV-3 regions (**Fig. 20.2**). Treatment can be varied according to whether treating a baby or somewhat older child; for the older child one often needs to apply additional treatment such as inserted needling (Shimizu 1975).

When working on the abdomen focus more on the upper abdomen and around the navel. On the back focus in particular on treating the lumbar region on the left side.

Additional tapping can be applied to the stomach channel in front of the shins, around the navel, and around GV-3, GV-4. Shimizu recommends additional tapping to ST-36, ST-37, and BL-60 (Shimizu 1975).

■ Recommendations for Symptomatic Treatment

Needling
Apply shallowly inserted needles at points such as BL-20, BL-21, BL-22 on the back, and CV-12, ST-25 on the abdomen (Yoneyama and Mori 1964). Palpate and treat the more reactive points. Often one finds tight bands along the bladder channel from around the level of BL-18 down to BL-22 or BL-17 down to around BL-21. More commonly these are stronger on the left side.

Shimizu (1975) comments that, for babies, if the contact needling (tapping, stroking) is not enough, inserting needles to ST-25 and BL-60 can be helpful. On older children (over age 2) we usually need to apply in–out needling technique to acupoints such as left SP-14, BL-23, and lateral to BL-25.

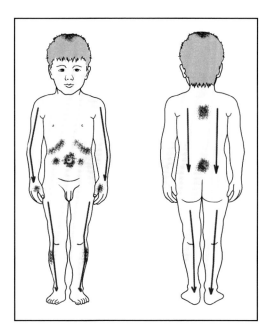

Fig. 20.2   Stroking:
- Down the arms (large intestine channels)
- Down the legs (stomach and bladder channels)
- Down the back (bladder channels)

Tapping:
- GV-20: 5 to 10 times
- GV-12:10 to 20 times
- GV-3 area: 10 to 20 times
- LI-4: 5 to 10 times each
- ST-25: 5 to 10 times each
- Subcostal areas: 5 to 10 times each
- Around navel: 5 to 10 times
- Around ST-36–ST-37: 5 to 10 times each

Okyu—Direct Moxa

To help reduce the symptoms of the diarrhea, heat can be applied around the navel. A simple way of doing this if the child will stay still is to use the large *chinetsukyu* moxa cones. Each cone is removed after the child starts to feel clear heat. Treatment points can include CV-9, CV-7, KI-16. In general one will tend not to use *okyu* much on babies and small children unless the symptoms are very heavy or resistant or part of a constitutional spleen weak pattern.

For strong symptoms of diarrhea, especially as part of the spleen weak constitution, apply moxa to BL-18, BL-20 contralaterally or bilaterally. For diarrhea in the nursing child apply moxa to GV-12 and CV-7 (Manaka, Itaya, and Birch 1995). For stronger, more stubborn symptoms or diarrhea, moxa can be applied to GV-

12 and BL-23 (Shimizu 1975). If there are clear food allergies involved in the development of the symptoms, applying moxa to the extra point *uranaitei* can be helpful.

Press-Spheres *(Ryu)*, Press-Tack Needles *(Empishin)*, and Intradermal Needles *(Hinaishin)*

For the child with strong or stubborn symptoms but who is too young to apply much, if any, moxa, I recommend starting by applying press-spheres or press-tack needles to acupoints such as BL-20, BL-18, CV-12, GV-3, or GV-4. After palpating these acupoints, examine to see which points are reactive. On a baby, if BL-20 is reactive on one side (usually more often on the left), place a press-sphere there. If there is not much change, increase the dose by leaving a press-tack needle there for a few hours with instruction for the parent to remove it and replace it with a press-sphere later that day at home. If still not enough, place the press-tack needle at the BL-20 reactive point and a press-sphere to, for example, CV-12 or GV-3, depending on which is reactive. In this way gradually increasing the dose can create change. If there is not enough change after this strategy you can then start thinking about how and whether the stronger, more difficult treatment of *okyu* can be applied. A similar strategy can be used on older children, starting with a stronger dose according to age and overall condition.

Bloodletting

Shimizu (1975) recommends that in stubborn cases of diarrhea one can bleed SI-1 or ST-45 and, if there is a vein visible between the distal and middle joints of the index finger this can also be bled.

■ **Other Considerations**

Dietary

Often one needs to discuss diet with the parents. Cow's milk sensitivity is a common trigger of such symptoms; thus one needs to have the parent test to determine whether it is involved in the development of the symptoms. Some children have more general dietary sensitivity and seem to react to many substances.

Home Treatment

Home treatment using a simple form of the core non-pattern-based root treatment is good for the parents to apply regularly at home. If the symptoms are strong and stubborn, it can also be helpful to apply heat around the navel. In the clinic we use moxa, but this is not good for the parents to apply. They can use something like a hot water bottle, or a small heated object that is wrapped in a towel and placed over the navel. When the area gets warm to the touch and turns red, stop applying the heat.

Abdominal Pain

Case 1
Andy, Boy Age 7 Years

Main complaints: Andy had daily abdominal pain that occurred especially in the evening, but it could also occur several times daily. It was distressing to him and caused him to withdraw to his room to go to bed and sleep to help control the pain. He had undergone various medical examinations, and the most recent diagnosis was irritable bowel syndrome. His parents were distressed because there was little they could do to help, and his condition seemed to be affecting his family and social life.

History: Problems with abdominal pain for around 18 months. He generally had a good appetite, slept well, and had a good mood. He seemed a little sensitive and emotionally distressed. He had a small hernia of the navel, which the doctors suggested leaving alone. His mother was an acupuncturist and was taking the *shonishin* class. She brought him to class to learn about what she could do at home to help him. The first two treatments were done in class, the next three in the 2 weeks afterward. After that she applied treatment on him at home on a regular basis.

Assessment: He showed a clear lung vacuity pattern based on skin texture (slightly thin), stiff shoulders, abdominal reaction in the lung reflex area, and weakness of the lung and spleen pulse positions with repletion of the liver (liver pulse position stronger and hard). He also had tight bands to either side of the spine around the level of BL-17 to BL-20, which are typical of chronic digestive problems.

Treatment: Using a *herabari*, tapping was applied to LI-4, over the abdomen, along the stomach channel below the knees, around GV-20, the supraclavicular fossa region, GV-12, GV-3 to GV-4 area.

Using an *enshin*, light stroking was applied down the arms, legs, abdomen, and back.

Using a *teishin*, left LU-9 and SP-3 were supplemented, right LR-3 drained.

Press-tack needles (0.3 mm) were placed on left BL-20, right BL-18.

A press-sphere was placed and retained on GV-12.

Second visit—next day

He was happy with the treatment because it was not painful and was quite relaxing. Otherwise there was not much to report.

Treatment: The dose of the whole treatment was slightly increased (more weight of contact with tapping and stroking, more strokes and taps).

Using a *herabari*, tapping was applied to LI-4, over the abdomen, along the stomach channel below the knees, around GV-20, the supraclavicular fossa region, GV-12, GV-3 to GV-4 area.

Using an *enshin*, light stroking was applied down the arms, legs, abdomen, and back.

Using a *teishin*, left LU-9 and SP-3 were supplemented, right LR-3 drained.

Press-tack needles (0.3 mm) were placed on left BL-20, right BL-18.

A press-sphere was placed and retained on GV-12.

The mother was taught to apply the basic core non-pattern-based treatment daily and to try treating the first two points of the lung vacuity pattern (normally parents are not taught the Meridian Therapy treatment as home treatment, but the mother was an acupuncturist who had come specifically to study how to treat children).

Third visit—3 days later

The pain had lessened over the last 3 days, and he was quite happy with this. Home treatment had gone well, but the mother was unsure yet about the lung vacuity pattern treatment.

Hyodo (1986) recommends needling or applying press-spheres to the following points for treatment of indigestion: BL-21, BL-20, CV-12, CV-6.

Press-Spheres (Ryu), Press-Tack Needles (Emp-ishin), and Intradermal Needles (Hinaishin)

In addition to checking the acupoints that Hyodo recommends (BL-21, BL-20, CV-12, CV-6) I also recommend examining the stomach channel on the legs around and below ST-36. It has been my experience that hard reactive knots are commonly found around BL-20 or slightly medial to BL-20. Focusing treatment to these knots is often helpful. On more stubborn or stronger symptoms on children who can tolerate an increased dose of treatment, place press-tack needles (0.6 mm) or intradermal needles (3 mm) to the most reactive acupoints, paying attention to dose needs and care instructions for the parent.

Okyu—Direct Moxa

Sometimes the symptoms are more stubborn, and the treatment approach has not created much change after a few sessions, in which case it can be helpful to apply moxa. For this it is generally better to use the 80% style of moxa (see Chapter 13)—let it get hot but not burn down too far. Manaka recommends for chronic indigestion applying moxa to CV-12, BL-20, and GV-12 (Manaka et al 1995). Irie (1980) has a slightly different recommendation for indigestion: BL-21, GV-12 (three to five moxa each). Palpate and choose the most reactive acupoints. For severe colic Shiroda (1982) also recommends KI-16, CV-12, CV-6, BL-50, and Sawada's GB-33 (extra point, 3 *cun* below GB-32).

Cupping, Bloodletting

In stubborn cases, especially on older children, it may be necessary to apply light cupping on the child. The treatment area should be on the back, focusing especially on the lumbar region, and, if the upper back and shoulder regions are stiff, these regions too. On older children, if vascular spiders appear on the lumbar region, these can be stabbed and squeezed to remove a few drops of blood. Pay attention that you do not cause pain with the technique. Sometimes bloodletting SP-1 can be useful for abdominal pain (Maruyama and Kudo 1982).

Case 2
Jos, Girl Age 7 Years

Main complaints: She had abdominal or stomach pain for more than a year. Pain focused around and below the navel. Pain can be worse with bowel movement, but not always. Pain is not daily but occurs every week at least one time per week.

History: She tried testing for lactose intolerance, but the results were inconclusive. Warmth seems to help the pain when it occurs.

The doctor performed several investigations but could not find any pathology. Further tests are planned to continue investigating the pain.

The doctor recommended a kind of abdominal massage, but this did not help.

Bowel movements are regular, appetite is good, sleep and mood in general seem to be good.

In the past she seemed to be tired easily but in the last months this problem is better.

No other significant medical history.

Assessment: Abdomen: a little stiffness and discomfort above and to the left and right of the navel (spleen, liver, and lung reflex areas).

Pulse: heart and spleen pulse weak, liver pulse replete.

Diagnosis: With the pulse, abdominal findings, and symptoms I diagnosed her as having spleen vacuity with liver repletion.

Treatment: Tapping was applied with the *herabari* to bilateral LI-4, GV-12, bilaterally around BL-17 to BL-20, GV-3, and the shoulder regions.

Using an *enshin*, light stroking was applied down the arms, legs, abdomen, and back.

Using a *teishin*, right SP-3 and PC-7 were supplemented, left LV-3 and then LI-6 were drained.

Press-tacks (0.3 mm) were left on bilateral BL-20.

Second visit –7 days later

She had pain the day of the first treatment and a little the next day, but since then no abdominal pain. Her mother reported that the pain after the treatment may have also been due to the stress of a swimming exam at school.

Treatment: Tapping was applied with the *herabari* to bilateral LI-4, GV-12, bilaterally around BL-17 to BL-20, GV-3, and the shoulder regions.
Using an *enshin*, light stroking was applied down the arms, legs, abdomen, and back.
Using a *teishin*, right SP-3 and PC-7 were supplemented, left LV-3 and then SI-7 were drained.
Press-tacks (0.3 mm) were left on bilateral BL-20.
The mother was taught to apply the core non-pattern root stroking treatment with a little extra tapping around GV-3, GV-12.

Third visit—50 days later

She is doing much better and has had no abdominal pain. Her mother has been doing the home treatment regularly over the holidays, which Jos likes. She is now back at school, and her mother thought it a good idea to treat preventively in case of stress reactive pain.

Treatment: Tapping was applied with the *herabari* to bilateral LI-4, CV-12, bilateral ST-25, GV-12, bilaterally BL-20, and the shoulder regions.
Using an *enshin*, light stroking was applied down the arms, legs, abdomen, and back.
Using a *teishin*, right SP-3 and PC-7 were supplemented, left LV-3 and then BL-58 were drained.
Press-tacks (0.3 mm) were left on bilateral BL-20.

Fourth visit—30 days later

She has occasionally had some abdominal pain, but this has generally been much better. She has mentioned having mild headache symptoms on a couple of occasions. The mother had forgotten to do home treatment during the last month.

Treatment: Tapping was applied with the *herabari* to bilateral LI-4, CV-12, bilateral ST-25, GV-12, bilaterally BL-20, and the shoulder regions.
Using an *enshin*, light stroking was applied down the arms, legs, abdomen, and back.
Using a *teishin*, right SP-3 and PC-7 were supplemented, left LV-3 and then BL-58 were drained.

Press-tacks (0.3 mm) were left on bilateral BL-20.

Fifth visit—19 days later

She has occasionally had some abdominal pain, but still remains much better. The mother had done home treatment regularly, and Jos did not complain of any headaches.

Treatment: Tapping was applied with the *herabari* to bilateral LI-4, CV-12, bilateral ST-25, ST-37 area, GV-12, bilaterally BL-17 to BL-20, and the shoulder regions.
Using an *enshin*, light stroking was applied down the arms, legs, abdomen, and back.
Using a *teishin*, right SP-3 and PC-7 were supplemented, left LV-3 and then SI-7 were drained.
Press-tacks (0.3 mm) were left on bilateral BL-20.

Sixth visit—20 days later

She has occasionally mentioned having some abdominal pain but has not complained about it. She has mentioned having mild headache symptoms on a couple of occasions. Her main complaint is that she has developed painful plantar warts on the bottom of both feet, probably from the swimming pool.

Treatment: Direct moxa (*okyu*) was applied to the center of the larger warts on the bottom of each foot (one on each foot).
Tapping was applied with the herabari to bilateral LI-4, bilateral ST-37 area, GV-12, bilaterally BL-17 to BL-20 and the shoulder regions.
Using an *enshin*, light stroking was applied down the arms, legs, abdomen, and back.
Using a *teishin*, right SP-3 and PC-7 were supplemented, left LV-was drained.
Press-tacks (0.3 mm) were left on bilateral BL-20.

Seventh visit—36 days later

No abdominal pain, no headaches, but still some discomfort from the plantar warts.

Treatment: Direct moxa (okyu) was applied to the center of the larger warts on the bottom of each foot (one on each foot).

Tapping was applied with the *herabari* to bilateral LI-4, bilateral ST-37 area, GV-12, bilaterally BL-17 to BL-20 and the shoulder regions.

Using an *enshin*, light stroking was applied down the arms, legs, abdomen, and back.

Using a *teishin*, right SP-3 and PC-7 were supplemented, left LV-3 and then TB-5 were drained.

Press-tacks (0.3 mm) were left on bilateral BL-20.

The mother was taught to apply moxa to the warts and to try to do this regularly, if possible daily.

No further treatments have been given. Jos remains better, with no complaints about abdominal pain or headaches. The plantar warts improved with the home moxa.

The following case from my colleague Paul Movsessian in the Blue Mountains outside Sydney illustrates how to take a straightforward and more direct treatment approach on a child with intestinal parasites. His use of a wide range of treatment tools is illustrative of how to take a broad approach once one has mastered the basic treatment models described in this book.

Case 3
Lisa, Girl Age 9 Years

Main complaints: She had parasitic gut dysfunction since the age of 5, with symptoms of abdominal cramps around the solar plexus region above the navel, especially at night, stomach pain, recurring worms, nausea and vomiting, constipation—regular but difficult-to-pass stool and stool soft with strong odor.

History: When she was 3 months old she had aseptic meningitis and a severe urinary tract infection treated with very strong antibiotics administered intravenously over 5 days and was hospitalized for 3 weeks. She has had chicken pox and suffers from asthma. Her teeth were slow to emerge. For the gut problem she has tried many different therapies, some of which helped with acute symptoms but none of which helped with the chronic problem. Besides various medically prescribed medications she has used a variety of homeopathic remedies, Australian bush flowers, salts, minerals, Western herbal remedies, kinesiology, naturopathy, heat packs, and pre-/probiotics.

Assessment: She looked quite frail and thin, her color was pale white with red patches and, dark blackish circles under the eyes, and her behavior was quite timid.

Her breathing was shallow, with no detectable odor. Her voice had quite deficient timbre with some slight whining.

She catches colds easily and regularly, sleep is disrupted by tossing and turning due to overheating, and she wakes quite tired. She also has recurrent ear infections and poor concentration.

On palpation the skin was found to be bumpy, hot, and sweaty over her body, with cold limbs and an overall poor luster.

Treatment: Due to some trepidation about treatment from the child and the very deficient constitution, on my initial visit I kept the treatment short and light to assess her response.

Using a copper *Yoneyama* and an *inrishin* light stroking and tapping were applied down the arms, legs, abdomen, back, and neck over a period of ~ 2 minutes.

Okyu moxa, rice grain size, was applied three times per point to GV-12, right BL-18, and left BL-20. *Okyu* was also applied to CV-12 and ST-26 bilaterally, once again three times per point.

I finished by making some recommendations regarding use of papaya seeds and honey and diatomaceous earth.

When treatment ended she seemed a bit more animated.

Second visit—6 days later

The evening after the treatment she was quite sleepy and tired; however, she reported having no abdominal cramps this week.

Treatment: Using a copper *Yoneyama* and an *inrishin* light stroking and tapping were applied down the arms, legs, abdomen, back, and neck over a period of ~ 2 minutes.

Okyu moxa, rice grain size, was applied three times per point to GV-12, right BL-18 and left BL-20, and bilateral *uranaitei*. *Okyu* was also applied to ST-34 bilaterally.[2]

The overall treatment dose was lower.

---

[2] This point can be used in acute gastric pain, and, because I felt her body would still need to eliminate the parasites, I chose to clear the stomach channel with this point.

Third visit—22 days later

She had been away for 3 weeks with school holidays. During the 3 weeks she had no cramps or digestive complaints. However, she did have a sore throat and cough.

Treatment: Using a copper *Yoneyama* and an *inrishin* light stroking and tapping were applied down the arms, legs, abdomen, back, and neck over a period of ~ 2 minutes.

Okyu moxa, rice grain size, was applied three times per point to GV-12, right BL-18 and left BL-20, and bilateral *uranaitei*. *Okyu* was also applied to CV-12 and ST-34 bilaterally.

Fourth visit—26 days later

Her gut symptoms have been much better. However, she had caught cold a few weeks ago, and now she has a lingering, barking cough with no expectoration and constantly needs to clear her throat.

The pulse and abdominal findings confirmed a lung vacuity with liver repletion pattern.

Treatment: Using a *tesihin*, right LU-8 and SP-5 were supplemented, left LV-3 was drained.

Okyu moxa was applied to GV-12, right BL-18 and left BL-20, bilateral asthma *shu* points.

Press-spheres were placed and retained at the stop coughing points in the elbows.

Lastly a kind of natural inhaler was recommended for the respiratory passages, and a light oil massage was recommended on the neck as home treatment.

Fifth visit—14 days later

Her mother reported that everything continues to improve. The gut is still fine, the cough is better, but there remains a little throat clearing.

Treatment: First ion-pumping cords (IPC) were applied for 2 minutes using surface electrodes with black at CV-22 and red at LI-4 bilaterally.

Using a *tesihin*, right LU-8, SP-5, and right I V-4 were supplemented.

Okyu was applied on the back three times per point at GV-12, BL-13, BL-17, and the asthma *shu* points.

A press-sphere was left on CV-12 for 3 to 4 days.

Sixth visit—7 days later

Her mother reported that everything had been improved until Lisa had a sleepover with a sick friend, and now once again the symptoms have returned of sore gut, with a stuffy and congested feeling in the head and another cough.

Treatment: Using a *teishin*, right LU-8 and SP-5 were supplemented.

Using an *enrishin*, right ST-40 was drained. Light stroking was also applied down the *yang* channels on the arms and legs.

Okyu moxa was applied to GV-12, CV-12, and the asthma *shu* points.

For the head congestion treatment finished with a 5-second application at 100 Hz with the Manaka ion beam device with only black on GV-23 and then a 5-second application at 100 Hz on LI-20 black and LI-4 red bilaterally.[3]

Seventh visit—6 days later

Her mother reported that Lisa had felt well from treatment and has been very well with the only complaint being a bit stuffy in the chest and having a slight cough.

Treatment: Due the stubbornness of clearing this condition it was decided to use only the *okyu* moxa as treatment. Her neck around the sternocleidomastoid muscle (SCM) was very tight. I used *okyu* three times bilaterally around the acupoint LI-10 for the neck and then applied a Thermie Warmer[4] to stroke the supraclavicular fossa region around the SCM. I also used the Thermie Warmer around the area of LU-1–LU-2. I then applied *okyu* to GV-12, BL-17, and the asthma *shu*

---

3   The ion beam device is an electrical device that generates bipolar fields such that a positively charged field is created at the red electrode and a negatively charged field at the black electrode. It is briefly described in Manaka's book (Manaka et al 1995, pp. 123–125).

4   The Thermie Warmer (Austin Medical Equipment Inc.) is a handheld metal instrument in which a thick piece of incenselike substance burns. The radiant heat of the incense warms the metal instrument, which is then massaged over the skin to give a mild warming massage.

points. On the front I applied *okyu* to CV-17 and CV-12.

Eighth visit—22 days later

Lisa has a slight mild cough lingering, but her overall immunity seems to have strengthened and everything else is feeling well. Abdominal palpation revealed a pattern indicating the use of KI-6–LU-7.

Treatment: A north magnet was applied to KI-6 and south to LU-7 for 2 minutes.[5]

Okyu was applied bilaterally to BL-13 and BL-42.

Press-spheres were applied to bilateral KI-26 (which was quite reactive).

Ninth visit—56 days later

Since the last treatment she has had no more gut or lung symptoms.

But now it is the end of school and she is a bit run down and has a bad flu. Thus she wanted to come in for treatment to help recover from that. She has swollen glands, lethargy, and feverishness and feels grumpy.

Treatment: IPC cords were applied using surface electrodes, with black at BL-62 and red at SI-3 bilaterally for 5 minutes.

Using a *Yoneyama* instrument, light tapping was applied around the occiput and stroking down the bladder channel on the back and stomach channel on the front.

Using a *teishin*, CV-12, ST-25 bilaterally, and CV-6 were supplemented.

Okyu was applied to GV-14.

Tenth visit—49 days later

She has been better and still no recurrence of the main complaints. But this week she twisted and sprained her right lateral ankle.

Treatment: Using something like Manaka's burn treatment, aluminum foil was placed over the sprained area with the black clip of the IPC attached and the red clip attached to a needle at left TB-5.[6] This was left for 15 minutes.

Using hot style *chinetsukyu*, moxa was applied around the sprain.

Treatment finished with a little gentle *sotai*[7] for the ankle.

Eleventh visit—35 days later

Her ankle had improved immediately after treatment. The original gut complaints are still okay with no recurrence of symptoms. Her glands and lungs are normal. She feels very healthy, her energy is good, her body temperature seems normal, and her immune system is feeling stronger.

Treatment: Using a *teishin*, right LU-9 and SP-3 were supplemented.

Using an *inrishin*, light stroking was applied down the *yang* channels on the arms and legs.

Three cones of *okyu* moxa were applied each to GV-12, right BL-18, left BL-20, and CV-12.

It was agreed to stop treatment here and that she would come back for treatment should the symptoms recur.

Stomach Problems

Case 1
Larry, Boy Age 9 Years

Main complaints: Over the last few years Larry had had a lot of problems with stomach upset and vomiting. He had stomach upset around six or seven times a month, often accompanied by

---

[5] The application of the two poles of a magnet at two different acupoints is a specialized field of study in Japan and Germany. In Japan it is part of what is called plus–minus acupuncture (Matsumoto and Birch 1986, pp. 143–145). These polarity treatment methods are labeled as polarity agents, which include the IPC. Manaka describes the use of certain polarity agents for testing and others for treatment (Manaka et al 1995). It is necessary to study the relevant systems of diagnosis and treatment in depth before attempting to apply polarity agents like north–south magnets in treatment.

[6] For a brief description of Manaka's burn treatment see Matsumoto and Birch (1988, pp. 355–358).

[7] *Sotai* is a gentle system of exercise to adjust body structure, see Hashimoto, Kawakami, 1983.

vomiting in the morning. The symptoms recovered by late morning. The cause of the problem was unclear; it had been diagnosed as chronic gastritis, possibly stress related.

Secondary complaints: He had a small problem with being very energetic, triggering sometimes uncontrolled behavior and big emotional swings. He was also very talkative and tended to think a lot.

Assessment: His appetite and sleep were generally good, his diet was okay, with no clear reactions to any particular foods. All other systems were normal. His abdominal tone was a bit poor, generally slightly weaker below the navel level and a full feeling above the navel on the *ren mai.* He could not do abdominal breathing and tended to breathe a little high in the chest. The left deep pulses were overall slightly weaker than the right, with weakness of the spleen pulse and repletion of the stomach pulse.

Diagnosis: He had a tendency toward *kanmush-isho*-type symptoms and had a liver vacuity pattern with spleen vacuity and stomach repletion.

Treatment: Since he was an older and relatively mature child the *shonishin* non-pattern-based treatment was not applied.

Regular needles were used to supplement CV-12, left LR-3, KI-3, right SP-3, drain right ST-40, left GB-37, and left SI-7.

Using a needle, contact needling was applied over the lower abdomen and in the area around ST-12.

Regular needles were used to supplement BL-18, BL-23, GV-6 (which felt spongy and weak).

Using an *enshin,* stroking was applied down the back.

Press-spheres were placed and retained on CV-12, GV-12, and right BL-20.

Second visit—1 week later

He had had a good week, the first part slightly better than the second. His emotions and energy were also a little calmer.

Treatment: Regular needles were used to supplement CV-12, left LR-3, KI-3, right LU-9, drain right TB-5, left GB-37, and left SI-7.

Using a needle, contact needling was applied over the lower abdomen and in the area around ST-12.

Regular needles were used to supplement BL-18, BL-23.

Using an *enshin,* stroking was applied down the back.

Press-spheres were placed and retained on GV-12, CV-6, and right BL-17.

A needle was used to supplement left KI-3.

Third visit—12 days later

Condition not as good as after the first treatment.

Treatment: Regular needles were used to supplement left LR-3, KI-3, right SP-3, drain right ST-40 and TB-5.

Using a needle, contact needling was applied over the lower abdomen and in the area around ST-12.

Regular needles were used to supplement BL-23.

Using an *enshin,* stroking was applied down the back.

Chinetsukyu mild warmth moxa was applied to GV-3 and BL-23.

Press-spheres were placed and retained on GV-3 and CV-6.

Fourth visit—9 days later

Overall he was better than before treatment started but not as good as after the first visit. The stomach symptoms had improved, and his energy and emotions were calmer.

Treatment: Regular needles were used to supplement CV-12, left LR-3, KI-3, right LU-9, SP-3, drain right TB-5, left GB-37, and right LI-6.

Using a needle, contact needling was applied over the lower abdomen and in the area around ST-12.

Chinetsukyu mild warmth moxa was applied to CV-12, CV-6, and ST-25.

Regular needles were used to supplement BL-18, BL-23.

Using an *enshin,* stroking was applied down the back.

Press-spheres were placed and retained on GV-12, CV-6, and right BL-17.

Fifth visit—12 days later

Overall better again and more stable.

known this earlier it could have been useful to add something further to address his problems, such as applying treatment to the thoracic spine, targeting the neck, shoulder, and upper back a bit more. But in general Larry did very well with treatment. His gastritis resolved after only a few treatments and his general *kanmushisho*-type problems also showed clear improvement. Because of his age I did not ask the parents to perform home treatment. On reflection, it could have been helpful to do this.

■ General Approach for Patients with Stomach Problems

Dietary

Obviously, one needs to examine dietary issues for patients with stomach problems; what the child eats and drinks is a common trigger for stomach problems.

Home Treatment

Another common problem is the role of stress. Often in children stomach problems like gastralgia and gastritis show a clear psychogenic component, with reactions to stress issues at home. One way of dealing with these stress issues is to see how to engage the parents in some home treatment.

■ Most Likely Pattern-based Root Diagnosis

With stomach problems the most likely patterns will be spleen vacuity pattern or liver vacuity pattern. The spleen vacuity pattern will show, for example, pain and distension. The liver vacuity pattern will show more in relation to stress reactions.

■ Typical Non-pattern-based Root Treatment

For babies and smaller children the core non-pattern-based root treatment with tapping and/or stroking is applied over the arms, legs, abdomen, back, shoulders, and head. If the child is older this treatment approach can be used but at a higher dose. Usually the shoulders and neck will show signs of stiffness; also stroke over these areas (**Fig. 20.4**).

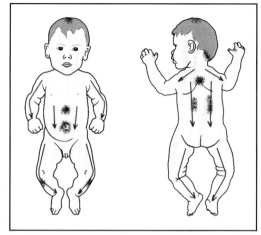

Fig. 20.4   Stroking:
- Down the arms (large intestine channels)
- Down the legs (stomach and bladder channels)
- Down the back (bladder channels)
- Down the abdomen (stomach channels)
- Across the shoulders

Tapping:
- GV-20: 5 to 10 times
- CV-12:10 to 20 times
- Around BL-18-BL-20:10 to 20 times
- Occipital area: 5 to 10 times
- LI-4: 5 to 10 times each
- Around CV-12: 5 to 10 times
- Around navel: 5 to 10 times
- Around ST-36–ST-37: 5 to 10 times each

Additional treatment can be targeted around the navel, CV-12, to the stomach channels on the leg, especially by the shins, and the areas around BL-18 to BL-20. If the child appears to have stress-related stomach problems, also tap around GV-20, GB-20, LI-4, and in general over the shoulders.

■ Recommendations for Symptomatic Treatment

Needling

For children with stomach problems, needling reactive points on the abdomen and back is usually quite effective. Reactive points include CV-12, CV-10, ST-21, ST-25, BL-17, BL-18, BL-20, and BL-22. On the younger child use the in–out needling technique; on the older child retain the needles for a while. If the stomach problems are due to stress or psychological factors, check around GB-20 and BL-10 and needle to release the tension there, using the in–out technique for younger children and the retained needle technique for older children. Additionally, if GV-20 or the area around GV-20 shows pressure pain reaction, especially with signs of puffiness/sponginess, this reactive point can also be needled. On children who show strong reaction on palpation of the abdominal points and are too nervous to let you needle these points, try palpating on the legs around ST-36 to ST-37 and needle the reactive points there.

Press-Spheres (*Ryu*), Press-Tack Needles (*Empishin*), and Intradermal Needles (*Hinaishin*)

Leaving press-spheres, press-tack needles, or intradermal needles for stomach problems is most easily targeted to acupoints on the back. It is common that strong reactions are found in the region of BL-17 to BL-20, especially around BL-20 and/or BL-18. Leaving something to treat these reactive points, either on one side or one point on each side of the spine can be very useful to help relieve the symptoms. On the abdomen, reactions on the *ren mai,* such as around CV-12 or CV-10, can be treated by leaving press-spheres or press-tack needles for stomach problems. On children with "nervous stomach"; that is, stomach problems that appear with stress, leaving a press-sphere on GV-12 can be helpful. Some children with this stress reaction can show a lot of stiffness in the upper back in the interscapular region, in which case direct treatment to reactions around BL-14 and BL-15.

Okyu—Direct Moxa

If the stomach problems are primarily due to food allergies or food sensitivities, apply moxa to the extra point *uranaitei.* In this case the point on both feet feels the heat, so apply the moxa to each foot so that heat is felt at least three times. If the symptoms are stubborn and you are treating an older child, this can be an acupoint used for home moxa therapy. If the child has problems due to constitution, such as the spleen weak constitution type, then sometimes stronger treatment is needed, such as moxa to BL-18, BL-20, and sometimes GV-12. The symptoms associated with this tend not to be limited to the stomach and tend to involve the whole digestive tract, but if the child is very run down and has a poor appetite

and stomach problems instead of loose stools or diarrhea, it could be useful to try this treatment. On smaller children it is better to start by treating these acupoints with press-spheres, or press-tack needles. If this is not working, then use moxa. On older children one can use moxa to these acupoints sooner. Remember that to minimize the number of points that we moxa, we apply the moxa to BL-18 and BL-20 contralaterally, usually boys left BL-18, right BL-20; girls, right BL-18, left BL-20. If the stomach problems are more due to stress, the "nervous stomach," examine the thoracic spine for reaction on the intervertebral spaces between T2 and T9. If there is reaction here apply moxa to the reactive points(s) in the style of Fukaya's "psychosomatic moxa treatment" (Irie 1980; Fukaya 1982).

Cupping

Meguro (1991, pp. 146–147) mentions the use of a more extensive cupping treatment for weak stomach in children. It is useful to remember that Meguro is a cupping specialist, meaning that his treatment exclusively involves the use of cupping for all patients. As acupuncturists, we can use this approach for some of our patients, but more likely we will be integrating the use of cupping into the overall treatment on each visit. When we do the following cupping treatment, it will probably be too much of a dose if all of it is applied in addition to the rest of the treatment. Thus the tendency is to use some of these treatment protocols or on occasion only to do the cupping as a separate treatment.

For children up to the age of 7 years, apply cups for 6 or 7 seconds over each of the following areas in the order presented:
- Over BL-20, BL-21, BL-23, and BL-51 (eight cups)
- Around ST-21, ST-27, and SP-14/SP-15 (six cups)

It is important to review the discussion of cupping methods in Chapter 14 to grasp the details of these cupping treatments. No cups should cause pain. We use only pumped cupping and not fire cupping.

Bloodletting

On an older child bloodletting SP-1 can be useful for stomach problems. Check the points for signs hence be careful of treatment dose. As the child with this *kanmushisho* tendency becomes older, his or her problems become more complex, with learned behavioral patterns built on top of the *kanmushisho* tendencies. I have had experiences treating children aged 6 to 9 years with ADHD who have reacted negatively to the first treatment because I misjudged the dose. It is better to do less and focus on building the treatment relationship at first. It is also advisable when treating a child with behavioral problems not to have the parent bring siblings into the room. Often the child does not want to stay still to receive treatment when a sibling is present. This can be much worse as the children seek to play with each other. It can be very difficult maintaining order and being able to do what you would like when the children are playing in your treatment room.

■ **Goals of Treatment**

Regulate the *qi* by moving it downward so as to help calm the child, and treat to restore balance to the channel system so as to help improve overall regulation of *qi* in the body. Release typical stiff areas that develop in relation to these behavioral problems.

■ **Most Likely Pattern-based Root Diagnosis**

Liver vacuity pattern is most commonly treated for this problem. On a baby or small child, where you cannot reliably get information from the pulse and abdomen, select and treat the liver vacuity pattern. To do this, supplement LR-8 and KI-10. An alternative point selection could be to use the fire/*ying*-spring points LR-2 and KI-2 if the child seems overheated; he or she would not only be very irritable, crying a lot, and so on, but would have a reddened appearance, almost looking feverish.

With older children where you can feel the pulse and abdomen, and you can understand what you are feeling, you have the possibility to treat with more discrimination. Liver vacuity pattern is still the more common pattern that shows, but you may find the liver involved in other ways, secondary to lung or spleen vacuity patterns. For example, you may find lung vacuity with liver repletion or lung vacuity pattern with liver vacuity or spleen vacuity pattern with liver repletion, or spleen vacuity pattern with liver vacuity. The method of discriminating repletion or vacuity of the liver is described in Chapter 19, p. 149, Urticaria—Most Likely Pattern-Based Root Diagnosis. In these cases apply treatment as follows:

- For lung vacuity with liver repletion pattern: supplement LU-9, SP-3, or LU-5, SP-9 on one side and drain LR-3 or LR-8 on the other side of the body.
- For the lung vacuity, liver vacuity pattern: supplement LU-9, SP-3, or LU-5, SP-9 on one side and LR-3 or LR-8 on the other side of the body.
- For the spleen vacuity with liver repletion pattern: supplement SP-3, PC-7, or SP-9, PC-3 on one side and drain LR-3 or LR-8 on the other side of the body.
- For the spleen vacuity with liver vacuity pattern: supplement SP-3, PC-7, or SP-9, PC-3 on one side and LR-3 or LR-8 on the other side of the body.

■ **Typical Non-pattern-based Root Treatment**

The treatment needs to be applied repeatedly. The *kanmushisho* pattern is typically part of the constitutional tendencies of the child, and thus symptoms will tend to repeat easily. To counter this, applying treatment regularly for a while is important. Shimizu (1975) mentions applying treatment on average three to five times per month, whereas Yoneyama and Mori (1964) state it is good to be patient—things improve with regular treatment. To aid consistency and frequency of treatment, it can be very helpful to have the parents apply a short, simplified, light form of the core non-pattern-based root treatment with stroking and tapping at home. This maintains the frequency and pushes the child to respond a little more quickly, which in many cases is very helpful. Chapter 8 describes the application of home treatments. It is important to pay attention to the issues of overtreatment and make sure you check carefully what to do and what you have the parents do at home.

For treatment, apply stroking down the arms, legs, back, and abdomen. If the shoulders are stiff, apply stroking across the shoulders. If the neck is

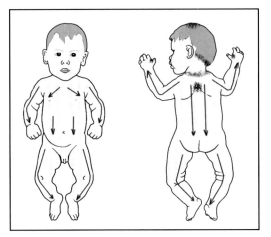

Fig. 21.1 Usual stroking plus tapping:
- LI-4: 10 to 15 times each
- GV-12: 20 to 30 times
- Shoulder area: 10 to 20 times
- Occipital area: 10 to 20 times
- GV-20: 10 times

stiff, apply stroking down the neck. Apply tapping to around GV-12 (**Fig. 21.1**).

Additional tapping or stroking can be applied to certain regions and acupoints depending on the severity of the *kanmushisho*. In general, focus more on the upper back, head, neck, and shoulders. Tapping around GV-12, the GB-20 to BL-10 area, across the occipital region, around GV-20 can be helpful. It can be helpful to start with tapping of the acupoints to which you may need to apply stronger treatment, such as needling in later treatment sessions. Check acupoints such as LI-4, LI-2, BL-10, BL-11 for stiffness of the muscles in these regions. Shimizu (1975) makes the following additional recommendations: lightly stroking distally over the webs between the fingers and toes. Apply additional tapping to the following acupoints: LU-5, LI-11, PC-4, ST-36, KI-6. The tapping of these acupoints can be useful as part of the core non-pattern-based treatment if the *kanmushisho* is strong. If the *kanmushisho* irritability manifests with abdominal bloating, focus especially on the abdomen, particularly the upper abdomen.

For the older child (5 years and older) with *kanmushisho*-type problems, it is my experience that tapping should be minimized and light stroking should be used. On the baby and young child the combination of stroking and tapping works

well. But it seems the tapping can be "stimulating," which can in some children be an irritant. Thus, on the older child, I recommend using stroking applied with slightly more contact and somewhat more slowly. Stroking is applied repetitively down the arms (all *yang* channels), down the back, down the neck, across the shoulders and down the legs (bladder and stomach channels). For the stroking it can be helpful to use a thicker instrument like the *enshin* that can warm up with the stroking movements. On subsequent visits, when you are more sure how the child is responding to treatment and what the appropriate dosage needs are, you can start adding other techniques (**Fig. 21.2**).

■ **Recommendations for Symptomatic Treatment**

Needling

If the *kanmushisho* symptoms are stubborn and do not respond enough to the light stroking and tapping, you may need to increase the dose ac-

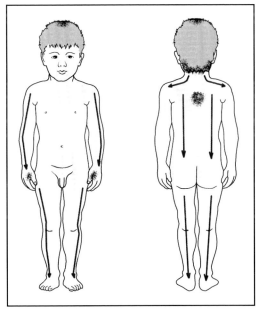

Fig. 21.2 Greater number and pressure of stroking plus additional stroking across the shoulders.
Light tapping around:
- LI-4
- GV-12
- Occipital area
- GV-20 area

Third visit—2 days later

When Colin came into the outer part of the office he calmed down. His mother said that he had been generally much better. It was easier to console him but he still had some difficulties, especially at night.

Treatment: The treatment from the second visit was repeated with the addition of very light stroking of SP-3.

Fourth visit—4 days later

His mother reported that he had generally been much happier and was showing signs of being more "normal," smiling and being playful rather than constantly in distress.

Treatment: Same as the previous visit with the addition of draining the stomach channel: stroking a little more heavily against the flow of the stomach channel over right ST-40.

Fifth visit—2 days later

His mother reported that she was so relieved that he was showing such signs of improvement. He had even stopped fussing when they were on the way to my office. Before, he would scream pretty much around the clock and was now having good periods of relief each day.

Treatment: Same treatment as on the last visit. Treatment continued like this, with him coming in on average twice a week for a while. He had some rough days but generally better periods. When the family went away for 10 days, he had more symptoms again after 6 days, so it seemed he was still reactive. His mother was taught to apply some gentle stroking while they were away but that had not worked much. So the treatment schedule of three treatments that first week was tried. The next week two treatments were given. Gradually, treatments were worked down to one treatment a week while maintaining the improvements.

Colin's mother was quite worried that when they went home to Europe for the summer he might regress. But he was doing well when they left and while away he had done extremely well with almost no symptoms. He was 4.5 months old when they left for the summer and so his diges-tion was getting stronger while he was away and he didn't need treatment when they returned. We arranged that they would call if further treatment was needed.

Case 3
Peter, Boy Age 15 Months

Main complaints: He was very irritable, becoming angry easily, crying and shouting a lot, and experiencing sleep disturbance. He had always had loose stools. At age 3 months he required hernia surgery, from which he recovered well, but an osteopath found a "cervical block" possibly related to head position during the surgery. It was suggested that this may be related to his irritability. He had always had loose stools and, as a small baby, had a big problem with regurgitation. He had had a few colds and after one of these his tonsils were found to be affected and his doctor had talked about the possibility of a tonsillectomy. He had just recovered from a cold and he had had a mild fever 2 days before.

Diagnosis: Based on his history, I diagnosed him with liver vacuity pattern.

The parents were concerned as they had a long drive back and forth to the clinic, and, because the roads were very congested, it might be difficult to do many treatments.

Treatment: Tapping was applied with a *herabari* to GV-20, GV-22, GV-12, neck area, and abdomen.

Stroking was applied with an *enshin* down the back, arms, and legs.

Using a *teishin*, left LR-8, KI-10, and right LU-9 were supplemented.

Press-spheres were left on GV-12 and bilateral BL-25.

Second visit—7 days later

He had slept better the first two nights, then his usual disturbed sleep pattern returned. There was no change in daytime behavior. His stools were a little better formed over the last few days.

Treatment: Tapping was applied with *herabari* to GV-20, GV-22, GV-12, CV-12, LI-4, and ST-36.

Stroking was applied with an *enshin* down the back, abdomen, neck, arms, and legs.

Using a *teishin*, left LR-8, KI-10, and right SP-9 were supplemented, left TB-5 drained.

Press-spheres were left on GV-12, bilateral BL-25, and behind *shen men* on the left ear.

Home treatment was taught to the parents: stroking down the arms, legs, back, and abdomen, with tapping around GV-12 and GV-3.

Third visit—6 days later

His stools were better formed over the week, but his behavior and sleep were a little worse. Home treatment went well.

Treatment: Needling was applied with in and out insertion to bilateral LI-4.

Retained needling was applied to bilateral GB-20 (~ 2 minutes).

Tapping was applied with a *herabari* to GV-20, GV-12, back, arms, and neck region.

Stroking was applied with an *enshin* down the back, abdomen, arms, and legs.

Using a *teishin*, left LR-8, KI-10, and right SP-3 were supplemented, left GB-37 was drained.

Press-spheres were left on GV-12, right BL-18, left BL-23.

Fourth visit—15 days later

His stools were generally better, but over the previous few days they had been loose and runny. Overall, his mood and behavior had been better these 2 weeks.

Treatment: Needling was applied with in and out insertion to bilateral LI-4.

Retained needling was applied to bilateral GB-20 (~ 2 minutes).

Tapping was applied with a *herabari* to GV-20, GV-12, back, and arms.

Stroking was applied with an *enshin* down the back, abdomen, arms, and legs.

Using a *teishin*, left LU-9 and SP-3 were supplemented.

Press-spheres were left on bilateral BL-25.

Fifth visit—7 days later

His mood, behavior, and sleep were all much better, but he had more problems with diarrhea.

Treatment: Retained needling was applied to bilateral GB-20 (~2 minutes).

Tapping was applied with a *herabari* to GV-20, GV-12, GV-3, abdomen, back, and LI-4.

Stroking was applied with an *enshin* down the back, abdomen, arms, and legs.

Using a *teishin*, left LU-9, SP-3, and right LR-3 were supplemented.

Press-spheres were left on CV-12 and bilateral BL-25.

Sixth visit—14 days later

His mood, behavior, and sleep remained much better. His bowels had been better and stools were normal during the last 5 days. Overall, his condition was much improved.

Treatment: Retained needling was applied to bilateral GB-20 (~ 2 minutes).

Tapping was applied with a *herabari* to GV-20, GV-12, GV-3, abdomen, back, and LI-4.

Stroking was applied with an *enshin*, down the back, abdomen, arms, and legs.

Using a *teishin*, left LU-9, SP-3, and right LR-3 were supplemented, right TB-5 was drained.

Press-spheres were left on CV-12 and GV-12.

The parents discussed how well he was doing but what a big burden it was to get to each treatment. They wanted to stop and to continue with simple home treatments a few times a week. They would call for a new appointment if his symptoms returned. We scheduled a follow-up visit for 2 months later, which they canceled because he was doing well, with sleep and behavior good and bowels normal.

Reflection: It is clear that starting to insert needles on the third visit was very helpful to improve his symptoms. This is the usual strategy for a child of his age. We try using only the stroking and tapping treatment approach, and if that is not working we start doing some inserted needling. I am unsure why the pattern changed from liver to lung. Perhaps the liver pattern was related to the hernia surgery and consequent symptoms of irritability, but his underlying constitutional tendency is shown in the digestive problems, which are usually suggestive of the spleen pattern. In his case the spleen is part of the lung pattern. It is too bad that travel made repeated treatments more difficult for Peter. I think in his case it would have been better to do a few infrequent but regularly scheduled follow-up visits for a while, to help counter underlying constitutional tendencies, but this was not possible.

Case 4
Maria, Girl Age 1 Year

Main complaint: Her sleep was restless. She did not have a significant problem with this, but, given her medical history, her parents were a little worried and very attentive. A few days after birth, she required surgery to repair her duodenum and spent 3 months in hospital, after which she required a lot of antibiotics. At first she had a restricted diet but now was able to eat everything. She was generally very energetic and active during the day, with a tendency to being a little restless. She had a tendency to catch cold easily and get mucus in the lungs. She had had an ear infection 10 days before, with fever, and required antibiotics. She had recovered from this. Everything else was good. She had a hard fibrous scar across the epigastrium (spleen reflex area). The lung reflex area also showed a reaction and her right deep weak pulses seemed weaker than the left.

Diagnosis: I diagnosed her with lung vacuity pattern, possibly with liver repletion.

Treatment: Using a *teishin*, a very light stroking action was applied down the arms (large intestine channel), legs (stomach and bladder channels), back (bladder channel), neck (bladder, gallbladder channels), and around the abdomen.

Using the *teishin*, right LU-9, SP-5 were supplemented, left LR-3 drained.

Tapping was applied using a *herabari* in the region over GV-12.

A press-sphere was placed and retained on GV-12.

Second visit—14 days later

She had been more restless, especially at night, for a couple of days following the treatment. She had had a fever without symptoms over the previous few days, which had stopped the day before.

Treatment: I decided that it was probably better to follow the medical history to select the pat-

tern rather than try to follow the pulse findings. I changed the diagnosis to spleen vacuity pattern. I also decided that an even lighter treatment would be better, so did not leave a press-sphere or apply any tapping.

Using a *teishin*, a very light stroking action was applied down the arms (large intestine channel), legs (stomach and bladder channels), back (bladder channel), neck (bladder, gallbladder channels), and around the abdomen.

Using the *teishin*, right SP-3, PC-7, left LR-3, GV-12, and GV-20 were supplemented.

Third visit—14 days later

She had been doing better, especially at night, following the last treatment. However, she had had irregularity of stools with alternating diarrhea and constipation, and given her history, was seeing the specialist within 2 weeks.

Treatment: Using a *teishin*, a very light stroking action was applied down the arms (large intestine channel), legs (stomach and bladder channels), back (bladder channel), neck (bladder, gallbladder channels), and around the abdomen.

Using the *teishin*, right SP-3, PC-7, and left GB-37 were supplemented.

Fourth visit—13 days later

She had been much better over the 2 weeks. Restlessness and especially sleep were better, as were the bowels. She saw the specialist who felt there was no need for concern and thought she was progressing very well.

Treatment: Using a *teishin*, a very light stroking action was applied down the arms (large intestine channel), legs (stomach and bladder channels), back (bladder channel), neck (bladder, gallbladder channels), and around the abdomen.

Using the *teishin*, right SP-3 and PC-7 were supplemented and left LR-3 drained.

Fifth visit—5 weeks later

She was very well, her sleep was good. A vaccination made her a little restless for a week with a mild skin rash, but she recovered from this.

Treatment: Using a *teishin*, a very light stroking action was applied down the arms (large intestine channel), legs (stomach and bladder channels), back (bladder channel), neck (bladder, gallbladder channels), and around the abdomen.

Using the *teishin*, right SP-3, PC-7, GB-37, GV-12, GV-20, and GV-23 were supplemented and left BL-58 drained.

Sixth visit—26 days later

She was good for the first 2 weeks but over the last couple of weeks her sleep had started to become disturbed again; she was especially having difficulty falling asleep. She had also had a reduced appetite, and during this period it was found that she had a strong reaction to sugar, which thus needed to be eliminated from her diet.

Treatment: Using a *teishin*, a very light stroking action was applied down the arms (large intestine channel), legs (stomach and bladder channels), back (bladder channel), neck (bladder, gallbladder channels), around the abdomen and chest, and down the *yin tang* area.

Using the *teishin*, right SP-3 and PC-7 were supplemented, and left LR-3, BL-58 drained.

Following this she was much better and remained so until after the summer holidays.

Seventh visit—3 months later

She had been much better until she returned from a vacation abroad (with a several-hour jet lag). This had triggered sleep disturbance for a while. Then during the last weekend everything at home was very busy and hectic, leaving her agitated, with difficulty falling asleep, crying, restlessness, and poor appetite.

Treatment: Using a *teishin*, a very light stroking action was applied down the arms (large intestine channel), legs (stomach and bladder channels), back (bladder channel), neck (bladder, gallbladder channels), around the abdomen and chest, and on the *du mai* GV-24 to GV-20.

Using the *teishin*, right SP-3 and PC-7 were supplemented and left LR-3, right ST-40 drained.

Following this she was much better again and has not had to return for treatment since.

Reflection: On the first visit I tried to use my diagnostic skills to select the pattern for treatment (pulse, abdominal findings, tends to catch cold) and chose the wrong pattern (lung instead of spleen). It was clear afterward that the spleen pattern was the correct one to treat; many later symptoms are typical spleen symptoms (alternating constipation and diarrhea, difficulty falling asleep, poor appetite). Her medical history also clearly indicated a constitutional pattern of spleen involvement. Also, I probably overtreated her on the first visit. The agitation and medical history could tend to create a greater sensitivity; thus a lower dose was needed. Usually a little tapping or the press-sphere is not a problem, but in her case it turned out better to avoid these methods. As already discussed, in treatment of older children with *kanmushisho* where the manifestations are of hyperactivity, I think tapping can be too stimulating and stroking to move *qi* downward is a better strategy; perhaps this was the case here as well.

Case 5
Marijke, Girl Age 2$^1/_2$ Years

Main complaints: She has had poor sleep since birth.

She has a tendency toward problems of constipation. She has daily abdominal pain. She was born almost full term but was small and remains slightly small for her age.

History: She has difficulty sleeping and frequently wakes up. She can become hysterical if she wakes and her mother is not present.

Her appetite used to be bad but improved over the last month.

She has used laxatives regularly for the last 10 months; the milder pediatric version was not effective so she uses a stronger version.

The abdominal pain is possibly related to the constipation problem and the need for laxatives.

Generally she has a good mood and no other health issues.

Assessment: Her overall condition is relatively good.

She allowed pulse diagnosis: her liver and kidney pulses are weak.

Diagnosis: The pulse and sleep disturbance symptoms indicate liver vacuity pattern. Possibly the abdominal pain and constipation problems are secondary to the liver pattern.

Treatment: Tapping was applied with the *herabari* to bilateral LI-4, GV-12, GV-20, and along the occipital margin.

Using an *enshin*, light stroking was applied down the arms, legs, abdomen, and back.

Using a *teishin*, right LV-8 and KI-10 were supplemented, as was right ST-36 (to counterbalance the perceived slight repletion of the spleen pulse).

Press-spheres were left on GV-12 and on the back of the left ear behind *shen men*.

Second visit—9 days later

Not much to report.

Treatment: Tapping was applied with the *herabari* to bilateral LI-4, GV-12, GV-3 area, bilateral ST-25, and along the occipital margin.

Using an *enshin*, light stroking was applied down the arms, legs, abdomen, and back.

Using a *teishin*, right LV-8 and KI-10 were supplemented, left SP-3 and TB-5 were drained (based on pulse assessment).

Press-spheres were left on GV-12 and on bilateral BL-25.

Third visit—7 days later

Her sleep has been better. The bowel movements have been the same, but she has had less abdominal pain, only a few times during the week rather than daily, and less intense.

Treatment: Tapping was applied with the *herabari* to bilateral LI-4, GV-12, bilateral ST-25, and along the occipital margin.

Using an *enshin*, light stroking was applied down the arms, legs, abdomen, and back.

Using a *teishin*, right LV-8 and KI-10 were supplemented, left LU-9 was supplemented, left ST-40 was drained (based on pulse assessment).

Press-spheres were left on GV-12 and on bilateral BL-25.

The mother was taught to apply the core non-pattern root stroking treatment with a little extra tapping around GV-3, GV-12, and bilateral ST-25.

Fourth visit—7 days later

She still resists going to bed but her sleep has been noticeably better, with less waking during the night and easier return to sleep when she does wake. She is still using the laxatives, but the bowel movements have been easier with less strain and pain. Abdominal pain is improved again. She enjoys the home treatment, which was done regularly during the week. She had a bit of a runny nose a few days before due to mild cold symptoms.

Treatment: Tapping was applied with the *herabari* to bilateral LI-4, GV-12, bilateral BL-25, GV-20, GV-23, and the supraclavicular fossa region.

Using an *enshin*, light stroking was applied down the arms, legs, abdomen, and back.

Using a *teishin*, right LV-8 and KI-10 were supplemented, left LU-9 was supplemented.

Press-spheres were left on GV-12 and on bilateral BL-25.

Fifth visit—7 days later

Her sleep has improved further, there is less abdominal pain again, and, although she is still using the laxatives, bowel movements are easier.

Treatment: Tapping was applied with the *herabari* to bilateral LI-4, GV-12, bilateral BL-25, GV-3 area, bilateral ST-25.

Using an *enshin*, light stroking was applied down the arms, legs, abdomen, and back.

Using a *teishin*, right LV-8 and KI-10 were supplemented, left LU-9 was supplemented.

Press-spheres were left on GV-12 and on bilateral BL-25.

Sixth visit—21 days later

Her sleep is much better, bowel movements are better and easier, almost no abdominal pain. She is now no longer using laxatives daily, but only if the day before there was no bowel movement.

Treatment: Tapping was applied with the *herabari* to bilateral LI-4, GV-12, bilateral BL-25, GV-3 area, bilateral ST-25, bilateral ST-36.

Using an *enshin*, light stroking was applied down the arms, legs, abdomen, and back.

Using a *teishin*, right LV-8 and KI-10 were supplemented, left LU-9 was supplemented.

Press-spheres were left on GV-12 and on bilateral BL-25.

Seventh visit—33 days later

Her sleep is still better but not quite as good as 5 weeks before, showing increased restlessness. Bowel movements are much better, and she uses much less laxative. We discussed that possibly it was too soon to put such a distance between treatments.

Treatment: Tapping was applied with the *herabari* to bilateral LI-4, GV-12, bilateral BL-25, GV-3 area, bilateral ST-25, and the supraclavicular fossa regions.

Using an *enshin*, light stroking was applied down the arms, legs, abdomen, and back.

Using a *teishin*, right LV-8 and KI-10 were supplemented, left ST-36 was supplemented.

Press-spheres were left on GV-12 and on bilateral BL-25.

Eighth visit—16 days later

She is doing very well. Her sleep is better, though there is a tendency to wake a bit early. Bowel movements are better, and she is still using less laxatives.

Treatment: Tapping was applied with the *herabari*, to bilateral LI-4, GV-12, bilateral BL-25, GV-3 area, bilateral ST-25, and bilateral ST-36.

Using an *enshin*, light stroking was applied down the arms, legs, abdomen, and back.

Using a *teishin*, right LV-8 and KI-10 were supplemented, left LU-9 was supplemented.

Press-spheres were left on GV-12 and on bilateral BL-25.

Ninth visit—28 days later

Her sleep is much better. Bowel movements are regular, and she hardly uses laxatives now.

Treatment: Tapping was applied with the *herabari* to bilateral LI-4, GV-12, bilateral BL-25, GV-3 area, bilateral ST-25, and bilateral ST-36.

Using an *enshin*, light stroking was applied down the arms, legs, abdomen, and back.

Using a *teishin*, right LV-8 and KI-10 were supplemented, left SP-9 was supplemented.

Press-spheres were left on GV-12 and on bilateral BL-25.

Tenth visit—56 days later

Her sleep and bowel movements are still much better. However, she just had a bad cold the week before with fever leading to pseudo-croup, all of which disturbed sleep and appetite. She still has problems with sleep, appetite, and coughing, with slight feverishness.

Treatment: Tapping was applied with the *herabari* to bilateral LI-4, GV-20, and GV-22.

Using a *teishin*, right LU-10 and SP-2 were supplemented.

Press-spheres were left bilaterally on the stop coughing points near LU-5.

Press-tacks (0.3 mm) were left on bilateral asthma *shu* points.

Comments: She was still slightly feverish; thus the basic *shonishin* treatment with stroking was not used, and slight tapping was applied only to points to help with congestion in the nose. The cold had been a bad one, and as can happen sometimes with acute severe symptoms, the pattern changed to a lung vacuity pattern. The *ying*-spring points were used instead of the regular lung vacuity pattern points to help with the fever. After this treatment she finished recovering more quickly from the cold. The problem of cough abated within 2 days, and her sleep improved. As of our last contact, she still sleeps much better and has regular bowel movements and is hardly using laxatives at all with no abdominal pain.

Case 6
Jelle, Boy Age 13 Years

Main complaints: He has problems with poor concentration and being a bit hyper. The problem is worse at school and less problematic at home. He has been diagnosed with attention deficit hyperactive disorder (ADHD). The doctor has prescribed Ritalin (Novartis) but both Jelle and his parents want to try an alternative approach and use the medication as a last resort.

History: He was born with only one kidney, but this has not resulted in any problems.

He generally eats well, and there is no clear relationship between the ADHD symptoms and dietary factors. He is busy at school and active with sports. He has a good appetite, and his sleep is okay. When younger he had a period of problems with chronic loose stools, but this gradually improved and has not been a problem for a while.

Assessment: There are signs of reaction in the lung and liver regions with palpation of the abdomen.

The lung and spleen pulses are weak.

Diagnosis: Based on the palpation and pulses, I diagnosed him with lung vacuity pattern.

Treatment: Using a 0.12 mm needle, in and out needling technique was applied to bilateral LI-4 and the stiff reaction just lateral to GB-20.

Using the *teishin*, left LU-9, SP-3 and then right LV-3 were supplemented. Left ST-40 and BL-58 were drained.

Supplementation was applied to soft-feeling regions in the supraclavicular fossa region and then to bilateral BL-13 and BL-20.

A press-sphere was applied to GV-12.

A press-tack needle (0.3 mm) was applied on the back of the left ear behind *shen men.*

Second visit—nine days later

Not much to report except that he slept deeply in the car after treatment.

Treatment: Using a 0.12 mm needle, in and out needling technique was applied to bilateral LI-4, BL-18, and around GB-21.

Using the *teishin*, left LU-9 and SP-3 were supplemented. Right LV-3 and left TB-5 were drained.

Needles were then inserted and retained at bilateral GB-20.

Supplementation was applied to soft-feeling regions in the supraclavicular fossa region and then to bilateral BL-13 and BL-20.

Press-tack needles (0.3 mm) were applied to GV-12 and on the back of the left ear behind *shen men*.

Third visit—six days later

Caught cold 2 days before and has felt tired with lack of energy for the last 2 days. Not much to report regarding the ADHD symptoms.

Treatment: Using a 0.12 mm needle, in and out needling technique was applied to bilateral LI-4.

Using the *teishin*, left LU-9, SP-3, and right ST-36 were supplemented

Needles were then inserted and retained at bilateral GB-20 and BL-18.

Chinetsukyu–cone moxa was applied to GV-14, GV-3, and the lateral *pigen* points (one cone per point).

Press-tack needles (0.3 mm) were applied to the lateral pigen points to center his energy by providing continuous but very gentle stimulation to the lateral *pigen* points. As we shall see, this strategy worked well.

A press-sphere was applied on the back of the left ear behind *shen men*.

Fourth visit—six days later

He has felt more relaxed in himself. His mother reports that his behavior and concentration have been a bit better.

Treatment: Using a 0.12 mm needle, in and out needling technique was applied to bilateral LI-4.

Using the *teishin*, left LU-9 and SP-3 were supplemented. Right LV-3, TB-5, and left BL-58 were drained.

Using the *teishin*, supplementation was applied to soft-feeling regions in the supraclavicular fossa region.

Needles were then inserted and retained at bilateral GB-20 and BL-18.

Using the *teishin*, bilateral BL-13 and BL-20 were supplemented.

Chinetsukyu–cone moxa was applied to GV-14, GV-3, and the lateral *pigen* points (one cone per point).

Press-tack needles (0.3 mm) were applied to the lateral *pigen* points.

A press-sphere was applied on the back of the left ear behind *shen men*.

Fifth visit—eight days later

He has been better but not as good as the previous week.

Treatment: Using a 0.12 mm needle, in and out needling technique was applied to bilateral LI-4.

Using the *teishin*, left LU-9, SP-3 and right GB-37 were supplemented (GB-37 was supplemented to counterbalance the slight repletion of the liver because I judged that the week had not been quite so good, possibly because I drained more points in the last session). Right ST-40 was drained.

Using the *teishin*, supplementation was applied to soft-feeling regions in the supraclavicular fossa region.

Needles were then inserted and retained at bilateral GB-20 and BL-18. In and out needling technique was applied bilaterally across the shoulders and at BL-15.

A press-tack needle (0.6 mm) was applied to GV-12.

Press-tack needles (0.3 mm) were applied to the lateral *pigen* points.

A press-sphere was applied on the back of the left ear behind *shen men*.

Similar treatments were applied another 10 times over the next 4 months. During this time he experienced a general improvement in his restlessness and concentration. His focus and performance in the classroom improved. In general he was happy with these changes, and he took over scheduling treatment sessions himself, even when he knew he was improved, to help him stay this way. For the next 6 months he received no treatments and generally had done well at school. But in the last few weeks he started developing some concentration problems again and decided to return for treatment.

Sixteenth visit

Treatment: Using a 0.12 mm needle, in and out needling technique was applied to bilateral LI-4.

Using the *teishin*, left LU-9 and SP-3 were supplemented. Right LV-3, TB-5, and left BL-58 were drained.

Using the *teishin*, supplementation was applied to soft-feeling regions in the supraclavicular fossa region.

Needles were then inserted and retained at bilateral GB-20 and BL-20. A heat lamp was applied to the region around the needles at BL-20.

Press-tack needles (0.3 mm) were applied to the lateral *pigen* points.

Seventeenth visit—6 days later

He has felt a bit calmer and more concentrated this week.

Treatment: Using a 0.12 mm needle, in and out needling technique was applied to bilateral LI-4.

Using the *teishin*, left LU-9 and SP-3 were supplemented. Right LV-3, TB-5, and left ST-40 were drained.

Using the *teishin*, supplementation was applied to soft-feeling regions in the supraclavicular fossa region.

Needles were then inserted and retained at bilateral GB-20, BL-18, and *josen*. A heat lamp was applied to the regions around the needles at *josen* and BL-18.

In and out needling method was applied bilaterally to stiff areas on the upper back and shoulders.

Press-tack needles (0.3 mm) were applied to the lateral *pigen* points.

Eighteenth visit—14 days later

Although his concentration has improved further, he still feels that he is a bit overall distracted.

Treatment: Using a 0.12 mm needle, in and out needling technique was applied to bilateral LI-4.

Using the *teishin*, left LU-9 and SP-3 were supplemented. Right LV-3, left ST-40, and TB-5 were drained.

Using the *teishin*, supplementation was applied to soft-feeling regions in the supraclavicular fossa region.

Needles were then inserted and retained at bilateral GB-20, BL-18, and GV-12. A heat lamp was applied to the regions around the needles at GV-12 and BL-18.

In and out needling method was applied bilaterally to stiff areas on the upper back and shoulders.

Press-tack needles (0.3 mm) were applied to the lateral *pigen* points.

Following this treatment Jelle has been much improved. He had a further eight treatments over the next 5 months and remained in a calmer, more concentrated state, able to perform better in the classroom and when doing homework. He has been very happy with treatment.

Stress

The following case is of a 10-year-old boy who was very stressed. The treatment is similar to that for *kanmushisho.*

Case 1
Paul, Boy Age 10 Years

Main complaints: He has frequent nasal sniffing and twitching, which he experiences as nasal itchiness. The problem has been continuous over the last several months.

History: He saw the doctor, who tested for and ruled out allergies. His mother reported that Paul was very stressed out due to the fact that his parents were separated, with ongoing conflicts and stresses. His studies at school were suffering. He was also having bad dreams. He tended to have somewhat sensitive skin, showing rashes relatively easily. The lung, spleen, and liver abdominal reflex showed reactions. The lung and spleen pulses were weak and the liver pulse hard.

Diagnosis: I diagnosed him with lung vacuity with liver repletion pattern.

Treatment: Tapping was applied using a *herabari* to LI-4, GV-20, GV-12, occipital region, the back, neck, shoulders, abdomen, arms, and legs.
  Using a *teishin*, left LU-9 and SP-3 were supplemented; right LR-3, ST-40, and left BL-58 were drained.
  A press-sphere was placed on GV-12.
  A 0.6 mm (Pyonex, Seirin-America) press-tack needle was left in the left ear at *shen men* with instructions to remove it in ~ 36 hours.

Second visit—8 days later

The symptoms stopped for the first 5 days and then started recurring, but less severely.

Treatment: Tapping was applied using a *herabari* to LI-4, GV-20, GV-12, occipital region, the back, neck, shoulders, abdomen, chest, arms, and legs.
  Using a *teishin*, left LU-9 and SP-3 were supplemented; right LR-3 and left BL-58 were drained.
  A press-sphere was placed on GV-12.
  A 0.6 mm (Pyonex) press-tack needle was left in the left ear at *shen men* with instructions to remove it in ~ 36 hours.
  Since his father brought him on the second visit, I did not teach the home treatment as I figured he would not be the one to administer it.

Third visit—6 days later

There are still some signs of nasal sniffing and twitching, but significantly less frequently and with less severity.

Treatment: Tapping was applied using a *herabari* to LI-4, GV-20, GV-12, occipital region, the back, neck, shoulders, abdomen, chest, arms, and legs.
  Using a *teishin*, left LU-9 and SP-3 were supplemented; right LR-3, ST40, and left TB-5 were drained; BL-13 and BL-20 were supplemented.
  A press-sphere was placed on GV-12.
  A 0.6 mm (Pyonex) press-tack needle was left in the left ear at *shen men* with instructions to remove it within ~ 36 hours.
  I taught the mother to do light tapping at LI-4, GV-12, GV-20, the back, arms, and legs daily.

Fourth visit—14 days later

He was much improved, with hardly any symptoms over the 2 weeks. Home treatment went well.

Treatment: Tapping was applied using a *herabari* to LI-4, GV-20, GV-12, occipital region, the back, neck, shoulders, abdomen, chest, arms, and legs.
  Using a *teishin*, left LU-9 and SP-3 were supplemented, right LR-3 and ST-40 were drained, BL-13 and BL-20 were supplemented.
  A press-sphere was placed on GV-12.
  A 0.6 mm (Pyonex) press-tack needle was left in the left ear at *shen men* with instructions to remove it within ~36 hours.

I scheduled to see Paul again in 3 weeks. His mother canceled close to the time of the appointment. Paul had had no symptoms, his work at school was much better, and he seemed calmer. She did not reschedule because of financial reasons, but insisted that she would call for an appointment should Paul need it. She was doing the home treatment several times per week.

Case 2
Timo, Boy Age 11 Years

Main complaints: He has been having nightmares over the last weeks, several times per week. The nightmares leave him feeling distressed, nervous, and fearful. They seem linked to the death of his grandmother just over 4 months earlier. He had been very close with and fond of his grandmother. They also seemed related to his mother's recent change of work schedule, which takes her occasionally abroad. During the last weeks he has also had some headaches, mostly frontal. Also in the last weeks he has had some eczema-like irritation around the eyes, which was treated by the general practitioner with steroid cream. This is better but still threatens.

History: As a toddler he had problems with pseudo-croup. He had frequent upper respiratory tract infections affecting the nose and lungs, which improved after having both tonsils and adenoids removed.

He has allergies to some animals, such as rabbits and horses.

He tends to get loose stools and in the past has had problems with abdominal pain, cramping, and diarrhea.

Diagnosis: He shows the kidney vacuity pattern on the abdomen and pulses.

Treatment: Using an *enshin*, light stroking was applied down the arms, legs, abdomen, and back.

Using a *teishin*, left KI-7 and LU-5 were supplemented; right SP-9, left TB-5, and BL-58 were drained.

Using the *teishin*, supplementation was applied to soft-feeling regions in the supraclavicular fossa regions and in the regions of the anterior-superior iliac spine on the abdomen.

Bilateral BL-13 and BL-23 were supplemented. Press-tacks (0.3 mm) were left on bilateral BL-23.

Recommendations were given to test for cow's milk sensitivity.

Second visit—7 days later

He had had no nightmares this week and no headaches. The skin irritation around the eyes looked better as well.

Treatment: Using an *enshin*, light stroking was applied down the arms, legs, abdomen, and back.

Using a *teishin*, left KI-7 and LU-5 were supplemented; right SP-9, left BL-58 and right TB-5 were drained.

Using the *teishin*, supplementation was applied to soft-feeling regions in the supraclavicular fossa regions and in the regions of the anterior-superior iliac spine on the abdomen. Bilateral BL-13 and BL-23 were supplemented.

Press-tacks (0.3 mm) were left on bilateral BL-23.

Using the *teishin*, CV-6 was supplemented.

Third visit—9 days later

He had some sleep-disturbed nights this week (not quite nightmares). The skin remained better. They have managed to eliminate cow's milk products from his diet.

Treatment: Using an *enshin*, light stroking was applied down the arms, legs, abdomen, and back.

Using a *teishin*, left KI-7 and LU-5 were supplemented; right SP-9, left BL-58, and right TB-5 were drained.

Using the *teishin*, supplementation was applied to soft-feeling regions in the supraclavicular fossa regions and in the regions of the anterior-superior iliac spine on the abdomen. Bilateral BL-13 and BL-23 were supplemented.

Press-tacks (0.3 mm) were left on bilateral BL-23.

Using the *teishin*, CV-6 was supplemented.

Fourth visit—5 days later

He reports still being fearful, and his sleep disturbance is better but still present. The skin remains better. He tried some milk to see if it irritated the skin around the eyes.

Treatment: Using an *enshin*, light stroking was applied down the arms, legs, abdomen, and back.

Using a *teishin*, left KI-7 and LU-5 were supplemented; right SP-9, left BL-58, and right TB-5 were drained.

Using the *teishin*, supplementation was applied to soft-feeling regions in the supraclavicular fossa regions and in the regions of the anterior-superior iliac spine on the abdomen. Bilateral BL-13 and BL-23 were supplemented.

Press-tacks (0.3 mm) were left on bilateral BL-23.

Using the *teishin*, CV-6 was supplemented.

Fifth visit—7 days later

Generally sleep is better but he had one nightmare and is still a bit fearful.

Treatment: Using an *enshin*, light stroking was applied down the arms, legs, abdomen, and back.

Using a *teishin*, left KI-7 and LU-5 were supplemented; right SP-9, left BL-58, and right LI-6 were drained.

Using the *teishin*, supplementation was applied to soft-feeling regions in the supraclavicular fossa regions and in the regions of the anterior-superior iliac spine on the abdomen. Bilateral BL-13 and BL-23 were supplemented.

In and out needling was applied to bilateral GB-20 using 0.12 mm needles.

Press-tacks (0.3 mm) were left on bilateral BL-23.

Sixth visit—19 days later

He had a headache the day that the needles were removed, but otherwise he has been *better*.

Treatment: Using a *teishin*, left KI-7 and LU-5 were supplemented; right SP-9, left BL-58, and GB-37 were drained.

In and out needling was applied around bilateral GB-20 using 0.12 mm needles.

Bilateral BL-13 and BL-23 were supplemented.

Press-tacks (0.3 mm) were left on bilateral BL-23.

Seventh visit—10 days later

He had confirmed having sensitivity to cow's milk products and determined to avoid them consistently from now on. His sleep had generally been okay the last few days.

Treatment: He now shows a lung vacuity pattern, which remained with him after this session.

Using a *teishin*, left LU-9 and SP-3 were supplemented; right LV-3, left LI-6, and TB-5 were drained.

Using the *teishin*, supplementation was applied to soft-feeling regions in the supraclavicular fossa regions and in the regions of the anterior-superior iliac spine on the abdomen.

Needles (0.12 mm) were inserted and retained for a few minutes at bilateral GB-20, BL-13, and a strong reaction at right TB-17.

Press-tacks (0.3 mm) were left on bilateral BL-17.

After this treatment a similar treatment approach with small variations was used. His fearfulness improved, becoming more acute at the top of a mountain and when his mother was away for a few days. The nightmares became infrequent and less bothersome because he generally was calmer. He received a total of 12 more treatments over the next 10 months, reporting that he really liked the treatments and would prefer to have occasional treatments as follow-up rather than stop the treatments. He was generally seen every 4 to 6 weeks.

The following case from my colleague Bhavito Jansch in Switzerland illustrates how a simple supportive treatment approach can help a shy, anxious child become more confident and active.

Case 3
Ralf, Boy Age 11 Years

Main complaints: Ralf was a skinny young boy from a farming family close to my town. He was shy, anxious, and worried too much. He had problems in school and he ended up in a special school for learning impaired children. He was afraid of animals, humans, and new situations.

History: I treated two of his brothers for a couple of months before his mother asked me for help. Ralf was the oldest of four sons. He was supposed to be the leader of the whole gang, but he was not at all a leader type. He was born 5 weeks premature. He had a hole in the foramen of the heart. He had also had two operations for inguinal hernia. His ears were always blocked and he had some difficulty hearing well. He was always tired and needed a lot of sleep. His energy was especially low in the morning and very low in the afternoon. As a young child he vomited a lot after eating. Recently he has been having on–off pain in the testicles, for which the doctors could find no cause. He needs to rise at least once per night to urinate.

Assessment: The abdomen was slightly moist. The lower abdomen was more deficient than the upper. There were signs of swelling on the liver channel. His feet were cool, and overall his skin was somewhat thin. He also had a lot of tension in the neck and shoulders. His pulse was rapid, somewhat soft with some hardness in some positions, slightly floating. The kidney and liver were the weakest positions.

Diagnosis: He displayed liver vacuity pattern.

Treatment: Using a *teishin*, left LV-8, KI-10, and right SP-3 were supplemented. Left TB-4 was also supplemented. Right ST-40 was drained.
    Using an *enshin*, light stroking was applied on the arms, legs, abdomen, and back.
    Chinetsukyu was applied on GV-14, bilateral BL-23, and CV-4.

Second visit—7 days later

There was not much to report.

Treatment: Using a *teishin*, left LV-8, KI-10, and right SP-3 were supplemented. Left TB-4 was also supplemented. Right ST-40 was drained.
    Using an *enshin*, light stroking was applied on the arms, legs, abdomen, and back.
    Chinetsukyu was applied on GV-14, bilateral BL-23, and CV-4.
    A press-sphere was retained on GV-12.

Third visit—14 days later

The pulse and abdomen were more or less the same. Although Ralf felt okay his condition was not very different from before. His energy was more or less the same.

Treatment: Using a *teishin*, left LV-8, KI-10, and right ST-36 were supplemented. Left GB-37 and BL-58 were drained.
    Using a Yoneyama instrument, light tapping was applied on the arms, legs, abdomen, and back to give a higher dose of treatment.
    Chinetsukyu was applied on GV-14, bilateral BL-23, and CV-4.
    A press-sphere was retained on GV-12.

Fourth visit—7 days later

This time his mother gave positive feedback. In small things he became a bit more confident. His energy was a bit better, especially in the afternoon.

Treatment: Using a *teishin*, left LV-8, KI-10, and right ST-36 were supplemented. Left GB-37 and BL-58 were drained.
    Using a Yoneyama instrument, light tapping was applied on the arms, legs, abdomen, and back to give a higher dose of treatment.
    Chinetsukyu was applied on GV-14, bilateral BL-23, and CV-4.
    A press-sphere was retained on GV-12.

Fifth visit—28 days later

His energy and appetite were clearly better. He started to argue with his brothers once in a while. His mother wanted me to continue, and I changed the pattern toward a kidney vacuity pattern because of the cool feet.

Treatment: Using a *teishin*, left KI-7, LU-5, and right ST-36 were supplemented.
    Using a Yoneyama instrument, light tapping was applied on the arms, legs, abdomen, and back to give a higher dose of treatment.
    Chinetsukyu was applied on GV-14, bilateral BL-23, and CV-4.
    A press-sphere was retained on GV-12.
    The 6th to 10th treatments were given every 2 weeks and followed the same pattern. During this time his energy and appetite improved further. He even asked his father if he could drive the tractor once. His feet were no longer cool, and

he started asking me about what I was doing and how the instruments were used.

On the 11th treatment, again 14 days later, I added use of the extraordinary vessels, the *du-mai-yangqiaomai* "to give him a spine" (i.e., to boost his confidence).[1]

At the 12th treatment 14 days later, his energy was quite normal. His hearing had improved, and he no longer needed to rise at night to urinate. His mother told me proudly that he started to bring the cows alone to the pasture and showed no more fear for animals or humans. Besides treating the kidney pattern I applied the *dumai-yangqiao-mai* treatment again.

We finished treatment for the moment because Ralf requested to do so. For me it felt alright to stop here and see what time will bring to his young life. I was happy to have been able to help him through this state of anxiety and give him a chance to become a normal boy.

Posttraumatic Stress Disorder

This condition is one whereby the child exhibits a lot of stress-related signs following a physically or emotionally traumatic event. The problem is commonly chronic and can be somewhat debilitating. For example, the child may be very withdrawn, unable to actively participate in usual daily activities, have fear of going out of the house, and so on. In many respects one can approach treatment of a child with this history and problems in the same way that one does for the stressed child, but emotional issues and vulnerabilities can be much stronger and the dose issues more complicated, and generally one may need a longer course of treatment to help produce longer-lasting results. As a result of this it is better to start out with very low dose treatment approaches while you map out the patient's responses to what you do.

Case 1
Jared, Boy Age 10 Years

Main complaints: He is very fearful and anxious and is afraid to go out. He has daily abdominal pain before going to school.

---

[1]   This was done using zinc–copper pellets in the manner that Toyohari employs treatment of the extraordinary vessels (Fukushima 1991); see also the next footnote.

History: The problems of anxiety, fearfulness, and abdominal pains started 2 and a half years before following an episode where a man tried to abduct him on the street. He was able to avoid being abducted but was very distressed and has had problems of posttraumatic stress disorder since then. He could not go out of the house without being accompanied by his mother or brother and thus could not go to school. He had seen a psychologist many times who helped him reduce the fearfulness and anxiety so that he can go out and go to school, but he still has daily pain in the morning before going to school. He was no longer seeing the psychologist. He often used mild analgesic medicine, such as acetaminophen, for the abdominal pain to help him prepare to go to school. He also still has some difficulties with anxiety before going out to play with friends and especially staying over with friends. The problems at school also improved after he changed schools and now has a much more understanding teacher who he finds more supportive.

The sleep problems have been better since seeing the psychologist but had been a big problem even before the anxiety problems started.

When younger he had the respiratory syncytial (RS) virus and needed to be hospitalized and intubated for the bronchiolitis. At the time he was ill with this, his parents started divorce proceedings and his grandmother died, causing severe additional stresses for him.

He also had problems with pneumonia several times and needed a lot of antibiotics.

He has cow's milk allergy and avoids cow-milk products.

He had many problems with constipation when younger. He had to see the doctor many times because of accompanying abdominal pain. This has been better for the last few years.

He is also dyslexic, which affects his performance at school.

He tends to sweat easily.

Assessment: The history of RS virus and pneumonia and constipation suggest a probable lung vacuity–type constitution. The history of sleep problems suggests a liver and spleen involvement. The history of chronic stressful events and the more recent abduction episode, with current problems of anxiety and fearfulness, daily abdominal pain associated with worry, and easily sweating suggests posttraumatic stress disorder with sympathetic activation.

It will be necessary to ensure very careful regulation of treatment dose.

Abdominal findings: There is some stiffness to the left and right sides of the navel and in the right subcostal region.

Pulse: The lung and spleen pulses are weak, but the kidney pulse is also slightly weak. The pulse overall is a little weak, and the presence of repletion is difficult to detect.

Tentative diagnosis: All the various signs and symptoms taken together seem to indicate a lung vacuity pattern.

Treatment: To help with the strong psychological symptoms, treatment was applied to right LV-3 and HT-5. This symptomatic treatment was accomplished by placing a small copper plate on LV-3 and a zinc plate on HT-5. The appropriateness of this was confirmed by monitoring the pulses and having the pulse quality improve.[2] It was decided to do this first because there are no needles involved, thus eliminating the risk of fearful responses to treatment; because it tends to be relaxing for the patient; and because it changes the pulse quality, thus allowing me to reassess the pulse afterward to more confidently confirm the selection of lung vacuity pattern.[3]

Using a *teishin*, supplementation was applied carefully to left LU-9 and SP-3. Then draining techniques were carefully applied to right LV-8 and left BL-58 (based on pulse reassessment). The region of the supraclavicular fossa was then treated using the same *teishin* applying supplementation to one or two softer areas on each side.[4] Bilateral BL-13 and BL-20 were supplemented using the *teishin* to support the root treatment.

Press-tack needles (0.3 mm) were placed at GV-9 (which was very sensitive) and on the left ear behind *shen men*.

---

[2] This kind of treatment usage is part of the Toyohari *kikei* (extraordinary vessel) treatment system (Fukushima 1991). In Japan several schools of acupuncture have extended the eight treatment points of the extraordinary vessels to 12 so that all 12 channels can be targeted, not just the eight associated with the treatment points for the extraordinary vessels. The application of polarity agents for point combinations such as the extraordinary vessels is common in Japan (Matsumoto and Birch 1986; Manaka, Itaya, and Birch 1995).

[3] This kind of preroot treatment procedure is often done in Toyohari, not only to address symptoms but to clarify the pulse when it is difficult to read.

[4] This is part of what is called *naso* treatment in Toyohari (Birch and Ida 2001).

Second visit—7 days later

He was a bit more irritable for several days following the treatment, but his abdominal pain had been better.

Treatment: HT-5 and LV-3 were treated using copper on right HT-5 and zinc on right LV-3 (based on pulse responses).

Using a *teishin*, supplementation was applied carefully to left LU-9 and SP-3. Then draining techniques were carefully applied to right LV-8 and left BL-58 (based on pulse reassessment). The region of the supraclavicular fossa was then treated using the same *teishin*, applying supplementation to one or two softer areas on each side. Bilateral BL-13 and BL-20 were supplemented using the teishin to support the root treatment.

Press-tack needles (0.3 mm) were placed at GV-12 (which was more sensitive than GV-9 this week) and on the left ear behind *shen men*.

Third visit—7 days later

He had a mild rash on the face for several days following the treatment, but his abdominal pain had been better again, as was his anxiety.

Treatment: HT-5 and LV-3 were treated using copper on right LV-3 and zinc on right HT-5 (based on pulse responses).

Using a *teishin*, supplementation was applied carefully to left LU-9 and SP-3. Then draining techniques were carefully applied to right LV-8, left BL-58, and right GB-37 (based on pulse reassessment). The region of the supraclavicular fossa was then treated using the same *teishin* applying supplementation to one or two softer areas on each side. Bilateral BL-13 and BL-20 were supplemented using the *teishin* to support the root treatment.

Using 0.12 mm gauge needles, in and out needling was applied to bilateral GB-20.

Press-tack needles (0.3 mm) were placed at GV-9 and on the left ear behind *shen men*.

Fourth visit—7 days later

He has generally been feeling better with less abdominal pain and anxiety. He had injured his right ankle, which was still a bit painful when walking.

Treatment: HT-5 and LV-3 were treated using copper on right HT-5 and zinc on right LV-3 (based on pulse responses).

Using a *teishin*, supplementation was applied carefully to left LU-9 and SP-3. Then draining techniques were carefully applied to right LV-8, left BL-58, and right TB-5 (based on pulse reassessment). The region of the supraclavicular fossa was then treated using the same *teishin*, applying supplementation to one or two softer areas on each side. Bilateral BL-13 and BL-20 were supplemented using the *teishin* to support the root treatment.

Using 0.12 mm gauge needles, in and out needling was applied to bilateral GB-20 and right BL-57.

Press-tack needles (0.3 mm) were placed at GV-12 and on the left ear behind *shen men*.

Fifth visit—14 days later

His foot is okay now. He injured his right knee in sport play with his friends and has some pain associated with this, but he is not using any acetaminophen for the pain. He has generally been feeling better with less abdominal pain and anxiety, although the more stressful time before going to school is still the main period of anxiety for him.

Treatment: HT-5 and LV-3 were treated using copper on right HT-5 and zinc on left LV-3 (based on pulse responses).

Using a *teishin*, supplementation was applied carefully to left LU-9 and SP-3. Then draining techniques were carefully applied to right LV-3, left BL-58, and right TB-5 (based on pulse reassessment). The region of the supraclavicular fossa was then treated using the same *teishin*, applying supplementation to one or two softer areas on each side. Bilateral BL-13 and BL-20 were supplemented using the *teishin* to support the root treatment.

Using 0.12 mm gauge needles, in and out needling was applied to bilateral GB-20, GB-21, and the upper part of the interscapular region.

Press-tack needles (0.3 mm) were placed at GV-12 and on the left ear behind *shen men*.

Sixth visit—7 days later

He has been checking out new schools for the next academic year, which has made him very anxious.

He has thus had more abdominal pain this week and increased difficulty falling asleep. But aside from this he still generally feels better.

Treatment: Using 0.12 mm gauge needles, in and out needling was applied to bilateral LI-4, the back of the shoulders, and bilateral BL-17 and BL-18.

Using a *teishin*, supplementation was applied carefully to left LU-9 and SP-3. Then draining techniques were carefully applied to right LV-3 and left BL-58 (based on pulse reassessment). The region of the supraclavicular fossa was then treated using the same *teishin*, applying supplementation to one or two softer areas on each side. Bilateral BL-13 and BL-20 were supplemented using the *teishin* to support the root treatment.

Press-tack needles (0.3 mm) were placed at GV-12 and on the left ear behind *shen men*.

Seventh visit—7 days later

He has been much better this week, but he is still a little delayed in falling asleep.

Treatment: Using 0.12 mm gauge needles, in and out needling was applied to bilateral LI-4, the back of the shoulders, bilateral BL-17, BL-18, and BL-20.

Using a *teishin*, supplementation was applied carefully to left LU-9 and SP-3. Then draining techniques were carefully applied to right LV-3 and left BL-58 (based on pulse reassessment). The region of the supraclavicular fossa was then treated using the same *teishin*, applying supplementation to one or two softer areas on each side. Bilateral BL-13 and BL-20 were supplemented using the *teishin* to support the root treatment.

Needles (0.16 mm) were inserted and retained at bilateral GB-20.

Press-tack needles (0.3 mm) were placed at GV-9 and on the left ear behind *shen men*.

Eighth visit—15 days later

He had been very good for the first week, but then he had a bad cold that turned into stomach flu, triggering a lot more abdominal pain with disturbed bowel movements.

Treatment: Using 0.12 mm gauge needles, in and out needling was applied to bilateral LI-4, the back of the shoulders, bilateral BL-17, BL-18, and BL-20.

Using a *teishin*, supplementation was applied carefully to left LU-9 and SP-3. Then draining techniques were carefully applied to right LV-3, left SI-7, and left BL-58 (based on pulse reassessment). The region of the supraclavicular fossa was then treated using the same *teishin*, applying supplementation to one or two softer areas on each side. Bilateral BL-13 and BL-20 were supplemented using the *teishin* to support the root treatment.

Needles (0.16 mm) were inserted and retained at bilateral GB-20.

Press-tack needles (0.3 mm) were placed at GV-9 and on the left ear behind *shen men*.

Unfortunately he experienced 3 weeks of increased abdominal pain after the stomach flu, missing school for several days due to this. But he reported this abdominal pain would come and go during the day and night regardless of stress, school, and other factors. He also experienced poor bowel movements and abdominal bloating and discomfort during the same period, which also disturbed his sleep. During this time he was also still checking out new schools for the next academic term, which was somewhat stressful and worrying for him.

I treated him three times during this period where the principle difference in treatment was to focus on the acute digestive symptoms. For this as well as the regular root treatment I used retained needling at bilateral BL-17, BL-18, and BL-20 (the six flowers) with a heat lamp over the area and 0.6 mm press-tacks retained at reactive points, such as BL-18 and BL-20. After this period of disturbed intestinal function, he returned to the condition he was in before the onset of the stomach flu. He generally felt better and less anxious, with almost no morning abdominal pain.

I treated him three more times over the next month with similar treatments before the summer holidays. During this time he felt better, no problem going to school, almost no anxiety or fearfulness. With the last treatment he agreed to come back after the summer if he was worried, experiencing abdominal pain, anxiety, and other issues, but so far, 18 months later he has not returned for treatment.

Reflections: I think that a very gently applied, nonstimulating, and not uncomfortable treatment is better for helping regulate the autonomic nervous system when it is dysregulated, especially as I thought was happening with him, when there is increased sympathetic tone. Except for the period when he had a bad cold/stomach flu, he did well, improving better than I had hoped would be possible. It is of course possible to have used other techniques that are more stimulating and stronger, but with a child that has been so anxious and fearful, use of techniques like *okyu*, direct moxa, which can be quite effective for the acute digestive symptoms, can be very difficult and not at all well tolerated, but perhaps I erred too much on the side of caution and could have improved the digestive symptoms more quickly. My experience treating patients with posttraumatic stress disorder is that less is generally better and that it is better to be more cautious and much gentler in one's treatment approach.

Obsessive Compulsive Disorder (OCD)

We do not generally see many children with this kind of problem, partly I think because parents and doctors don't think of acupuncture for obsessive compulsive disorder (OCD) and will much more likely have pursued a pharmacological treatment approach, perhaps combined with psychotherapy. Thus, when patients do come to us with OCD they are likely to be taking medication for the problem. The use of pediatric acupuncture will come up if there are side effects from the medicine that the parents are concerned about, or if there are other symptoms not affected by the medication, or if the parents anticipate possible problems and would like to try an additional treatment as support and potentially as a preventive approach to try to offset potential side effects, given that patients often need to take the medication over extended periods of time. The following case from my colleague Dan Zizza in Seattle is a case in point. The patient had just started taking Effexor (Pfizer Inc.), a potent serotonin–norepinephrine reuptake inhibitor, which can have adverse effects over extended use,[5] and which is likely to have been a motivator for starting acupuncture treatment.

---

[5] See, for example, http://www.drugs.com/sfx/effexor-side-effects.html, and http://www.webmd.com/drugs/2/drug-4896/effexor-xr-oral/details/list-sideeffects.html.

Case 1
Ben, Boy Age 8 Years

Main complaints and history: Ben presented with multiple psychological and behavioral problems. His problems began to appear at age 7, one year prior to seeing me. His mother reported that he is the last of five children and that she suffered from postpartum depression following his birth.

His main symptoms involved having the feeling that he always *had* to do things in a certain way or he would get upset. He had repeated behaviors, such as going up and down steps or sitting down and standing up in a particular way. He would repeat rhyming words in his head over and over. This word repetition in his head he found the most disturbing. He had a head movement tic of tucking his chin toward his shoulders two times each side. He could hold grudges and become very oppositional and argumentative. He was very set in his ways, and he got very upset with distractions. He was also very conscientious, caring, affectionate, and a deep thinker.

He was always afraid of looking stupid in school, and he worked hard at schoolwork. Having a very strict teacher during that particular school year made these symptoms worsen and come to the forefront. Later that year his mother pulled him out of that school.

He was given a Western psychiatric diagnosis of obsessive compulsive disorder (OCD) and put on 37.5 mg of Effexor 1 week prior to his first visit with me.

He had some difficulty falling asleep, and he could have his sleep disturbed by noises in the house. His appetite was generally good, and he didn't complain of any problems with digestion.

Appearance: Ben's skin was pale with poor luster. He had a darkened appearance around the eyes. His build was muscular and solid, and he was of average height for his age. He avoided eye contact, mostly looking down to the floor. He spoke with a soft voice and halting speech.

Examination: Ben's abdomen felt rough with poor luster overall, and was particularly puffy under the navel. His kidney and lung channels felt rough and weak upon palpation. His pulse was sinking, of moderate rate, and weak. The kidney and lung pulse positions felt the weakest, and there was a hardness deep in the spleen position.

Diagnosis: I diagnosed him as having kidney vacuity with spleen repletion pattern.

Treatment: Using a *teishin*, supplementation was applied to left KI-10 and LU-5 points, with draining needling technique to right SP-9, right LI-6, and left BL-58.

Using an *enshin*, light stroking was then applied to the kidney, lung, spleen, stomach, large intestine, and bladder channels on the arms and legs.

Using the *Yoneyama zanshin*, a light scraping was applied over the scalp followed by light tapping around the occiput, down the neck, trapezius region, and down the upper back.

Using the *teishin*, treatment was also applied to GV-12, BL-15, BL-21, BL-23, and *josen* on the back and CV-4 on the abdomen.

Press-spheres were placed and retained on GV-12 and GV-3.

Second visit—5 days later

Ben did well with the first treatment, reporting that he liked it and felt calmer immediately after the treatment.

Treatment: Using a *teishin*, supplementation was applied to left KI-10 and LU-5 points, with draining needling technique to right SP-9 and left GB-37.

Using an *enshin*, light stroking was then applied with the flow of the kidney and lung channels and against the flow of the spleen and gallbladder channels. Light stroking was also applied on the abdomen and back.

Using the *Yoneyama zanshin*, a light scraping was applied over the scalp followed by light tapping around the occiput, down the neck, trapezius region, and down the upper back.

Using the *teishin*, treatment was also applied to GV-12, CV-4, GV-3, and left ST-12.

Third visit—6 days later

Ben reported that he was doing very well, feeling happy and calmer inside.

Treatment: Using a *teishin*, supplementation was applied to left KI-10 and LU-5 points, with draining needling technique to right SP-9, left LI-6, and right ST-40.

Using an *enshin*, light stroking was then applied to the kidney, lung, spleen, stomach, and large intestine channels on the arms and legs.

Using the *Yoneyama zanshin*, a light tapping was applied over the scalp, around the occiput, upper back, BL-12, and GV-12.

Using the *teishin*, treatment was also applied to BL-23, the sacral region, and CV-4.

Additionally, I included the extraordinary vessel treatment of *yin wei–chong* mai by placing a copper disc on the right SP-4 and a zinc disc on the left PC-6 for about half a minute.[6]

Fourth visit—eight days later

Ben reported continuing to do well, feeling happy and only occasionally repeating words in his head anymore, only doing so out of boredom when he had to sit in the car for longer periods of time.

Treatment: Using a *teishin*, supplementation was applied to left KI-10 and LU-5 points, with draining needling technique to right SP-9, left GB-37.

Using an *enshin*, light stroking was then applied to the kidney, lung, spleen, stomach, and large intestine channels on the arms and legs.

Using the *Yoneyama zanshin*, a light tapping was applied over the scalp, around the occiput, upper back, BL-12, and GV-12.

Using the *teishin*, treatment was also applied to BL-23, the sacral region, and CV-4.

Additionally, I included the extraordinary vessel treatment of *yin wei–chong mai* by placing a copper disc on the right SP-4 and a zinc disc on the left PC-6 for about half a minute.

Fifth visit—19 days later

All OCD-like symptoms have ceased. The repeating rhyming words, his particular way of sitting and standing up, and the head movement tic have all stopped occurring since Ben's last treatment. Ben's pulses felt far more balanced, and the quality was more like what would be expected in a boy of his age, floating,

a little rapid, and with good strength and vitality. His root pattern shifted to kidney vacuity with spleen vacuity.

Treatment: Using a *teishin*, supplementation was applied to left KI-10, LU-5, and right SP-3. Using an *enshin*, light stroking was then applied to the kidney, lung, and spleen channels on the arms and legs. Stroking was also applied on the bladder channels on the back and legs.

Using the *Yoneyama zanshin*, a light scraping was applied along the large intestine and gallbladder channels with light tapping around the occiput, upper back, and GV-12.

Using the *teishin*, treatment was also applied to BL-23, the sacral region, and CV-4.

Sixth visit—60 days later

I didn't hear from Ben or his mother for another 2 months. After 60 days his mother called to say that Ben had developed a new tic of opening his eyes wide and looking up to the left repeatedly. No other repeated behaviors were reported. The new tic was attributed to a new stressful event in Ben's life, and to his tendency to be a perfectionist. Abdominal and pulse findings revealed a different pattern, lung with liver vacuity pattern.

Treatment: Using a *teishin*, supplementation was applied to left LU-9, SP-3, and right LV-3. Draining technique was applied to left BL-58.

Using an *enshin*, stroking was applied along the lung and spleen channels.

Using the *Yoneyama zanshin*, light tapping was applied over the large intestine, stomach, and bladder channels.

Using a *teishin*, a light stroking method (*sanshin*) was applied over the scalp, face, GB-20, and BL-10 areas, with further tapping with the *Yoneyama zanshin* to the upper back, to GV-12, and down the back to *josen*.

The *enshin* was used to rub over rough skin on the abdomen in the right subcostal area, and CV-4 was supplemented.

The extraordinary vessel pair of *yang wei–dai mai* was applied with a copper disc to left GB-41 and a zinc disc to left TW-5. These were retained for only a few seconds.

---

[6] This is in the Toyohari style of extraordinary vessel treatments. Dan is both practitioner and instructor of Toyohari.

Seventh visit—2 days later

He was feeling better, but the nervous eye tic continued.

Treatment: Using a *teishin*, supplementation was applied to left LU-9, SP-3, and right LV-8, KI-10. Draining technique was applied to left BL-58.

Using an *enshin*, stroking was applied along the lung and spleen channels.

Using the *Yoneyama zanshin*, light tapping was applied over the large intestine, stomach, and bladder channels.

Using a *teishin*, a light stroking method (*sanshin*) was applied over the scalp, face, GB-20, and BL-10 areas, with further tapping with the *Yoneyama zanshin* to the upper back, to GV-12, and down the back to *josen.*

The *enshin* was used to rub over rough skin on the abdomen in the right subcostal area, and CV-4 was supplemented.

The extraordinary vessel pair of *yang wei–dai mai* was applied with a copper disc to left GB-41 and a zinc disc to left TW-5. These were retained for only a few seconds.

Press-spheres were placed at GV-12 and GV-3.

Eighth visit—7 days later

Ben felt a lot better after the last treatment, and the eye tic had completely stopped.

Treatment: Using a *teishin*, supplementation was applied to left LU-9, SP-3, and right LV-8. Draining technique was applied to left BL-58.

Using an *enshin*, stroking was applied along the lung and spleen channels.

Using the *Yoneyama zanshin*, light tapping was applied over the large intestine, stomach, and bladder channels.

Using a *teishin*, a light stroking method (*sanshin*) was applied over the scalp, face, GB-20, and BL-10 areas, with further tapping with the *Yoneyama zanshin* to the upper back, to GV-12, and down the back to *josen.*

The *enshin* was used to rub over rough skin on the abdomen in the right subcostal area, and CV-4 was supplemented.

Ninth visit—31 days later

The eye tic did not return, and no OCD-like behaviors occurred. A treatment similar to the one given on the eighth visit was used.

I did not see Ben again for treatment for another year and a half. His psychological and behavioral problems never recurred, although he still tended to be a perfectionist, and he would become overwhelmed with school stresses at times. His chief complaints after this point were related to seasonal allergies, headaches, athletic injuries, and food sensitivities. He did continue on the Effexor for another few years, and I don't know of any further psychiatric evaluations other than to suggest he stay on the Effexor primarily because he would feel the effects of stressors in his life so acutely even though his OCD-like symptoms were resolved.

Anxiety—Fearfulness

The following case is from my colleague Paul Movsessian who lives in the Blue Mountains outside Sydney, Australia. It is probable that the combination of the basic *shonishin* treatment with Bach flower remedies produced such a dramatic change in Nellie's symptoms.

Case 1
Nellie, Girl Aged 6 Years

Main complaints: She had oversensitive fear reflexes.

History: The cause appears to be birth trauma. Her mother worked while pregnant right up to delivery. She had suffered severe reflux throughout pregnancy. She had planned to have a water birth and started in the water. Contractions and dilation came on quickly, the baby got her right shoulder stuck during delivery, and the mother had to leave the water and be taken into the emergency room. Once delivered Nellie needed oxygen. At 1 month old she had been a very unsettled baby and went to a cranio-osteopath that found her sphenoid bone was shifted, and she was treated using craniosacral osteopathy. She was also born with a birth rash that lasted

1 and a half years. At age 2 she had a severe urinary tract infection and needed strong antibiotics. She does not take any prescribed medications, but her mother gives her a variety of Australian bush flower essences and tissue salts. She is using minerals, essential fatty acids (EFA), and vitamin supplements. She has tried occupational therapy, retained primitive reflex kinesiology, Brain Gym (Brain Gym International), and the vega testing method. Everything has helped to a degree but nothing has held and she seems to be getting worse.

She shows many fear reflexes and is hypersensitive to smells, sounds, and touch. She exhibits hypervigilance leading to insecurity, anxiety, and breathing difficulties. She exhibits poor adaptability to change. She is clinging and crying when having to go to school or under different circumstances at school with interactions between her and other children or teachers. She shows insecurity and anxiety reactions when exposed to new people or new circumstances. She also has problems with frontal headaches, hearing problems, and aches and pains in her wrists and ankles, but she sleeps well. Her condition is affecting her learning at school and her general home and social life. Two years ago her mother had to go overseas for 6 weeks and leave her behind, and this seemed to have had a worsening effect on the situation.

Appearance: She is quite small but with a strong-looking body. Her color is reddish. She is anxious and quiet. Her eyes are open wide in an alert state, constantly looking at her mother for reassurance.

She shows somewhat heavy, labored breathing. There is no detectable odor. Her voice is sing-song like, and strong. Her skin is cold overall with good luster.

Treatment: Using the *Yoneyama zanshin* for tapping and an *enshin* for stroking a combination of light tapping and light stroking was applied down the arms, legs, abdomen, back, and neck over a period of ~2 minutes.

Points on the upper spine that show light reaction to touch are used for psychosomatic disorders (Fukaya 1982), the following showed reaction and one *okyu* rice grain size moxa was applied each to GV-14, GV-12, GV-11, GV-10, and GV-9.

Press-spheres were applied to the auricular points point zero and *shen men* bilaterally. The mother was instructed to retain them for 1 day and then remove them.

Finally, since the mother had been using Australian bush flower essences I made a home recommendation for a Bach flower combination of rock rose and walnut or aspen and mimulus, depending on how she responded. Starting with the first combination and using two drops twice a day.

We ended the treatment here with the child looking a bit more relaxed and the mother feeling hopeful.

Second visit—8 days later

Her mother reported a tremendous shift in her response. Nellie was much more joyful and relaxed. There were no tears when leaving her to go to school. It was a very good week with big improvements.

Treatment: Using the *Yoneyama zanshin* for tapping and an *enshin* for stroking a combination of light tapping and light stroking was applied down the arms, legs, abdomen, back, and neck over a period of ~2 minutes.

One *okyu* rice grain size moxa was applied each to GV-14, GV-12, GV-11, GV-10, and between GV-12 and GV-11.

Press-spheres were applied to the auricular points point zero and *shen men* bilaterally. The mother was instructed to retain them for 1 day and then remove them.

Third visit—7 days later

Nellie had another good week. Her mother had been able to take her to school without any clinging or crying or even needing support from the teachers. She was much happier and coming out of that fear state but starting to be a bit more defiant in her behavior, which was very unlike her. I decided to now start treating with the Meridian Therapy pattern-based root treatment approach. The pulse and abdomen findings confirmed a lung vacuity with liver repletion pattern.

Treatment: Using a *teishin*, right LU-9 and SP-3 were supplemented, which also settled the liver pulse.

Using an *inrishin*, light tapping and light stroking were applied down the arms, legs, abdomen, back, and neck.

One *okyu* rice grain size moxa was applied each to GV-12, GV-11, and between these two points, and to CV-12 and CV-6.

Fourth visit—6 days later

Nellie was pretty much the same. She was doing very well and was also less defiant. The teachers made comments about the change in her behavior. Today she has a bit of an upset stomach. The pattern-based treatment shifted to the spleen vacuity pattern.

Treatment: Using a *teishin*, right SP-3 and PC-7 were supplemented.

Using an *inrishin*, light draining techniques were applied to right ST-40 and left GB-37.

Using an *enshin*, light stroking was applied down the arms, legs, abdomen, back, and neck.

One *okyu* rice grain size moxa was applied each to GV-12, GV-11, and between these two points, and three times to CV-12.

Fifth visit—7 days later

Her mother reported that everything is continuing to improve. Her gut was fine the same afternoon of the treatment. Her daughter is feeling very comfortable in her body and able to take more risks without fear or anxiety.

Treatment: Using the *Yoneyama zanshin*, light tapping was applied around the occiput.

Using an *enshin*, light stroking was applied down the arms, legs, abdomen, back, and neck.

One *okyu* rice grain size moxa was applied to GV-12, GV-11, and between these two points, one time per point. *Okyu* was also applied three times to CV-12.

Sixth visit—15 days later

Her mother reported that everything has improved and cleared up, and all that seems to remain is the inability to get a deep breath.

Treatment: Using the *Yoneyama zanshin*, light tapping was applied around the occiput.

Using an *enshin*, light stroking was applied down the arms, legs, abdomen, back, and neck.

One *okyu* rice grain size moxa was applied each to GV-12, GV-11, and between these two points, and three times to LU-4 and CV-6.

Seventh visit—56 days later

Nellie has been doing very well. The treatment effects have been sustained, and teachers reported at school that it is like she is a completely new girl. She is less fearful and clingy. Since the last treatment she has had the flu with 1 day of fever, but she recovered very quickly.

Treatment: Using the *Yoneyama zanshin*, light tapping was applied around the occiput.

Using an *enshin*, light stroking was applied down the arms, legs, abdomen, back, and neck.

One *okyu* rice grain size moxa was applied each to GV-14, GV-13, GV-12, and between GV-12 and GV-11.

Treatment finished by using a *teishin*, to supplement CV-12, KD-16 bilateral, and CV-6.

Eighth visit—49 days later

During October she went camping with her father, and there was a tremendous thunder and lightning storm that triggered her fear reflexes. Up until this time she had been completely fine. At present the fear remains but she has not reverted to the clinging behavior.

Treatment: Using the *Yoneyama zanshin*, light tapping was applied around the occiput and GV-20.

Using an *enshin*, light stroking was applied down the arms, legs, abdomen, back, and neck.

One *okyu* rice grain size moxa was applied each to GV-14, GV-13, GV-12, GV-11, and between GV-12 and GV-11, and additionally for shock to BL-23.

Treatment finished by using a *teishin* to supplement CV-12, KD-16 bilateral, and CV-6.

Ninth visit—35 days later

After the last treatment all her fear reflexes settled again, and she is once more doing very well. She exhibits only a small amount of anxiety; otherwise she is feeling much better.

Treatment: Using an *enshin*, light stroking was applied over right KI-7 and LU-8 (to supplement the kidney), and then down the arms, legs, abdomen, back, and neck.

Turning her over, a mild warming massage was applied over UB-23 and UB-52 bilaterally.[7]

Using the *enshin* again, light stroking was applied to ST-36, ST-37, and ST-39 to strengthen the stomach, large and small intestine via the lower he-sea points, and then to CV-12 and LU-1–LU-2 area.

Treatment was finished by using an *enshin* to apply light stroking over the supraclavicular region to complete the treatment.

Further Emotional/Behavioral Problems

Yoneyama and Mori (1964) discuss treatment of night terrors and a condition called "allotriophagy."

Night Terrors
This is generally seen in children from age 2 years upward to when they start school, and is seen especially in children who show the *kanmushisho* pattern. The child will suddenly show very strange behavior at night (without waking up, and with no recollection of it). This behavior can last up to 15 minutes, and can be seen several nights in a row.

To treat, apply the same *shonishin* core non-pattern-based root treatment as for *kanmushisho*. However, since the child is generally a little older, it is usually good to add thin, shallowly inserted needles to points such as BL-10, GB-20, and BL-11. If the symptoms are stronger (and more stubborn), add points such as LI-2, LU-11, and SP-1 as well. (A less painful method of stimulating points such as SP-1 or LU-11 is to apply pressure to them with a *teishin* or, if your technique is good, to apply low-dose bloodletting to them.)

Allotriophagy
This is a disorder characterized by pathological interest in and efforts to swallow anything that comes to hand, and is therefore categorized as an emotionally unstable condition.

The *shonishin* core non-pattern-based root treatment as described under *kanmushisho* is generally sufficient for this disorder, especially for acute or recent episodes. However, if this problem is caused by extreme hunger resulting from the presence of some intestinal parasite, such as a worm, it is necessary to eliminate the worm as well.

---

[7]   This was applied using the Thermie Tiger Warmer (Austin Medical Equipment, Inc.).

22 Urinary Disturbances

This chapter includes not only the more common problem of bed-wetting but also a case study of the less common problem of the child who loses control during the day as well.

Case 1
Simon, Boy Age 10 Years

Main complaints: Bed-wetting, which always occurred after 5 a.m. at a frequency of about three times a week. The problem had been intermittent for years, with no more than 6 months' remission at a time.

History and other problems: Simon was asthmatic. Since age 4 he had taken medication for the asthma. He was using the weakest kind of steroid inhaler twice every day. He had never been hospitalized for the asthma. Since infancy he had had severe problems with eczema. At age 5 he received acupuncture for ~18 months, which helped the eczema considerably, but the problem persisted, especially on the hands. He had clear food allergies causing the asthma and/or the eczema to flare up. For example, he would have very severe asthma attacks after eating foods containing certain food dyes. He avoided cow's milk products and was in general very careful about what he ate. He had problems with seasonal allergies, such as hay fever. The previous year, for example, it had been particularly bad, with severe irritation of the nose and ala nasi. These allergies could irritate the asthma. As a small child he was never able to sweat. Then by about age 5 he was able to sweat a little in a few places, such as the head and face. But he still did not sweat normally like other children. Other systems were good. Appetite, sleep, bowel movements, and energy were generally good. He was on his school soccer team. He had mood swings. He always had cold feet. Occasionally he suffered mild stomach pain. He occasionally had frontal headaches.

Assessment: Simon's facial complexion was off-white, with dark sunken eyes (kidney sign). The luster of his skin, especially around his eyes, was not so good. His posture was not very good; he had sloping shoulders (lung sign). Over the whole abdomen the skin was rough. There was some tightness in the subcostal region. The skin on the upper back was soft and empty. The muscles on the lower back were a little tight. The lung, spleen, liver, and kidney pulses were all weak.

Diagnosis: In this case the signs and symptoms supported several possibilities. It was decided to start with a lung vacuity pattern and see how he responded to this treatment.

Treatment: A silver needle was used to supplement left LU-9, SP-3, and right LR-3, KI-3, drain left BL-58, and supplement bilateral TB-4.[1]

Sanshin[2]/contact needling was applied over the area of ST-12[3] bilaterally.

Bilateral BL-13 and BL-20 were supplemented.

Tapping was applied with a *herabari* over the back of the head and neck.

Chinetsukyu/warm moxa was applied around GV-14, BL-13, GV-3, and BL-25.

Press-spheres were applied to GV-4 and CV-4.

---

[1] On older children we try, if possible, to use techniques that we might use on adults, but modified slightly to make them easier to accept by children. On smaller children it is normal to use the *teishin* for the pattern-based root treatment. However, on most adults the use of a silver needle is more normal in Toyohari-style Meridian Therapy. The use of the silver needle instead of the *teishin* increases the treatment dose. I have not described this needling technique in the book because it is not possible to learn it without taking at least a 1-year specialized training program, and it is not taught outside that program.

[2] *Sanshin*, contact needling, is similar to the treatment methods using tapping and stroking, but instead of using special tools to apply the method, one uses a regular needle. It is held at the skin surface for short periods or moved quickly over the skin surface. It is a technique used on adults by many traditional acupuncturists in Japan. Because the patient was 10 years old, it was selected as suitable for him. If he had been younger, supplementation with a *teishin* could have been used instead.

[3] Treatment of this area is a specialized Toyohari method called *naso* (Birch and Ida 2001; Yanagishita 2001a).

Second visit—6 days later

The skin seemed a little better, the healing time a little shorter. With regard to the asthma, he had a more productive cough. He had had one incidence of bed-wetting. He also had an increased appetite this week but was very tired on the day of the treatment. It was now much clearer that the primary pattern to focus on was a kidney vacuity pattern. The third deep left (kidney) and first deep right (lung) pulses were the weakest pulses, and there was a little more softness on the abdomen in the lower portions below the navel.

Treatment: A silver needle was used to supplement CV-12, left KI-7, and LU-5, drain right SP-5, TB-5, and left BL-58.

The *sanshin*/contact needle technique was applied over the inguinal/lateral abdomen region, ST-12 region, and to left BL-10.

Bilateral BL-13, BL-23, and around GV-6 were supplemented.

Chinetsukyu[4]/warm moxa was applied to GV-14, GV-3, and bilateral BL-23.

Press-spheres were applied to bilateral BL-23 and bilateral asthma *shu* points.

Third visit—8 days later

The skin had improved further. His emotional state was more stable. There were some asthma symptoms, but they were milder than usual. He had had three episodes of bed-wetting. His mother speculated that, because he had more energy than usual, he was much more active; consequently he was exhausted at the end of the day, sleeping more deeply than usual, and this could have contributed to the increase in bed-wetting.

Treatment: A silver needle was used to supplement CV-12, left KI-7, and LU-5, drain right SP-3, TB-5, and left BL-58.

The *sanshin*/contact needle technique was applied over the inguinal/lateral abdomen region,

---

[4] This is another technique used within the Toyohari treatment approach. Although the *chinetsukyu* method where heat is clearly felt is used more generally in Japan, its use with almost no sensations of heat is more specific to the Toyohari system as a general form of supplementation (Birch and Ida 1998, pp. 133–137).

ST-12 region, and to left BL-10.

Bilateral BL-13, BL-23, and around GV-6, GV-8 were supplemented.

Chinetsukyu/warm moxa was applied to GV-14, GV-3, and bilateral BL-23.

Press-spheres were applied to bilateral BL-23, asthma *shu* points, and CV-4.

Yin tang was supplemented using the silver needle.

Fourth visit—1 week later

The asthma symptoms were better. There had been no incidents of bed-wetting. He had more energy, but with more balanced behavior, and so was not as exhausted at night. His appetite was good.

Treatment: A silver needle was used to supplement CV-12, left KI-7, and LU-5, drain right SP-5, TB-5, and ST-40.

The *sanshin*/contact needle technique was applied over the inguinal/lateral abdomen region and the ST-12 region.

Bilateral BL-13, BL-23, and around GV-5, GV-6 were supplemented.

Chinetsukyu/warm moxa was applied to GV-14, GV-3, and bilateral BL-23.

Press-spheres were applied to bilateral BL-23 and bilateral asthma *shu* points and CV-4.

Fifth visit—1 week later

He was in a soccer game, which his team won, and he was the man of the match. In celebration he ate some candy with the wrong food dye in it and suffered a very severe asthma attack, which was not responsive to the normal inhaler treatment. This also triggered incidents of bed-wetting. Prior to this he had been doing very well. Since the start of the attack the bed-wetting had slowly subsided, and he was almost back to his usual state. His energy levels were slightly lower, his skin was better, and he was also beginning to show some of his seasonal allergies (hay fever).

Treatment: A silver needle was used to supplement CV-12, left KI-7, and LU-5, drain right SP-5, LI-6, and left GB-37.

The *sanshi*/contact needle technique was applied over the ST-12 region.

Tapping with a *herabari* was applied over the upper back.

Bilateral BL-13, BL-23, and around GV4, GV-6 were supplemented.

Chinetsukyu/warm moxa was applied to GV-14, GV-3, and bilateral BL-23.

Press-spheres were applied to bilateral BL-23 and CV-4.

Intradermal needles were placed to the asthma *shu* points (with instructions to remove them after 2 days and replace them with press-spheres).

Sixth visit—6 days later

He was doing much better, both physically and mentally, and his energy levels were good. He was a little wheezy, but generally his asthma symptoms seemed better, and he had forgotten to take his inhaler medicine that day (something he did not generally do).

Treatment: A silver needle was used to supplement CV-12, left KI-7, and LU-8, drain right SP-5, TB-5, and left BL-58.

The *sanshin*/contact needle technique was applied over the upper back and ST-12 region.

Bilateral BL-13, BL-23, and around GV-6 were supplemented.

Chinetsukyu/warm moxa was applied to GV-14, GV-3, and bilateral BL-23.

Press-spheres were applied to bilateral BL-23 and CV-6.

Intradermal needles were placed to the asthma *shu* points (with instructions to remove them after 2 days and replace them with press-spheres).

Seventh visit—8 days later

He was doing very well. He had forgotten to take his inhaler medicine several times, with no symptoms. He was a little wheezy at the time of treatment. He had had one small incident of bed-wetting, during which he woke up.

Treatment: A silver needle was used to supplement CV-12, left KI-7, and LU-8, drain right SP-5, TB-5, and ST-40.

The *sanshin*/contact needle technique was applied over the upper back and ST-12 region.

Bilateral BL-13, BL-23 were supplemented.

Chinetsukyu/warm moxa was applied to GV-14, GV-3, and bilateral BL-23.

Press-spheres were applied to bilateral BL-23 and CV-6.

Intradermal needles were placed to the asthma *shu* points (with instructions to remove them after 2 days and replace them with press-spheres).

Left KI-7 was supplemented again.

Eighth visit—1 week later

He had had a very good week with one very short-lived asthma attack. He had again forgotten to take his inhaler medicine several times this week. His mother noticed that his gait was better and his torso looser; he seemed to be walking more evenly. He also reported that when he played soccer or played with his friends he was now sweating in areas he had never been able to sweat before.

Treatment: A silver needle was used to supplement CV-12, left KI-7, and LU-5, drain right SP-3, TB-5, left BL-58, and GB-37.

The *sanshin*/contact needle technique was applied over the ST-12 region.

Using silver spike point (SSP) surface electrodes, ion-pumping cords were briefly applied bilaterally to PC-6 (black) and SP-4 (red).[5]

Bilateral BL-13, BL-23, and around GV-6 were supplemented.

Chinetsukyu/warm moxa was applied to GV-14, GV-3, and bilateral BL-23.

Press-spheres were applied to bilateral BL-23 and CV-4.

Intradermal needles were placed to the asthma *shu* points (with instructions to remove them after 2 days and replace them with press-spheres).

Ninth visit—1 week later

His mother noticed that he was having virtually no seasonal allergy or hay fever symptoms, and that, although he had very mild asthma symptoms in the morning on waking, they

---

[5]   For use of the "ion-pumping (IP) cords" see Manaka, Itaya, and Birch (1995). The IP cords are wires with a diode in each so as to create a polarity effect within the wire.

were much better then before for this time of year (mid-May). His facial complexion was now much better too. He had clear luster around the eyes. The dark sunken appearance of his eyes had been replaced by a vaguely dark ring around the eyes.

Treatment: Using SSP surface electrodes, ion-pumping cords were briefly applied to right PC-6 (black) and left SP-4 (red), with right KI-6 (black) and left LU-7 red.

A silver needle was used to supplement CV-12, left KI-7, and LU-8, drain right SP-3, TB-5, left BL-58, and GB-37.

The *sanshin*/contact needle technique was applied over the ST-12 region.

Stroking down the back was applied with an *enshin*.

Bilateral BL-13, BL-23 were supplemented.

Press-spheres were applied to bilateral BL-23 and CV-5.

Intradermal needles were placed to the asthma *shu* points (with instructions to remove them after 2 days and replace them with press-spheres).

Left KI-7 was supplemented again.

Tenth visit—2 weeks later

He had had a very good week with no asthma symptoms at all. He was using the inhaler at less than 50% of the normal dose. He had no seasonal allergy symptoms, which had not occurred before at this time of year.

Treatment: Using SSP surface electrodes, ion-pumping cords were briefly applied to right PC-6 (black) and left SP-4 (red), with right KI-6 (black) and left LU-7 (red).

A silver needle was used to supplement left KI-7 and LU-8, drain right SP-3, and left BL-58, SI-7.

The *sanshin*/contact needle technique was applied over the ST-12 region.

Light stroking was applied down the back with an *enshin*.

Bilateral BL-13, BL-23 were supplemented.

Press-spheres were applied to bilateral BL-23 and CV-4.

Intradermal needles were placed to the asthma *shu* points (with instructions to remove them after 2 days and replace them with press-spheres).

CV-12 was supplemented again.

Eleventh visit—2 weeks later

He had had almost no asthma symptoms, only very mild wheezing on waking in the morning. He was taking the inhaler medicine about three or four times per week rather than twice a day. He had virtually no allergy symptoms. He had not had a problem with bed-wetting for several weeks now. He also reported that the extent of areas that were now sweating normally on active exertion had increased again.

Treatment: Using SSP surface electrodes, ion-pumping cords were briefly applied to right PC-6 (black) and left SP-4 (red), with right KI-6 (black) and left LU-7 (red).

A silver needle was used to supplement CV-12, left KI-7, LU-8, and right SP-3, drain right TB-5, ST-40, and left BL-58.

The *sanshin*/contact needle technique was applied over the ST-12 region.

Light stroking was applied down the back with an *enshin*.

Bilateral BL-13, BL-23, and around GV-4 were supplemented.

Press-spheres were applied to bilateral BL-23 and CV-4.

Intradermal needles were placed to the asthma *shu* points (with instructions to remove them after 2 days and replace them with press-spheres).

The patient discontinued treatment at this time because the family was moving out of town and it would not be possible to continue treatment.

Reflection: Although this case is listed under "bed-wetting," the patient clearly had a more complex condition. The history of allergic constitution with asthma, food allergy components, and eczema makes this a complicated case. Most likely he started with a lung vacuity pattern constitution, but the protracted use of steroids for his lung problems gradually weakened the kidney, so that he showed a kidney vacuity pattern, which eventually gave rise to the bed-wetting symptoms. As a 10-year-old boy it was possible to apply more treatment than on a younger child and also to treat him in a similar manner to an adult (the use of a silver needle rather than a *teishin*). The complexity of his condition and history of eczema made me hesitate to teach home treatment to the parents. I decided to wait and see how he

(1964) state that the best results are obtained with deeper insertion to the acupoint GV-1, but that this is difficult to do, so they suggest alternative points, such as CV-3, ST-28 on the abdomen and BL-25, BL-32 on the back.

Shimizu (1975) has a more detailed discussion of treatment with needling for this problem.

For younger children (below age 6) after applying the core non-pattern-based root treatment one can insert needles to acupoints such as CV-3, BL-32, LR-8 or LR-1, GV-20, and GV-12.

For the school-age child (age 6 and older) insert needles to the following acupoints: CV-12, KI-10, CV-3, KI-12, *josen* (extra point between L5 and SI),[6] BL-32, GV-2, BL-23, BL-18, GV-20, GV-12, LU-7, LR-8, or LR-1.

Hyodo (1986) recommends the following acupoints to be needled or have press-spheres placed on them: GV-1, BL-25, BL-32, CV-3.

Selection of which acupoints to needle is based as usual on palpation; select those that show more reaction on palpation (a knot, stiffness, discomfort, pressure pain).

Okyu—Direct Moxa

Similar to what we find with the recommendations for needling, we see several different recommendations by different authors over how and where to apply *okyu* for bed-wetting.

Yoneyama and Mori (1964) suggest that *okyu* can be applied instead of needling to the same points that can be needled: CV-3, ST-28, BL-25, and BL-32.

Shimizu (1975) recommends that, on school-age children (age 6 and older), moxa should be applied to some of the following acupoints in addition to the needling of the other points: GV-20, GV-12, CV-3, KI-12, BL-32, and LR-1, using five half rice grain cones on each. Do not apply moxa to the same points that have been needled; one has to select which technique to use on those points if they are reactive.

Irie (1980) recommends the following points for treatment with moxa: CV-3, GV-12, and an extra point, the "moving LR-1 point"—palpate between LR-1 and LR-2, treat the more reactive point (one to five moxa each).

Manaka (Manaka, Itaya, and Birch 1995) recommends using moxa on the following acupoints after applying the core non-pattern-based root: GV-12, BL-32, CV-4, and KI-7.

The extra point, "moving LR-1," is treated with moxa if a reaction is found. Generally this will be a better target than the LR-1 mentioned by Shimizu. This is a difficult area to needle, but *okyu* here is easier to apply provided you do not let the moxa become too hot.

Sometimes it is helpful to apply heat over the lower abdomen and/or lower back. In Asia, moxa poles are recommended for this. It depends on your preferences and which tools are available to you as to what you recommend the parent apply at home. The moxa pole can become very hot quite quickly, so you need to explain carefully how to use it so that no one is accidentally burned by it. It is also possible to use lit incense sticks instead of the moxa pole to warm the areas around the selected acupoints. Thicker incense sticks are better for this. Typical targets for such treatment include any cool regions on the lower abdomen, the lower back, and the reactive points on the lower abdomen or lower back.

Integrating the Pattern-based and Core Non-pattern-based Root Treatments with Needling and Moxa Symptomatic Treatments

I would like to suggest a basic approach that can help process and integrate the information from the various authors whose works I have cited. This will give you a more integrated and flexible approach. The different authors cited above have helped us understand which acupoints typically show reactions when the child has a problem with night urination, and thus can be treated for the problem. We need a strategic approach for choosing among these acupoints and deciding what techniques to apply to them, and a way of doing this systematically. Some of the acupoints that show reaction are typically used in the pattern-based root treatment (e.g., LR-8, KI-10, KI-7) and thus can be given double duty. Some of the points are not feasible for needling, such as GV-1

---

[6]   *Josen* is better treated with an intradermal needle or press-tack needle rather than by simple needling.

and LR-1. Some of the points may be good to retain needles or press-spheres to give a sustained treatment effect. For example, if *josen* shows a reaction this is most commonly treated with an intradermal needle (Akabane 1986) or a press-tack needle.

The following steps show how to construct a basic treatment approach. On the first visit(s) you will do less, and then gradually increase the dose as needed on future visits:

1. On all children up to the age of 10, apply the core non-pattern-based root treatment. When feasible, teach the parents to do some simple form of this regularly at home.
2. Apply the basic pattern-based treatment, usually the kidney, liver, or lung pattern. If you are able to obtain enough pulse information to determine additional steps, such as treating a secondary pattern (liver secondary to the primary lung pattern, spleen secondary to the primary kidney pattern, etc.) and relevant *yang* channels, do so. On very young children use the noninserted needling methods to the relevant treatment points. On older children, once they are used to you applying needling techniques, apply inserted needling techniques to the relevant points, leaving the needles for a few minutes while you apply the symptomatic needling of relevant points before turning the child over to work on the back.[7]
3. Palpate all the points accessible that are mentioned as being good for treatment by needles or moxa (excluding the pattern-based root treatment points), while the patient is lying face up. Based on what you find, decide whether to only use needling or to apply needling to some points and moxa to others.
4. Insert needles to a few reactive points that are not used in the pattern-based root treatment or indicated as to be treated with moxa. If you decide to apply moxa to some points, do this now on the selected acupoints.
5. Have the patient turn over onto the abdomen and then either needle or needle and moxa reactive points on the posterior half of the body as per those listed earlier by the different authors.

6. Additional measures can be used, such as press-spheres, press-tack needles, intradermal needles, and, occasionally, cupping or bloodletting, according to need.

Press-Spheres *(Ryu)*, Press-Tack Needles *(Empishin)*, and Intradermal Needles *(Hinaishin)*

It is often very helpful to leave something like the press-spheres, press-tack needles, or intradermal needles to extend the treatment effects between visits. You have to judge by age, dose, and responsiveness of the child which are better to use for which child on which acupoints, and for how long to leave the items you have placed on the acupoints.

Usually, we apply these treatment techniques to the reactive points on the abdomen or back that remain reactive after treatment. We do not apply any of these methods to points where moxa

Example

Whole Treatment of an 8-Year-Old Boy
First visit:
Stroking is applied down the arms, legs, back, and abdomen.
Using a *teishin*, supplementation is applied to left KI-10, LU-5 with draining to right SP-9.
Tapping is applied over the lower abdomen, GV-12, occipital, GV-3, and lumbar–sacral regions.
Press-spheres are placed at GV-12, BL-25 (most stiff points found).

Later visit—for example, fifth visit:
There has been some improvement in the symptoms, but not enough. The parents are regularly applying a simple stroking and tapping core non-pattern-based root treatment at home.
Stroking is applied down the arms, legs, back, and abdomen.
Thin needles are inserted carefully to left KI-10, LU-5 for the pattern-based root treatment.
Needles are inserted for a couple of minutes to CV-3, ST-28.
Needles are inserted for a couple of minutes to BL-32, BL-23.
Moxa is applied lightly to BL-25.
Press-sphere is placed at GV-12.
Press-tack needles are placed at BL-23.

has been burned, but it is all right to apply them over a point that was needled earlier in the treatment. Common points to palpate and leave the press-spheres, press-tack needles, or intradermal needles are CV-3, CV-4, KI-11, KI-12, ST-28, BL-23, BL-32, BL-25, GV-2, and GV-3. But if other very reactive points in these areas are found, they can be treated instead.

If the child is anxious, it can be helpful to treat GV-12 and the point *shen men* in the ear or the point on the back of the ear directly behind *shen men*.

Cupping, Bloodletting

Cupping and/or bloodletting can be applied for this condition. The typical bloodletting treatment involves bleeding of vascular spiders on the lumbar–sacral region, if they are found. This only makes sense if the vascular spiders are clearly of the more pathological variety—darker and thicker. Carefully stab the vascular spiders (see Chapter 15, p. 103 for a discussion of this) and then squeeze out a few drops of blood. It is important to pay attention to the dose of treatment when applying this technique.

Meguro (1991, pp. 170–171) mentions the use of a more extensive cupping treatment for night urination. It is useful to remember that Meguro is a cupping specialist, meaning that his treatment exclusively involves the use of cupping for all patients. As acupuncturists, we can use this approach for some of our patients, but more likely we will be integrating the use of cupping into the overall treatment on each visit. When we do the following, cupping treatment will probably be too high a dose if all of it is applied in addition to the rest of the treatment. Thus the tendency is to use some of these treatment protocols or, on occasion only, to do the cupping as a separate treatment.

For children up to the age of 7 apply cups for 3 to 4 seconds over each of the following areas:

Around ST-23/ST-24, around ST-28 and SP-15 (six cups).

Over BL-23, BL-21, and BL-51 (six cups) and over the sacrum and sacroiliac joint upper region and lower region (four cups) and lateral to this over the middle of the gluteus (two cups).

For children over the age of 7, cup the same regions and also add cupping over BL-57.

Leave the cups a little longer according to age and strength of the child (longer for the older child). Leave the cups especially a little bit longer over the sacrum and side of the sacrum regions.

It is important to review the discussion of cupping methods in Chapter 14 to grasp the details of these cupping treatments. No cups should cause pain. We use only pumped cupping and not fire cupping.

Other Considerations

It is important to train the child well in urination habits; often the child needs to be instructed to go to the toilet to urinate more regularly during the day and especially to go to the toilet just before going to bed. It is said that the best approach is to wake the child up ~1 hour after falling asleep and take the child to the toilet to urinate. Shimizu (1975) suggests that the parents need to make sure that the child wakes up enough to experience urinating and remember doing so. Having the child urinate when only half awake generally does not work as well.

With the problem of night urination the child very often loses confidence, often develops anxiety, and can develop an inferiority complex. An important part of the treatment is thus to help the child develop more self-confidence and reduce anxiety. It is thus important to instruct the parents about not scolding the child for having an accident, and not to tease or hold the problem over the child for any reason. Instead, it is better to just change the child in the event of an accident. Every morning that the child gets up without an accident it is good for the parents to give praise.

Dietary

Obviously it is important to instruct the child and parents about dietary habits. It is important for the child not to drink much after dinner and especially not before going to bed. It can also be important for the child to not eat much (if anything) after dinner and before going to bed.

Home Treatment

It can be very helpful to have the parents start doing some form of the core non-pattern-based root treatment at home on a regular basis for most children with bed-wetting problems. However, if the child is older, you need to also instruct the parents in the application of more targeted treatment, focusing on acupoints specifically indicated for the problem using tapping of those points, heat to those points (perhaps using a moxa pole or a thick incense stick), changing the press-spheres on those points, and so on.

Further Case Histories

Case 2
Edward, Boy Age 4½ Years

Main complaints: Edward was having difficulty controlling his urination. At night he had bed-wetting episodes, but if the parents woke him a couple of hours after going to bed to make him urinate, he would have a dry night. During the day, however, he was having daily accidents.

History: He had had some issues with bed-wetting, but this was almost completely eliminated by taking him to the toilet after he had fallen asleep. The daytime episodes of loss of bladder control did not occur at school, where he was careful to ask to go to the toilet, but would instead occur after school when he was playing with friends, or at the weekend during playtime. It seemed that he was so occupied with playing that he would lose awareness of his bladder fullness, leading to what were now daily occurrences. His father brought him for treatment. It was clear that his father was quite worried and stressed out about this problem, and with a little inquiry it became clear that there was tension between Edward and his father over the issue. In the past he had had problems with congestion in the lungs but this was fine now. The kidney, lung, and spleen pulse all felt weak, which could be either a kidney vacuity pattern or a lung vacuity pattern.

Treatment: It seemed like a good idea to teach the father to do the treatment daily at home. This would not only treat Edward but could also help resolve the tension between the father and his son, which could be contributing to Edward's problem. Thus, on this visit, I decided only to apply the basic *shonishin* method and to

make sure I explained the daily home treatment clearly.

Using a *teishin*, very light stroking was applied down the arms (large intestine channel), legs (bladder and stomach channels), back, abdomen, and around the abdomen clockwise.

Tapping with a *herabari* was applied over the lower abdomen, GV-3, GV-12, and GV-20.

Small press-tack needles (0.6 mm) were retained at bilateral BL-52 (with instructions to remove them in ~30 hours).

A press-sphere was left on GV-12.

The father was taught how to do the stroking and tapping treatment.

Second visit—6 weeks later

The summer holidays had made treatment before this time impossible. For the first 4 weeks after the treatment and with daily home treatment, Edward had no accidents. In the last couple of weeks he had had a couple of minor episodes.

Treatment: Using a *teishin*, very light stroking was applied down the arms (large intestine channel), legs (bladder and stomach channels), back, abdomen, and around the abdomen clockwise.

Tapping with a *herabari* was applied over the lower abdomen, GV-3, GV-12, GV-20, and LI-4.

The *teishin* was used to supplement left KI-7, LU-5, drain right SP-9.

Small press-tack needles (0.6 mm) were retained at bilateral BL-52 (with instructions to remove them in ~30 hours).

A press-sphere was left on GV-12.

Third visit—13 days later

He was doing well, with no symptoms.

Treatment: Using a *teishin*, very light stroking was applied down the arms (large intestine channel), legs (bladder and stomach channels), back, abdomen, and around the abdomen clockwise.

Tapping with a *herabari* was applied over the lower abdomen, GV-4, GV-12, and GV-20.

The *teishin* was used to supplement left KI-7, LU-5, and right ST-36.

Press-spheres were left on GV-12, bilateral BL-23.

Fourth visit—19 days later

Edward was doing well; he had had only one accident. The father reported that he was much more relaxed about the problem and that he noticed that his increased relaxation also seemed to help Edward.

Treatment: Using a *teishin,* very light stroking was applied down the arms (large intestine channel), legs (bladder and stomach channels), back, abdomen, and around the abdomen clockwise.

Tapping with a *herabari* was applied over the lower abdomen, GV-3, GV-12, GV-20, LI-4, and over the occipital area.

The *teishin* was used to supplement left KI-7, LU-5, and right SP-9, drain right LI-6.

Small press-tack needles (0.6 mm) were retained at bilateral BL-52 (with instructions to remove them in ~30 hours).

A press-sphere was left on GV-12.

Fifth visit—3 weeks later

No accidents. Edward was doing very well.

Treatment: Tapping with a *herabari* was applied over the lower abdomen, GV-3, GV-12, GV-20, LI-4, ST-12, and occipital regions, arms, legs, and back.

The *teishin* was used to supplement left LU-9 and SP-3.

Small press-tack needles (0.6 mm) were retained at bilateral BL-23 (with instructions to remove them in ~30 hours).

The father discussed how he would like to stop treatment and call if the problem returned. It seemed that his doing the simple daily treatment at home was good for both him and Edward.

Reflection: It can, of course, be more difficult to help children retain awareness of the state of their bladder when they are busy with other things. The tactics I tried here do not always work, but it is a very good idea to always try this. There can be a variety of reasons why children lose their sense of bladder fullness and then have problems of involuntary urination. You have to try to figure out why and target that issue separately along with the general pattern and non-pattern-based root treatments. On the last treatment with Edward, his pattern had changed, the kidney pulse was no longer weak, and I judged that he had returned to his more constitutional state, the lung vacuity pattern.

The following case is from my colleague Sue Pready, who practices in Cardiff and Swindon in the United Kingdom. It describes treatment of an older child who had never gained proper control of her bladder. She was still bed-wetting regularly at age 12. The doctors had performed many different examinations but could find no obvious problem. She had tried many different treatments for the problem but without much success. She responded very well to the acupuncture treatment. I also used Bach flowers which probably contributed to the results (see Chapter 30 for a brief discussion of Bach flowers).

Case 3
Karen, Girl Age 12 Years

Main complaints: She has persistent bed-wetting. Her symptoms are intermittent, but she has never gained control of her bladder at night.

History: She has had many investigations to determine why she has the ongoing problem of bed-wetting. No pathology or problems were identified. Although she seems a well-adjusted child it is suspected that the fact that her parents separated and divorced probably created a background stress that is related to the problem.

She has tried many different techniques and interventions. Medication that the doctor prescribed was temporarily helpful, but would not work when she was more tired. She stopped this medicine because she did not like how it made her feel and because it didn't always work. Other therapies and techniques have not helped.

She tends to have stiff and painful shoulders, which worsened after starting high school 2 months before.

Assessment: On questioning further she and her parent report that she is very active during the day, and when she returns home from school she is very tired. By the time she goes to bed she is "dead to the world" and falls asleep quickly and very deeply.

Her feet are somewhat cool to the touch, but she is not aware of having cold feet.

Abdomen: the lower abdomen is slightly softer and cooler than the upper abdomen.

Pulse: liver and kidney pulses are weak, lung

pulse slightly weak, spleen-stomach pulse position slightly hard.

Diagnosis: With the pulse, abdominal findings, and symptoms I find she has liver vacuity.

Treatment: She was advised to try to regulate her activities during the day so that she would not come home so tired. It was explained that she was probably so tired and slept so deeply that she couldn't register signals that the bladder was full.

Tapping was applied with the *herabari* across the lower abdomen.

Using a *teishin*, right LV-8 and KI-10 were supplemented. After reassessing the pulse, left SP-9 and right TB-5 were drained.

Using the *teishin*, supplementation was applied to slightly soft feeling regions in the lower abdominal/inguinal areas and the regions above the clavicle.

Needles (0.16 mm) were inserted and retained at bilateral GB-20. Needles (0.16 mm) were also inserted with a heat lamp applied over the region to bilateral BL-23 and BL-28.

Press-tacks (0.6 mm) were left on bilateral BL-23 and CV-3.

Second visit—7 days later

While the press-tacks were retained for 3 days, she had no episodes of bed-wetting, and after they were removed she had one episode of bed-wetting.

Treatment: Needles (0.16 mm) were inserted and retained to bilateral ST-28.

Using a *teishin*, supplementation was applied to right LV-8, KI-10, and left SP-9. Right TB-5 and left GB-37 were drained.

Using the *teishin*, supplementation was applied to slightly soft-feeling regions in the lower abdominal/inguinal areas and the regions above the clavicle.

Needles (0.16 mm) were inserted and retained at bilateral GB-20 and bilateral BL-23 and BL-28 with a heat lamp over the low back region.

Press-tacks (0.6 mm) were left on bilateral BL-23 and CV-3.

She was advised to start using a 40°C saltwater footbath before going to bed.

Third visit—8 days later

No episodes of bed-wetting. She has been doing the footbath regularly. She is working on trying to regulate her activities during the day.

Treatment: Needles (0.16 mm) were inserted and retained to bilateral ST-28.

Using a *teishin*, supplementation was applied to right LV-8, KI-10, and left SP-9. Left BL-58 and ST-40 were drained.

Using the *teishin*, supplementation was applied to slightly soft-feeling regions in the lower abdominal/inguinal areas and the regions above the clavicle.

Needles (0.16 mm) were inserted and retained at bilateral GB-20 and bilateral BL-23 and BL-27 with a heat lamp over the low back region.

Press-tacks (0.6 mm) were left on bilateral BL-23 and CV-3.

Fourth visit—6 days later

She had three episodes of bed-wetting and reported that she had been very busy at the end of the week and more tired when the episodes started.

Treatment: Needles (0.16 mm) were inserted and retained to bilateral ST-28.

Using a *teishin*, supplementation was applied to right LV-8, KI-10. Left SP-9, right TB-5, and left BL-58 were drained.

Using the *teishin*, supplementation was applied to slightly soft-feeling regions in the lower abdominal/inguinal areas.

Using a *herabari*, tapping was applied over the shoulder and upper back.

Needles (0.16 mm) were inserted with a heat lamp applied over the region to bilateral BL-23 and BL-32.

Press-tacks (0.6 mm) were left on bilateral BL-23 and CV-3.

While the needles and heat lamp were applied on the back, her father was asked to select Bach flower remedies for her to start taking. She argued with her father about two of the remedies that he had selected and reluctantly agreed to two others. She left with a mix of Bach flowers to take.

Fifth visit—8 days later

No episodes of bed-wetting. Her father also reported that she was a bit less exhausted at the end of the day.

Treatment: Needles (0.16 mm) were inserted and retained to bilateral ST-28.

Using a *teishin*, supplementation was applied to right LV-8, KI-10. Left SP-9 and right TB-5 were drained.

Using the *teishin*, supplementation was applied to slightly soft-feeling regions in the lower abdominal/inguinal areas and the regions above the clavicle.

Needles (0.16 mm) were inserted with a heat lamp applied over the region to bilateral BL-23 and BL-32.

Press-tacks (0.6 mm) were left on bilateral BL-23 and CV-3.

Sixth visit—20 days later

No episodes of bed-wetting. She had now gone more than a month with no episodes and felt very good about this.

Treatment: Needles (0.16 mm) were inserted and retained to bilateral ST-28.

Using a *teishin*, supplementation was applied to right LV-8, KI-10, and left LU-9. Left BL-58 was drained.

Using the *teishin*, supplementation was applied to slightly soft-feeling regions in the lower abdominal/inguinal areas and the regions above the clavicle.

Needles (0.16 mm) were inserted with a heat lamp applied over the region to bilateral BL-23 and BL-32.

Press-tacks (0.6 mm) were left on bilateral BL-23 and CV-3.

Seventh visit—20 days later

No episodes of bed-wetting. She had now gone approximately 7 weeks with no episodes and felt very good about this; it was the longest she had ever managed.

Treatment: Needles (0.16 mm) were inserted and retained to bilateral ST-28. While the needles re-

mained inserted, using a *teishin*, supplementation was applied to right LV-8, KI-10, and left LU-9. Left BL-58 was drained.

Using the *teishin*, supplementation was applied to slightly soft-feeling regions in the lower abdominal/inguinal areas and the regions above the clavicle.

Needles (0.16 mm) were inserted with a heat lamp applied over the region to bilateral BL-23 and BL-32.

Press-tacks (0.6 mm) were left on bilateral BL-23 and CV-3.

Eighth visit—27 days later

She had had two episodes of spotting but no bed-wetting. On both nights they occurred she had stayed up later than usual and was more tired than usual. She had fallen and cut her chin, requiring several stitches, but it was healing okay.

Treatment: Needles (0.16 mm) were inserted and retained to bilateral ST-28. While the needles remained inserted, using a *teishin*, supplementation was applied to right LV-8, KI-10, and left LU-9. Left TB-5 was drained.

Needles (0.16 mm) were inserted with a heat lamp applied over the region to bilateral BL-23 and lateral to BL-28.

Needles (0.16 mm) were inserted and retained at GB-20.

In and out needling was applied over the shoulder region and interscapular region.

Press-tacks (0.6 mm) were left on bilateral BL-23 and CV-3.

Ninth visit—39 days later

She had had three bed-wetting episodes while on holiday. She agreed that on each occasion she was very tired from having a very hectic and busy day with late nights.

Treatment: Needles (0.16 mm) were inserted and retained to bilateral ST-29. While the needles remained inserted, using a *teishin*, supplementation was applied to right LV-8, KI-10, and left LU-9. Right TB-5 was drained.

Needles (0.16 mm) were inserted with a heat lamp applied over the region to bilateral BL-23 and lateral to BL-28.

Needles (0.16 mm) were inserted and retained at GB-20.

In and out needling was applied over the shoulder region and interscapular region.

Press-tacks (0.6 mm) were left on bilateral BL-23 and CV-3.

I advised her to pay more attention again to her energy regulation, to use the warm salty foot bath before going to bed, and to spend a few minutes each day trying to find a quiet space doing something like a very short meditation.

Following this treatment she stopped bed-wetting again. After this we agreed to a regular schedule for doing treatments ~3 to 4 weeks apart. She has maintained her improvements and has not had an episode for over 4 months.

The following case is from my colleague Sue Pready, who practices in Cardiff and Swindon in the United Kingdom.

Case 4
Greg, Boy Age 8 Years

Main complaint: He had been dry during the day since the age of 18 months but always had problems of wetting at night. This never improved or changed, and he had very few dry nights in a month. He described how the urge to urinate sometimes woke him but generally the bed-wetting was worse with stress (going back to school, writing tests, etc.). He underwent medical tests to check that his bladder was big enough, which it was. He was prescribed Desmopressin to stimulate hormones from the kidney. He had been taking it for 4 months with no effect on the symptoms, and the pediatrician subsequently prescribed another 4 months' worth of the medication. If the wetting episode woke him early, he usually had difficulty falling back to sleep; thus he was often tired in the morning.

History: He was born with pyloric stenosis, which required surgery at the age of 1 month. He sometimes had headaches in the morning across the forehead, probably because of his disturbed nights; he also tended to sleep lightly. He had broken his little right toe 2 months before, which had to be set in the hospital.

Assessment: He had a wiry, slim, and muscular build. Everything else seemed normal. He had a good appetite and a good mood, but he tended to speak with a very quiet voice. The lower abdo-

men was cool to the touch; there was a scar from the surgery around CV-12. He was very ticklish. His pulse was slightly weak, rapid, and of normal depth. The weakest pulses were the kidney, lung, and spleen pulses.

Diagnosis: His pulses indicate kidney vacuity pattern with spleen vacuity as a secondary pattern.[8]

Treatment: Using a *teishin*, supplementation was applied to left KI-7, LU-5, and right SP-3.

Draining technique was applied to right BL-58. Supplementation was then applied to CV-3, BL-13, and BL-23.

Light stroking was applied down the back and bladder channel on the legs with an *enshin*.

Light tapping was applied with a *herabari* to the occiput and around GV-12.

A press-sphere was placed at GV-12.

The mother was taught to change the press-sphere at GV-12 and apply light tapping around GV-12 and over the occiput as a daily home treatment.

Second visit—10 days later

The symptoms were better; he had had 4 dry nights. He was much more talkative. He was quite tired after the treatment. They decided he should stop taking the DesmoMelt because it had not affected the symptoms at all after 4 months of continuous use. Examination showed similar findings as on the first visit.

Treatment: Using a *teishin*, supplementation was applied to left KI-7, LU-5, right SP-3, and right TB-4.

Supplementation was also applied to CV-3, BL-13, BL-23, BL-25, and BL-32.

Heat was applied over BL-23 and the heels using a moxa pole.

Press-spheres were applied to GV-12 and CV-3.

Home treatment was extended with the addition of a very light stroking of the lung channel.

Third visit—4 days later

He had dry nights following the last treatment. However, he also had some morning headaches,

---

8   In Toyohari this is called kidney–spleen *sokoku* pattern.

probably due to sleep disturbance following two nightmares.

Treatment: Using a silver needle, supplementation was applied to left KI-7, LU-5, right SP-3, and right TB-4.[9] Supplementation was also applied over the abdominal scar and to CV-3, ST-28, the area around ST-12, and BL-23.

Heat was applied using a moxa pole over BL-23 and over the heels.

Fourth visit—2 days later

He had slept better without nightmares and was a bit happier in the morning. However, he had not had a dry night the last 2 nights. His mother thought this was because of worrying about a test at school this week.

Treatment: *Chinetsukyu*/warm moxa was applied to CV-3 and ST-28.

Using a *teishin*, supplementation was applied to left KI-7, LU-5, and right SP-3.

Supplementation was also applied around ST-12, BL-13, and BL-23.

Chinetsukyu/warm moxa was then applied to BL-13, BL-23, and BL-28.

Fifth visit—6 days later

It was clear that the main issue was his self-confidence. He had had 2 dry nights during this week. His sleep was better, and he had no headaches in the morning.

Treatment: Using the silver needle, supplementation was applied to left KI-7, LU-5, right SP-3, and bilateral TB-4, ST-36.

Using a *teishin*, supplementation was also applied to CV-3, ST-28, the area around ST-12, BL-13, and BL-23.

Chinetsukyu/warm moxa was applied to CV-3 and ST-28.

Light stroking was applied down the back using an *enshin*.

Heat was applied over the low back using a moxa pole.

---

9   The switch from *teishin* to a silver needle is normal in the Toyohari style of Meridian Therapy. It represents a way of increasing the dose and strength of the treatment.

Sixth visit—6 days later

He had been better, with no headaches, no nightmares, and 2 dry nights.

Assessment showed that his pattern seemed to have changed; he now showed the liver vacuity pattern.

Treatment: Using a *teishin*, supplementation was applied to left LR-8, KI-10, right SP-3, and PC-7.

Supplementation was also applied to CV-3, ST-28, the area around ST-12 and low abdomen, and to BL-18, BL-23, BL-28, and GV-12.

Chinetsukyu/warm moxa was applied to BL-28 and BL-23.

Seventh visit—7 days later

His condition was similar to the previous week.

Treatment: Using a *teishin*, supplementation was applied to left LR-8, KI-10, right LU-9, and SP-3.

Supplementation was also applied to CV-3, the area around ST-12 and low abdomen, and to BL-23 and BL-28.

Chinetsukyu/warm moxa was applied to ST-28 and CV-3.

Light stroking was followed by heat with a moxa pole and press-spheres to SP-6.

Eighth visit—7 days later

He had 5 dry nights this week.

Treatment: Treatment was the same as the last visit.

Ninth visit—7 days later

Every night was dry. His sleep was good, and there were still no headaches.

Treatment: Treatment was the same as the last visit.

Tenth visit—6 days later

Every night was dry. He was doing well.

Treatment: Treatment was the same as the last visit.

Eleventh visit—19 days later

He was wet the first night on holiday, all other nights were dry.

Treatment: Treatment was the same as the last visit with the addition of heat by a moxa pole to CV-3, ST-28, and BL-23, and press-spheres retained at SP-6, CV-3, and GV-12.

Twelfth visit—20 days later

One night was wet, all others were dry.

Treatment: Treatment was the same as the last visit.

Thirteenth visit—4 days later

He was wet the last 3 nights and dreamt about it, but he was not worried about anything. Generally he was much calmer.

Treatment: Using a silver needle, supplementation was applied to left LR-8, KI-10, right SP-3, and PC-7.
    Chinetsukyu/warm moxa was applied to TB-4 and SP-6.
    Okyu/direct moxa was applied on the heels at the extra point *shitsumin* in the center of the heel.

Heat with a moxa pole was applied over BL-18 and BL-23.

Fourteenth visit—8 weeks later

He has had no wet nights and has been doing well, with no other symptoms. His mother reported that since the last treatment he had had no wet nights; even if he had been late to bed or had had a drink close to bed time, he would even wake in the night to go to the toilet. His general mood was better, he slept better, and he was waking up refreshed. He had grown in confidence over the last few months and was a much happier child. He had friends for sleepovers and wanted to go to Cub Camp this year, none of which he would ever have considered before treatment.

Treatment: Treatment was the same as the last visit.
    While he had done well with treatment and had continuously improved, I felt that it would have been better to have a few more follow up visits to make sure of the changes, scheduled once every 2-4 months. But his mother thought it was better to stop due to increasing scheduling and financial issues. She agreed to bring him back if there were any setbacks, he has not returned.

vacuity pattern. If the child is young and the pulse and other signs for distinguishing the pattern are not clear, one needs other signs to distinguish them. If the hands tend to be cold, it is likely to be a lung vacuity pattern, and one should start treating this. Having generally stiff shoulders is also a sign of lung vacuity type. However, if the feet tend to get cold easily (but not the hands) this is more likely to be a kidney vacuity pattern. You may also notice some small temperature variations on the abdomen to support the choice of kidney pattern, such as slightly cooler below the navel compared with above the navel. Also, if the ear infections have triggered changes in hearing, you can suspect the kidney vacuity pattern.

For the lung vacuity pattern supplement LU-9 and SP-3. If the ear infection has arisen out of catching cold and there are still signs of the cold, such as cough, congested lungs, and alternating fever and chills, try treating the metal *jing*-river points LU-8 and SP-5 instead. If the child has a fever with the ear infection, you need to check the temperature. If it is 37.8°C or higher, the core non-pattern-based root treatment is contraindicated. In this case try using the *ying*-spring points for the lung vacuity pattern, LU-10 and SP-2. For the kidney vacuity pattern supplement KI-7 and LU-8. If with fever, try the *ying*-spring points KI-2 and LU-10.

Case 2 illustrates an alternative strategy for treating the relevant acupoints, using a very light stroking along the flow of the channels over the target acupoints for supplementation, and light stroking against the flow of the channel over the target acupoint for draining.

■ **Typical Non-pattern-based Root Treatment**

One can apply either the core non-pattern-based treatment with stroking and some tapping or tapping alone. For treatment apply stroking down the arms, legs, back, and abdomen. If the shoulders are stiff, apply stroking across the shoulders. If the neck is stiff, apply stroking down the neck. Apply tapping around GV-12 (**Fig. 23.1**).

Additional Areas for Treatment

It has been my consistent experience that children with otitis media develop an area of stiffness that is usually painful on pressure below the ears. This

hardened area usually starts around TB-17 and extends downward from there. Sometimes it extends backward from there toward GB-12, sometimes

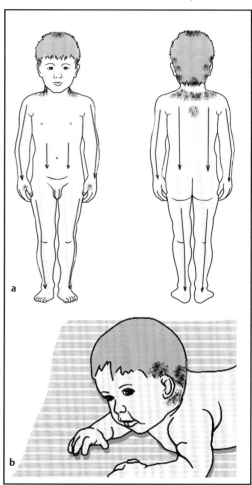

Fig. 23.1a, b Usual stroking plus:
- Below, above, and behind the ear(s): 10 times each
- Occipital area: 10 to 20 times
- Across the shoulders: 10 to 20 times
- GV-20 area: 10 to 20 times
- CV-12 area: 10 to 20 times
- LI-4: 10 to 20 each
- ST-12 area (supraclavicular fossa region): 5 to 10 times each

forward slightly from there. I feel that this area of stiffness is probably associated with blockage of the lymphatic drainage, and that it is thus an important area to target. Thus I always apply tapping to this area as well as the areas above and below the ears that are suggested by Yoneyama and Mori

(1964) and Hyodo (1986). I give a consistent focus to soften and break up this congested, hardened area. If the tapping alone does not make enough change I start applying stronger techniques to it, such as press-spheres, needling, and/or press-tack needles. See the following discussions.

■ Recommendations for Symptomatic Treatment

Needling
Whether one inserts needles and immediately removes them or inserts and retains them for a short while, needling can be helpful in the treatment of otitis media. The area of hardness and pressure pain below the ears can be a useful place to needle. The area around GB-12 can also become stiff and reactive, and this responds well to light needling.

Press-Spheres (Ryu), Press-Tack Needles (Empishin), and Intradermal Needles (Hinaishin)
It is useful to leave press-spheres on the hardened sensitive area(s) below the ear(s). If these areas do not sufficiently change I recommend switching soon to a stronger technique, such as leaving press-tack needles and maybe needling during the session. To help the child settle (ear infections can be quite painful and distressing) it can be helpful to also leave a press-sphere on GV-12. The main area for leaving the small press-tack needles (0.3 or 0.6 mm long) is the area below the ear(s), around TB-17 or below that point. On older children, where it is generally safer to leave intradermal needles, I leave them at the stubbornly reactive points, such as the area of reaction below the ears.

Okyu—Direct Moxa
The application of small direct moxa cones is recommended at points such as KI-2, KI-3, with KI-2 being especially effective (Yoneyama and Mori 1964). The following points are recommended on adults; they can be palpated and the most reactive one or two points treated with moxa for nonresponsive otitis media (KI-3 is strongly recommended): SI-19, TW-17, GB-12, HT-3, KI-3, BL-23, BL-11, and BL-12 (Shiroda 1986). If you are afraid to moxa these points because it is too difficult you can try applying needling, press-spheres,

press-tacks, or intradermal needles to the reactive points from this list (keeping in mind the issue of treatment dose).

Cupping
Cupping can be helpful over the upper back and backs of the shoulders to help relax the area when it is chronically stiff in the child with recurrent otitis media. As discussed in Chapter 14, be careful about the dose; applying the cups repeatedly for less time can be helpful.

Bloodletting
Bloodletting of the *jing* point GB-44 is recommended for ear pain (Birch and Ida 1998, p. 240), TB-1 could also be indicated (Birch and Ida 1998, p. 283). It can be very difficult to apply this technique on small children, and even on older children. You must have a painless technique. If the child with recurrent otitis media shows vascular spiders on the upper back in the GV-14 area or back of the shoulders, it can on occasion be useful to apply vascular spider bloodletting. This is usually easier to do than *jing* point bloodletting on a child, but your technique must be very good; otherwise do not apply it. If you do this, apply only the stabbing and squeezing method; do not also apply cupping.

You might choose to try the bloodletting because the child's problem is not changing and you have already tried other stronger techniques, such as needling or direct moxa. As discussed in Chapter 15, it will be important to make sure that the child will stay still for you and that you have a clear agreement with the child's parent to proceed.

■ Other Considerations

Dietary
It can be a good idea to examine the diet of the child. With repeat infections, cow's milk products can often be an irritant. Testing for and stopping the intake of cow's milk products can be important for some children, and so I always check this out.

Home Treatment
It is wonderful to have parents who have children with repeated infections start to apply treatment

at home. It not only makes the overall treatment more effective, it also gives the parents a sense of being able to help and contribute.

■ Further Case Histories

The following case is from the practice of my colleague Zoe Brenner in Bethesda, Maryland, United States.

Case 2
Clare, Girl Age 4 Years

The mother had been a long-time patient and mentioned that her 4-year-old was having chronic ear infections, resulting in difficult speech development because her hearing was impaired. She wanted to bring her in for treatment.

Main complaints: Clare had had many ear infections, and they were treated with antibiotics. The problems would usually start as a cold and then progress to the ears. Speech development was slow, which was attributed to the chronically congested ears. She was seeing a speech therapist to help with the problem. All other systems were unremarkable.

Diagnosis: Both the fact that she had ear problems with hearing difficulties and that she exhibited so much fear suggested the kidney vacuity pattern.

First visit

When the mother brought Clare, she hid behind her mother. She seemed disproportionately fearful.

Treatment: It was not possible to take her pulses that first time. With gentle coaxing it was possible to lightly stroke with the *enshin* down her legs on the *yang* channels and up on the *yin* channels then down her arms on both the *yin* and *yang* channels.[1] Light stroking with the *enshin* was also given down her back, stroking through her clothes as she would not remove them. She was a bit more relaxed but still quite wary.

Second visit—1 week later

Clare's mother reported that she had been very happy after the previous visit.

Treatment: The same *enshin* light-stroking core non-pattern-based root treatment was applied. After this she was less fearful, and it was possible to take her pulses. The kidney pulse was quite weak with relative repletion on her spleen pulse. To treat this, light treatment was applied using an *enshin* by stroking along the kidney channel near KI-3. After rechecking the pulses, the spleen pulse was still replete, so gentle stroking was applied against the flow of the spleen channel over SP-9.

Third visit—1 week later

Clare had been doing well, no problems. Her mother said that the speech therapist had noticed that Clare's enunciation was getting clearer, and her hearing had improved 20 dB.

Treatment: The treatment from the second visit was repeated, with the exception that gentle stroking with the *teishin* in the direction of flow of the lung channel over LU-9 was added after treating KI-3.

Fourth visit—1 week later

She had mild cold symptoms (runny nose, mild cough), otherwise no ear problems. Her mother was excited to report that Clare had gone to a party and did not hide for the first hour. This was a huge change for her to go in and be able to engage in play right away.

Treatment: The same treatment as on the third visit was repeated, with the exception of adding a mild pressing over the cheeks and neck below the ears to promote drainage and help with recovery from the cold.

Treatment was continued for a few more sessions, spreading them apart more as she continued to improve. The issue with the chronic ear infections, hearing, and speech completely resolved. One of the key signs that she was better came when she had a *Streptococcus* infection affecting the throat

---

[1]   Stroking like this on the *yin* channels will apply a light supplementing effect on the kidney and lung channels, which are treated for the kidney vacuity pattern.

with no ear involvement at all. Additionally, her fearfulness was quite improved, as everyone noted.

Case 3
Greg, Boy Age 21 Months

Main complaints: He had had over 15 ear infections in the past. As treatment, he had had grommets inserted into both ears and nasal surgery to help unblock the nasal passages where the infection started. Despite these measures he still developed ear infections, which were treated with fresh rounds of antibiotics. He had had multiple bouts of bronchitis, had been on albuterol (Ventolin, GlaxoSmithKline) since the age of 6 weeks, and taken many rounds of antibiotics for the bronchitis. There was almost continuous congestion in both the nose and the lungs. He was a restless sleeper and tended to wake early. He could become moody and irritable and tended to have loose stools and occasionally diarrhea. He had a good appetite and no skin problems.

Diagnosis: He had a lung weak constitution (see Chapter 26, Weak Constitution). The ear infections were secondary to the recurrent upper respiratory tract and lung infections.

Treatment: Using the *herabari*, tapping was applied to LI-4, around the ears, below the ears, and down toward the ST-12 area, on the back of the neck, especially along the occipital border, at GV-12 and GV-22.

Light stroking was applied with an *enshin* down the arms, legs, abdomen, and back.

Using a *teishin*, left LU-9 and SP-3 were supplemented.

Press-spheres were retained at GV-12 and the asthma *shu* points.

Testing for reaction to and discontinuing cow's milk was discussed with the parents, who agreed to start this immediately.

Second visit—5 days later

Greg had been on soy milk since the first visit. The phlegm in his nose and lungs seemed better. He had been calmer, less moody, and was relaxed after the treatment.

Treatment: Tapping was applied with the *herabari* to LI-4, around the ears, below the ears down toward ST-12, along the occipital border, GV-20, GV-12, and GV-22.

Light stroking was applied with an *enshin* down the arms, legs, abdomen, and back.

Using a *teishin*, left LU-9 and SP-5 were supplemented and right LR-3 drained.

Press-spheres were retained on GV-12 and the asthma *shu* points.

His parents were instructed to apply light tapping to the same points and areas and light stroking over the same regions.

Third visit—9 days later

He was doing much better. He had no nasal or lung congestion. His parents had stopped using the Ventolin. His mood and sleep were much better, and his loose stools were better. His home treatment was going well.

Treatment: I discussed with the parents whether he should come off the Ventolin so quickly and that they should discuss this with the prescribing doctor.

The same treatment was applied as on the last visit with the exception that left BL-58 was also drained, and the asthma *shu* points were not treated with the press-spheres because the points were slightly irritated.

Fourth visit—6 weeks later

Generally he had been good, there were no symptoms of the lungs or ears, and his nasal congestion was not bad despite catching cold and having mild on–off cold symptoms over the last 3 weeks (which would normally have triggered either ear infections, bronchitis, or both). But his sleep was not as good as on the last visit, and he had been a little more moody. The parents reported that they waited this long to return because the trip to the clinic took at least 90 minutes each way, and on the last visit they had been stuck in traffic for a long time, thus they wanted to make visits less frequent. They had been able to do some home treatment almost every day and felt that

Fourth visit—5 days later

He had had one good day with less nasal stuffiness. His appetite was better and he was eating more. His mother had been able to do home treatment with greater frequency.

Treatment: Using a *teishin*, very light stroking was applied down the large intestine, stomach, and bladder channels, down the abdomen and back.

Using a *teishin*, supplementation was applied to left LU-9, SP-3, draining to right LR-3.

Tapping was applied with a *herabari* over GV-12, occipital, and GV-22 to GV-23 areas.

Press-spheres were applied to BL-13 and CV-12.

Fifth visit—16 days later

His mother had been able to keep to the improved frequency of home treatments. His sense of smell was much improved, but the nose was quite stuffy and he seemed to still have a diminished sense of taste.

Treatment: Using a *teishin*, very light stroking was applied down the large intestine, stomach, and bladder channels, down the abdomen, back, and neck.

Using a *teishin*, supplementation was applied to left LU-9, SP-3, draining to right LR-3 and left LI-6. Supplementation was also applied to *yin tang* and bilateral LI-20.

Tapping was applied with a *herabari* over GV-12, occipital, and GV-22 to GV-23 areas.

Press-spheres were applied to BL-12 and CV-12.

Sixth visit—2 weeks later

The nasal symptoms were the same, but eating was better, and he had clearly started to gain weight.

Treatment: A needle was inserted and retained for a few minutes at GV-22.

Using a *teishin*, very light stroking was applied down the large intestine, stomach, and bladder channels, down the abdomen, back, and shoulders.

Using a *teishin*, supplementation was applied to CV-12, left LU-9, SP-3, draining to right LR-3 and left TB-5. Supplementation was also applied

to *yin tang* and bilateral LI-20.

Tapping was applied with a *herabari* over GV-12, occipital region, and on the head.

Press-spheres were applied to BL-13 and CV-12.

Seventh visit—2 weeks later

The nose had been less stuffy, the appetite was better again, and he had gained more weight.

Treatment: Using a *teishin*, very light stroking was applied down the large intestine, stomach, and bladder channels, down the abdomen, back, shoulders, and neck.

Using a *teishin*, supplementation was applied to left LU-9, SP-3, draining to right LR-3, and supplementation to bilateral LI-20.

Tapping was applied with a *herabari* over GV-12, occipital, and GV-22 to GV-23 areas.

Press-spheres were applied to BL-13 and CV-12.

Eighth visit—2 weeks later

He was generally doing well, the nasal symptoms were much better. He had been in contact with a dog and had no allergic reactions for the first time. He had had a cold and recovered quickly without it progressing and triggering many symptoms.

Treatment: Using a *teishin*, very light stroking was applied down the large intestine, stomach, and bladder channels, down the abdomen, back, shoulders, and neck.

Using a *teishin*, supplementation was applied to left LU-9, SP-3, draining to right LR-3, left BL-58 with supplementation to *yin tang*, bilateral LI-20, and bilateral BL-20.

Tapping was applied with a *herabari* over GV-12, occipital, and GV-22 to GV-23 areas.

Press-spheres were applied to BL-13 and CV-12.

Ninth visit—11 days later

The nasal stuffiness, appetite, and eating had all been better overall.

Treatment: Using a *teishin*, very light stroking was applied down the large intestine, stomach, and bladder channels, down the abdomen, back, and neck.

Using a *teishin*, supplementation was applied to left LU-9, SP-3, draining to right LR-3 and left LI-6 with supplementation to *yin tang* and bilateral LI-20.

Tapping was applied with a *herabari* over GV-12, occipital, and GV-22 to GV-23 areas.

Press-spheres were applied to BL-12 and CV-12.

Tenth visit—3 weeks later

The last 2 weeks were worse, with more nasal congestion, and his eating was not as good.

Treatment: A needle was inserted and retained for a few minutes at GV-22.

Using a *teishin*, very light stroking was applied down the large intestine, stomach, and bladder channels, down the abdomen and back.

Using an *enshin*, light stroking was applied down the back.

Using a *teishin*, supplementation was applied to left LU-9, SP-3, draining to right LR-3 and left LI-6.

Tapping was applied with a herabari over GV-12, occipital, and GV-22 to GV-23 areas.

Press-spheres were applied to CV-12.

Intradermal needles were placed for 2 hours and replaced by press-spheres at bilateral BL-13.

Eleventh visit—2 weeks later

The nose was still stuffy, but his eating was better, and he had gained weight again.

Treatment: A needle was inserted and retained for a few minutes at GV-22.

Using a *teishin*, very light stroking was applied down the large intestine, stomach, and bladder channels, down the abdomen and back.

Using an *enshin*, light stroking was applied down the back.

Using a *teishin*, supplementation was applied to left LU-9, SP-3, draining to right LR-3 and left LI-6.

Tapping was applied with a *herabari* over GV-12, occipital, and GV-22 to GV-23 areas.

Press-spheres were applied to CV-12 and bilateral BL-20.

Cupping was gently applied over the upper back.

He came for a further 16 treatments over the next 15 months. These treatments were relatively similar or modified slightly to match current complaints. Over this 15-month period he showed further improvements in his allergic sensitivities and nasal congestion. He maintained a healthier appetite and taste for food so that he was no longer underweight. His parents also discovered that he was quite allergic to gluten, and cutting this out of the diet and adding a little extra treatment targeted to food allergy problems—such as cupping around the navel—also contributed to the improvements in his condition.

Some children with an allergic-type constitution require a lot of treatment to improve substantially. One can usually get a good sense within a few treatments that the treatment approach is helping. In Michael's case it was the improved appetite and eating habits, despite the minimal change in nasal symptoms and sense of smell and taste. When working with a child with such an allergic constitution it is a good idea to help the parents understand that a longer course of treatment is necessary. Use home treatments as much as you can, schedule to less frequent treatments as soon as is realistic, and plan for regular but infrequent visits over a long time.

■ General Approach for Patients with Nasal Congestion

Treating children with chronic nasal congestion requires several targeted approaches. It is good to strengthen the child with both pattern-based and non-pattern-based root treatments so that the child's ability to overcome the problem improves. It is also important to try to identify potential irritants that either continually trigger the symptoms or hinder the child from recovery, such as dietary problems, airborne irritants, and so on. Teaching the parents to do some simple home treatment will be helpful and will involve attention to the last issue and probably teaching a simple form of the non-pattern-based root treatment. Finally, you need to work out which symptomatic treatment methods are best at which locations for the particular symptoms of each child.

■ Most Likely Pattern-based Root Diagnosis

The most likely pattern of treatment will be the lung vacuity pattern since the nose is the opening of the lungs, and nasal congestion problems often result from exposure to irritants (allergic constitution) or recurrent infections, both of which are typical signs of the lung vacuity pattern. In some cases the nasal congestion can progress to become the kidney vacuity pattern (look for signs of cool feet, with pulse and abdominal signs of this) or the spleen vacuity pattern (look for signs of recurrent digestive symptoms).[3]

■ Typical Non-pattern-based Root Treatment

One can apply either the core non-pattern-based treatment with stroking and some tapping, or tapping alone. For treatment apply stroking down the arms, legs, back, and abdomen. If the shoulders are stiff, apply stroking across the shoulders. If the neck is stiff, apply stroking down the neck. Apply tapping to around GV-12 (**Fig. 23.2**).

Additional tapping to target the symptoms can be applied around GV-22 to GV-23, the occipital region, especially around GB-20, GV-12, and the upper back region (including the BL-12–BL-13 region). Additional points to tap include LI-4, LI-11, ST-36, and sometimes *yin tang*. Applying a light stimulation around the nose is useful, and probably more comfortable with a light pressing using, for example, a *teishin* on acupoints such as LI-20 and BL-2.

■ Recommendations for Symptomatic Treatment

Needling
Yoneyama and Mori (1964) state that shallowly inserted needles to points such as BL-10, GB-20, and GV-23 can be very effective. However, on the acupoint GV-23, do not insert needles before the age of 2 years because the anterior fontanel is still

open. On the young child these acupoints can be treated using a retained needling method, making sure that the technique is painless so the child is unaware of the needles. The acupoint LI-4 can be helpful for nasal congestion: treat it with an in–out needling method rather than a retained needling method. In older children if the nasal problems are very stubborn and resistant, palpate *yin tang* and BL-2. You may need to use the retained needling method on these acupoints, provided the child will stay still for you.

Press-Spheres *(Ryu)*, Press-Tack Needles *(Empishin)*, and Intradermal Needles *(Hinaishin)*
A press-sphere to GV-12 is helpful. If BL-12 or BL-13 shows a distinctive knot that makes the child flinch or jump when touched, use press-spheres on younger children and if there is no response, on older children, use press-tack needles. These points are more likely to show reactions because of the symptoms and/or the lung vacuity pattern. If there are additional spleen signs (digestive problems, food allergies, or sensitivities), pal-

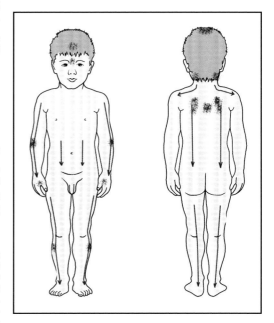

Fig. 23.2 Usual stroking plus tapping:
- GV-22-GV-23 area: 10 to 20 times
- GV-20 area: 10 to 20 times
- GB-20 area: 20 to 30 times
- LI-4: 10 to 20 times each
- Sometimes soft tapping around *yin tang*: 5 to 10 times

---

[3]   TCM tells us that cold affects the kidneys and dampness the spleen (Wiseman and Ellis 1985). Thus symptoms that are worsened by cold will lead one to think of the kidneys, and signs of dampness, such as mucus, lead one to think of the spleen. However, this is a simplification. Although the *Huang Di Nei Jing Su Wen (The Yellow Emperor's Inner Classic—Basic Questions)* makes these associations, the *Nan Jing (Classic of Difficulties)* makes other associations, both of which seem clinically useful. The *Nan Jing* says that cold injures the lungs, damp injures the kidneys, and overeating, overdrinking, overworking injures the spleen (Fukushima 1991). It is more useful to look at both sets of correspondences and be more flexible in one's approach. This is discussed briefly in Chapter 10.

pate around BL-20 and medial to it. If there is a clear reactive point, leave either a press-sphere (younger, more sensitive child) or a press-tack (older, less sensitive child).

On some older children if the symptom is not responding much, you can try leaving 0.3 or 0.6 mm press-tack needles on acupoints such as *yin tang* or BL-2, depending on the reactions in these points. You need to be sure that the child will not play with the needles or try to remove them. Often you place these needles with instructions to remove them by the next morning. The child may be willing to leave the needles untouched, but it is not so clear that friends or classmates will leave them alone because they are quite visible on the face. Another acupoint that can show strong reactions is the extra point *bi tong* at the juncture of the bone and cartilage on the nose. This is a good point to treat if the symptoms are stubborn and unchanging.

Okyu—Direct Moxa

Manaka recommends for nasal congestion of the newborn applying moxa to GV-12, GV-23, and/or the extra point near LI-4 (located at the distal heads of the first and second metacarpals) (Manaka, Itaya, and Birch 1995). It is probably not good to start doing this treatment because moxa is difficult on babies and small children. If, after tapping these points, you increase the dose with inserted needles and there is still no response, then you can think about this treatment.

Cupping

For children with food-related sensitivities that are related to the nasal congestion, cupping around the navel can be helpful. For children with airborne allergies contributing to the nasal congestion, cupping on the upper back can be helpful, using low-dose stimulation around GV-14, GV-12, or BL-12 regions.

Bloodletting

In general, for chronic nasal congestion, especially if the symptoms are strong and stubborn and not changing easily, bloodletting of vascular spiders on the upper back may be helpful. Examine the area around GV-14 to BL-13 for vascular spiders. If clear vascular spiders are found, these can be stabbed and bled using the squeezing method. Be careful about dosage.

■ Other Considerations

Dietary

It is not uncommon that you will need to test for cow's milk sensitivity. This is a common problem, but other dietary allergens may also be involved, which can take time to identify and eliminate.

Other Allergens

For the child with airborne allergies (dust, mites), if the symptoms are not responding well you may need to discuss the idea of having the parents buy a good air filtering system to be run continuously at home. Such a system can help minimize exposure to the allergens for the child in the space where he or she is most commonly exposed (bedroom, rooms they play in). While working at a symptomatic level, by reducing exposure and thus symptomatic reactions, it also aids the overall treatment of the allergic constitution. In many patients, the continuous triggering of allergic reactions with symptoms seems to keep the whole system sensitized so that the child more easily has further reactions. It can be difficult for normal functioning of the tissues to return because they are continuously in an irritated state. Your root treatment, both the core non-pattern-based root treatment and the pattern-based root treatment, will also be somewhat undermined by the continuous need to focus on symptom relief and control measures. However, when the symptoms are kept quieter (through reduced exposure to the allergens), not only do the irritated tissues of the nasal passages settle down, become less inflamed and swollen (allowing for more normal functioning to occur), but your root treatment can become the dominant aspect of the treatment that will help create changes to a greater degree and more quickly in the underlying allergic constitution. In such cases, this is often the most important part of treatment. Relieving symptoms for a while may not be too difficult, but creating a change so that there are fewer or no future symptoms can require a lot more work.

Home Treatment

Home treatment can be very helpful for speeding up improvement in chronic conditions. Generally

There are also hard painful areas found on palpation below each ear, around and extending downward and behind TB-17.

Abdominal findings: the kidney area is slightly softer.

Pulse findings: the kidney and lung pulses are weak.

Diagnosis: Her pulses and other findings indicate kidney vacuity.

Treatment: Using a *herabari*, tapping was applied to bilateral LI-4, GV-12, the supraclavicular regions, the occipital and neck regions.

Using an *enshin*, light stroking was applied down the arms, legs, abdomen, and back.

Using a *teishin*, supplementation was applied to right KI-7 and LU-5, draining to right TB-5.

A press-sphere was left at GV-12.

Second visit—22 days later

After the treatment, her headaches stopped, and she had no ear pain until she went swimming last week.

Treatment: Using a *herabari*, tapping was applied to bilateral LI-4, GV-12, the supraclavicular regions, the occipital and neck regions.

Using an *enshin*, light stroking was applied down the arms, legs, abdomen, and back.

Using a *teishin*, supplementation was applied to right KI-7 and LU-5, draining to right BL-58.

A press-sphere was left at GV-12.

Third visit—13 days later

She has had some acute gastrointestinal symptoms (abdominal pain, loose stools) the last couple of days and started a headache today. Prior to this she has had no headaches or ear pain.

Treatment: Using a *herabari,* tapping was applied to bilateral LI-4, GV-12, GV-20, the supraclavicular regions, the occipital and neck regions.

Using an *enshin*, light stroking was applied down the arms, legs, abdomen, and back.

Using a *teishin,* supplementation was applied to right KI-7, LU-5, and left ST-36, draining to right BL-58.

A press-sphere was left at GV-12.

Her mother was taught to apply the stroking and tapping as home treatment.

Fourth visit—14 days later

She has had no headaches for the last 2 weeks. She has had some discomfort but not pain around the ears. She has been enjoying the home treatment.

Treatment: Using a 0.12 mm needle, needling was applied in an in and out technique to bilateral TB-17.

Using a *herabari*, tapping was applied to bilateral LI-4, GV-12, the supraclavicular regions, the occipital and neck regions.

Using an *enshin*, light stroking was applied down the arms, legs, abdomen, and back.

Using a *teishin*, supplementation was applied to right KI-7, LU-5, and left SP-3, draining to right BL-58.

A press-sphere was left at GV-12.

Fifth visit—27 days later

She had 3 days with mild headache the week before accompanied by some ear discomfort. Otherwise she has been free of headaches and ear pain. Her mother reported that she is happier and more energetic and expressive and seems to be in a growth spurt.

Assessment of the abdomen and pulses showed that the kidney region of the abdomen and the kidney pulses were firmer. She now showed a lung vacuity pattern.

Treatment: Using a 0.12 mm needle, needling was applied in an in and out technique to bilateral TB-17.

Using a *herabari*, tapping was applied to bilateral LI-4, GV-12, the supraclavicular regions, and the occipital and neck regions.

Using an *enshin*, light stroking was applied down the arms, legs, abdomen, and back.

Using a *teishin*, supplementation was applied to right LU-9 and SP-3, draining to right LV-3 and BL-58.

A press-sphere was left at GV-12.

Sixth visit—21 days later

She had some ear pain the previous week with the cold weather, which was accompanied by a brief mild headache. Otherwise she has had no other headaches or ear pain.

Treatment: Using a 0.12 mm needle, needling was applied in an in and out technique to TB-17 and to stiff areas at the top of each sternocleido-mastoid muscle.

Using a *herabari*, tapping was applied to bilateral LI-4, GV-12, and the supraclavicular regions.

Using an *enshin,* light stroking was applied down the arms, legs, abdomen, and back.

Using a *teishin,* supplementation was applied to right LU-9 and SP-3, draining to right LV-3.

A press-sphere was left at GV-12.

Seventh visit—64 days later

She has been doing very well. No headaches or ear pain. But yesterday she fell on her back while playing in the playground at school. Her back and neck were sore, and she had a headache. Today she feels better with no headache, but she has pain in the back and neck. Her mother is concerned that this could trigger more headaches and felt it better to bring her in for treatment immediately.

Treatment: Using a 0.12 mm needle, needling was applied in an in and out technique to bilateral TB-17 and to stiff areas at the top of each sterno-cleidomastoid muscle.

Using a *herabari*, tapping was applied to bilateral LI-4, GV-12, the supraclavicular regions, and the occipital and upper back regions.

Using an *enshin,* light stroking was applied down the arms, legs, abdomen, and back.

Using a *teishin,* supplementation was applied to right LU-9 and SP-3, draining to right LV-3 and BL-58.

Press-tack needles (0.3 mm) were retained at GV-12 and bilateral GB-21.

Eighth visit—5½ months later

She has been doing very well and has had no headaches or ear pain. She banged her face around her left eye 2 months previously and still experiences a little tenderness from that, but otherwise is doing well. She came for a fol-low-up visit.

Treatment: Using a 0.12 mm needle, needling was applied in an in and out technique to bilateral GB-21 and left TB-17.

Using a *herabari*, tapping was applied to bilateral LI-4, GV-12, the supraclavicular regions, the occipital region, and around the eyes.

Using an *enshin,* light stroking was applied down the arms, legs, abdomen, and back.

Using a *teishin,* supplementation was applied to right LU-9, SP-3, and left LI-20, draining to right LV-3, ST-40, left BL-58, and right LI-20.

Press-tack needles (0.3 mm) were retained at GV-12 and right BL-18.

Ninth visit—3 months later

She has been doing very well, with no headaches or ear pain, except when she caught cold a few weeks before, at which time she had a mild head-ache (which could have been normal for the cold). She came for a follow-up visit.

Treatment: Using a 0.12 mm needle, needling was applied in an in and out technique to right TB-17 and the top of each sternocleidomastoid muscle.

Using a *herabari*, tapping was applied to bilateral LI-4, GV-12, the supraclavicular regions, and the occipital region.

Using an *enshin,* light stroking was applied down the arms, legs, abdomen, and back.

Using a *teishin,* supplementation was applied to right LU-9 and SP-3, draining to left LV-3, right SI-7.

Press-tack needles (0.3 mm) were retained at GV-12 and right BL-18.

She came for five more visits over the next year. Her ears were occasionally a bit sore or sensitive, but she did not have the ear infections and pain. On a couple of occasions she had some mild headaches that resolved quickly and easily. For these five visits treatments were similar.

Comments: She responded to treatment from the first visit. It was therefore not necessary to add a lot of extra techniques, and we could manage with light, quick treatments to help rid her of chronic headaches and ear pain. If she had not responded this quickly to treatment I had considered treating the extraordinary vessels, probably in the style of my teacher notice this as you examine the pulses to identify the pattern, liver repletion always occurs secondary to a lung or spleen vacuity pattern. Chapters 9 and 10 describe the details of the four primary vacuity patterns.

For the younger child use of the spring-loaded *teishin* or *tsumoshin* is sufficient for treatment of the pattern of vacuity that is found and for the repletion that is found in the pulses. But in the older child (here this can mean the emotionally older or more mature child), the spring-loaded *teishin* may not be very effective. In which case use 0.12 mm needles inserted painlessly to the primary treatment points for the vacuous channels. For the channels that you find to be replete, use the 0.16 mm needle with the appropriate needle technique. Chapter 10 describes the needling methods.

As the child becomes older it becomes easier to identify problems in *yang* channel pulses as well. The more common being that one or more *yang* channel pulses feel replete (as you touch that pulse position the pulse wave strikes your finger earlier—closer to the skin—than in other positions, and the pulse wave that strikes the finger feels somewhat stronger and has some hardness). Apply the draining needle technique to those *yang* channels in which you can clearly identify such repletion signs in the pulse. Be aware that this repletion of the *yang* channel pulses may not be obvious on initial examination of the pulses, but becomes apparent as you start to supplement the *yin* channel vacuity pattern. It is also important to not assume that the *yang* channel which feels replete relates to the channels in which the headache appears. The repletion of the *yang* channels that we end up treating very often appears to have no obvious relation to the patient's affected channels or location of symptoms.

If the child shows signs of counterflow *qi*, reddened complexion, flushing of the neck, face, emotional lability, cool or cold feet, use the *he*-sea points for treatment of the primary and secondary pattern rather than the standard points for that pattern.

Typical Non-pattern-based Root Treatment

If the child is younger, for example 6 to 10 years old, you might choose to apply this treatment

---

Examples of treatment

The child is diagnosed with liver vacuity pattern. Supplement LV-8 and KI-10 on one side of the body. On reexamination of the pulses, the spleen is found to be replete, SP-3 is drained on the other side of the body. On reexamination of the pulses, the triple burner pulses is found replete, TB-5 is drained on the side that feels more replete when touched.

The child is diagnosed with lung vacuity pattern and has some signs of counterflow *qi*. LU-5 and SP-9 are supplemented on one side. On reexamination of the pulses the liver pulse is replete. LV-8 is drained on the other side of the body. On reexamination of the pulses the bladder and stomach pulses are replete. BL-58 and ST-40 are drained each on the side that feels more replete on palpation.

---

regularly. Light stroking is applied in the usual pattern. Light tapping can be applied to LI-4 (unless needle insertion is used instead) and around GV-12 and the occipital regions.

If the child has clear signs of counterflow *qi*, regardless of the age of the child it is probably a good idea to apply the gentle stroking technique treatment pattern. This treatment applies stroking down the arms, legs, back, and abdomen; that is, it makes *qi* flow downward.

Recommendations for Symptomatic Treatment

There are many options for treatment of headaches[8] and often the patient shows many reactive points on palpation of the body. It is thus important to select points carefully so as not to overtreat the patient. If the child has been using a lot of medications, this can precipitate a lot of sensitive points, palpate carefully to identify the more reactive.

---

8   Textbooks on acupuncture for adult patients usually give a lot of detail in the treatment of headaches, some of which might be appropriate for the child, but we need to be more selective and focused to select simple treatment strategies and approaches.

Press-Spheres *(Ryu)*, Press-Tack Needles *(Emp-ishin)*, and Intradermal Needles *(Hinaishin)*

On the younger child a press-sphere or 0.3 mm press-tack can be helpful applied to GV-12. If the child is under a lot of stress, applying the press-sphere or 0.3 mm press-tack to the back of the ear behind *shen men* can also be helpful.

Also, if there is a lot of stress and/or the shoulders are very stiff, apply 0.3 mm press-tack needles (0.6 mm on older children) to the most reactive points on the shoulders, usually around GB-21. Treat to keep the shoulders more relaxed. If the pain or stress is causing sleep disturbance, palpate BL-17. If the point is reactive (stiff and jumpy or painful), place 0.3 mm press-tack needles to help with the sleep disturbance.

Bunkei Ono lists GB-40 as a good treatment point for migraines when treated with an intradermal needle (Ono 1988). In my experience on adult patients the reaction at GB-41 occurs in most migraine patients and is found along the anterior-inferior face of the malleolus, usually in the slight depression in front of the malleolus. On adults I start with the 3 mm intradermal needle. On children, if this point is reactive, I recommend using a 0.3 mm press-tack needle. If not strong enough try the 0.6 mm press-tack. If still not much change occurs, try the 3 mm intradermal needle. On some adult patients with migraine this GB-40 point shows no clear reaction, in which case I have been using LV-3 instead, which usually does show a clear reaction. If this is the case on the child, use press-tack needles the same way. If the child has either migraines or general headaches as a result of medication overuse, I recommend the use of the press-tack needle to this reactive LV-3 as part of the treatment for both the liver itself and the headache.

On some patients there is a very tender point on the neck found by palpation and often related to the start of the headache. If you ask the patient if there are signs that indicate the start of the headache and if those signs are in the neck, the patient will often point to the place where you find the very sensitive point on palpation. It can be useful in some patients to leave a press-tack needle on this reactive point.

Needling—the *Chishin* or Retained Needling Method

It is more likely that you will see older children who have problems of headaches. As a consequence it is usually easy to use needling for these children. As with adults there are typical areas and acupoints to which it is good to direct attention for treatment. The occipital margin, most commonly around GB-20, can show strong reactions; these should be needled. Sometimes the reactions are more lateral around GB-12, in which case needle those reactions. In many patients with headaches there are very stiff and painful regions on the shoulders around for example GB-21, TB-15, SI-14. If the child feels stress, these are very commonly found. The interscapular region is often stiff in children with headaches; points such as BL-43, BL-16, and BL-17 often show reaction. Chronic headaches often manifest with palpable stiffness and jumpiness/pressure pain around BL-18, needle this if present. If the child seems to be a bit more run down or tired, there may also be clear reactions at BL-23. In the child in whom the headaches appear to be related to the signs of counterflow *qi* that are present (reddened appearance of the face, signs of flushing up, cool feet, emotional lability) then it can be good to apply a heat lamp over the mid- and lower back points.

The in and out needling method at LI-4 can be useful in chronic headaches.

Okyu—Direct Moxa

Okyu can be used for the treatment of headaches. Adult literature detailing treatments by *okyu* list various treatment options for headache. *Chasing the Dragon's Tail* (Manaka, Itaya, and Birch 1995) gives treatment lists from Manaka and Shiroda-Sawada for various headache treatments. I have not had to apply *okyu* specifically for headaches in children and thus have no recommendations beyond checking the points listed and seeing if they are reactive. As already discussed, use of *okyu* can be more difficult on a child than on an adult and shouldn't be used unless all other treatment options have failed.

Cupping

If the muscles of the shoulders and upper back are very stiff and change little with general

Press-tack needles (0.6 mm) were retained at bilateral LV-3.

Sixth visit—9 days later

He had a mild headache after the infusion of the infliximab, but not a migraine. Otherwise he has been well and reports some stiffening of the neck with stress.

Treatment: Using a *teishin,* supplementation was applied to left LU-9 and SP-3, draining was applied to right LV-3 and left BL-58, TB-5.
  Needles (0.16 mm) were then inserted to bilateral GB-20, BL-18, and left GB-21, and the in and out needling technique was applied in a few locations over the shoulder regions.
  Press-tack needles (0.6 mm) were retained at bilateral LV-3.

Seventh visit—5 days later

No headaches; he is doing well.

Treatment: Using a *teishin,* supplementation was applied to left LU-9 and SP-3, draining was applied to right LV-3 and left TB-5.
  Needles (0.16 mm) were then inserted to bilateral GB-20, BL-18, and left GB-21, and the in and out needling technique was applied in a few locations over the shoulder regions.
  Press-tack needles (0.6 mm) were retained at bilateral LV-3.

Eighth visit—22 days later

He had several mild headaches and one stronger headache that caused him to miss school for a day during the previous week. He reported that he thought 3 weeks was too long a gap between treatments, but scheduling problems had been unavoidable.

Treatment: Using a *teishin,* supplementation was applied to left LU-9 and SP-3, draining was applied to right LV-3 and left TB-5.
  Needles (0.16 mm) were then inserted to bilateral GB-20, BL-18, and left GB-21, and the in and out needling technique was applied in a few locations over the shoulder regions.

Press-tack needles (0.6 mm) were retained at bilateral LV-3.

Ninth visit—14 days later

He has had some daily headaches but no migraine, even after the infusion of the infliximab. When he saw his doctor the doctor advised him to increase the dose of daily tricyclic medication.

Treatment: Using a *teishin,* supplementation was applied to left LU-9 and SP-3, draining was applied to right LV-3, TB-5, and left BL-58.
  Needles (0.16 mm) were then inserted to bilateral GB-20, BL-18, and left GB-21, and the in and out needling technique was applied in a few locations over the shoulder regions.
  Press-tack needles (0.6 mm) were retained at bilateral LV-3.

Tenth visit—13 days later

He had a severe headache one day and saw the doctor, who ordered a scan. The scan showed that he might have sinusitis and the doctor prescribed a nasal spray to help with that and ordered further tests to examine the sinuses more closely. The nasal spray seems to help relieve the headaches. The patient and his parents along with the doctor are suspecting that the headaches are actually sinus headaches and that the reason for the bad headaches diagnosed as migraines is the immune suppressant action of the infliximab infusion every 6 weeks.

Treatment: Using a *teishin,* supplementation was applied to left LU-9 and SP-3, draining was applied to right LV-3 and left BL-58, right TB-5 and GB-37.
  Needles (0.16 mm) were then inserted to bilateral GB-20, BL-18, and GB-21, and the in and out needling technique was applied in a few locations over the shoulder regions.
  Press-tack needles (0.6 mm) were retained at bilateral LV-3 and at pressure pain points close to ST-1.

Eleventh visit—9 days later

He has had no headaches, but today has had some mild early signs of Crohn's-like symptoms with some abdominal pain.

Treatment: Using a *teishin,* supplementation was applied to left LU-9 and SP-3, draining was applied to right LV-3 and left BL-58, TB-5.

Needles (0.16 mm) were then inserted to bilateral GB-20, BL-18, and BL-23. A heat lamp was applied on the back over an area covering BL-18 and BL-23.

Press-tack needles (0.6 mm) were retained at bilateral GB-21.

Twelfth visit—7 days later

The abdominal pain stopped after the last treatment. He has had some very mild headache but nothing bothersome.

Treatment: Using a *teishin,* supplementation was applied to left LU-9 and SP-3, draining was applied to right LV-3, TB-5 and left SI-7.

Needles (0.16 mm) were then inserted to bilateral GB-20, BL-18, and BL-23. A heat lamp was applied on the back over an area covering BL-18 and BL-23.

Press-tack needles (0.6 mm) were retained at bilateral LV-3 and GB-21.

Thirteenth visit—8 days later

He has had no migraines and no daily headaches. The scan did not find a problem with the sinuses. The doctors now suspect that the migraines may be a side effect of the infliximab and have started to lower the dose of the tricyclic medication to stop it in a few weeks.

Treatment: Using a *teishin,* supplementation was applied to left LU-9 and SP-3, draining was applied to right LV-3, TB-5, and left BL-58.

Needles (0.16 mm) were then inserted to bilateral GB-20, BL-18, and BL-23. A heat lamp was applied on the back over an area covering BL-18 and BL-23.

Press-tack needles (0.6 mm) were retained at bilateral LV-3 and GB-21.

Fourteenth visit—15 days later

He has had no headaches, even following the administration of the infliximab infusion. He reported that in general he has noticed that his neck and

shoulders are much looser and more comfortable than before.

Treatment: Using a *teishin,* supplementation was applied to left LU-9 and SP-3, draining to right LV-3 and TB-5.

Needles (0.16 mm) were inserted to bilateral GB-20, GB-21, BL-18, and BL-23, with a heat lamp over the back covering the area of BL-18 to BL-23.

Press-tack needles (0.6 mm) were retained at bilateral LV-3 and BL-18.

Treatment has been very helpful, and Jan and his parents are very happy to continue treatments, which continue at a frequency of one to three times per month. He does not miss much school anymore and thus also feels less stress due to that. He also feels that he is able to handle everything better, which is important since he has had a very significant medical history and is very afraid of any recurrence of the Crohn's symptoms. I hope over time to develop treatment options to first try to improve the condition of his liver, using Manaka's IP-cord hepatitis treatment. Then I hope to be able later to explore the use of *okyu* to try to affect the bigger problem of the Crohn's disease because *okyu* has the reputation of helping immune-related disorders and helps regulate immune functioning in cases of autoimmune disease. His Crohn's disease doctor is planning to increase the dose of the infliximab to adjust to the fact that he is much larger than he was when it was first prescribed. The plan is to do this to further decrease the risk of experiencing symptoms of the Crohn's. At the same time he will be finishing the tricyclic medication, with potential reactions from this as well. Our plans are to monitor the effects of the increased infliximab and elimination of the tricyclic medication since it could cause problems triggering more headaches and to stick with the treatment that has been so helpful to date. Thus the plans for the liver and moxa treatments are on hold while we bring him through the current planned changes.

Case 3
June, Girl Age 13 Years

Main complaints: She has frequent headaches, three to seven times per week. She is very stressed and tired.

Despite the problem of being dyslexic, June had gotten into a good school, but found she had to work harder than before to maintain her grades. This created stress that was a clear trigger for the headaches. The lung vacuity pattern can generally result in bilateral stiffness of the shoulders. Stress often causes the shoulders and neck region to become more stiff as well. Thus an important focus for her treatment was to try to coax her neck and shoulder muscles, which are naturally a bit stiff, to become less stiff. Having tenderness along the cervical spine on palpation and having headaches when she awakes were signs that using a more supportive pillow would be good to try. Thus my main foci of treatment were to treat the underlying lung vacuity pattern, while treating to release tension in the neck and shoulder regions. In addition, she is a more replete type of person, and can easily show signs of repletion. In her case this manifests as repletion in the liver channel, which was always present and repletion in one or more yang channels. Making sure to treat this each time is also important. With follow-up treatment to help her cope with stress better and keep the tension in her neck and shoulders reduced, June can cope with school better, approach her studies feeling less stressed, and miss fewer days of school due to pain.

25 Developmental Problems

This is a broad category that includes children who, from birth, have had developmental problems, such as growth abnormalities (limbs, organs that do not develop properly or at all, spina bifida, etc.), genetic mutations, mental development problems (autism, Down syndrome, mental retardation), or complications of intrauterine growth or birthing (e.g., cerebral palsy). It also includes children who have an accident or disease that leaves them damaged (e.g., mental development problems due to head trauma, loss of locomotor function due to viral infection, such as polio). The text by Yoneyama and Mori (1964) discusses the treatment of polio sequelae. Although we hardly ever see such patients today, we can apply some of the same principles of treatment more generally.

Many of the children with these types of problems usually need special care. Most commonly we see children with these problems who are not institutionalized and live at home with their parents. They are often receiving special medical care or go to special schools that cater to their needs. In some children there is a single problem, such as nonuse of the legs; in others a broad spectrum of problems affects multiple developmental and functional systems. In some children the treatment helps create real substantial change and improvements. In others, the treatment helps lessen difficulties and improves function, mood, performance, and the child's quality of life. It can also create a better environment and improve the child's interaction with his or her environment.

Case 1
Catherine, Girl Age Almost 3 Years

Just 3 weeks before going on a summer-long study trip to Japan I received a phone call from a mother in New York, a 1-hour flight away. She had gotten my name because she was looking for an acupuncturist who treated children, and she had not been able to find anyone closer. Her daughter Catherine had been born with cerebral palsy. At that time she was around 33 months old.

Main complaints: She had no use of her legs. If she was laid down she could not push herself into a sitting position. She was unable to walk, even with assistance. Catherine was under care at the local children's hospital. She was primarily managed by a pediatric neurologist and was seeing a pediatric physical therapist to see what else could be offered. The neurologist had recently indicated that, because there was no change in Catherine's condition, he was projecting that she would probably end up either in a wheelchair or, if lucky, she might be able to walk wearing metal braces as support, but that did not seem likely. The mother was not happy to hear this; it indicated that the doctors could not offer much more help for Catherine. The mother reported that Catherine had no problems with the arms, head, or neck. She had normal control of bladder emptying and bowel movements. Her appetite was good, and she was quite a quick-minded, concentrated child. Could I help, and if so, how should we proceed?

We arranged for the mother to bring Catherine up to Boston by plane early the next week to come for a 1-hour appointment where we would start treatment. Once scheduled, I thought about what could realistically be done. In cases such as this, the literature in Japan suggests regular *shonishin* can be helpful, but that one often needs to use *okyu*/direct moxa on the lower back to help trigger change. I was concerned about the lack of time we had to schedule many treatments, given that I was leaving soon for Japan. Also, while I wanted to have the mother start doing home treatment as soon as possible, I felt I could not apply direct moxa without the ability to be present at follow-up and certainly could not imagine having the parent try home moxa without my supervision. Thus I planned to do a short core non-pattern-based root treatment, apply minimal light symptomatic treatment, and spend the rest of the hour teaching the mother how to do treatment daily at home. I saw Catherine before I had properly learned Meridian Therapy and thus was unable to add any specific pattern-based add in and out insertion to acupoints such as LI-4, LI-10, and LI-11. If the shoulders or interscapular regions are very stiff and there are knots in those regions, you can apply in and out needling on these knots on older children. For problems of the lower limbs, if additional tapping has not been helpful, you can add in and out insertion to acupoints such as ST-36, GB-34. You may also find knots on the low back/buttock regions, such as lateral to the sides of the sacrum. Needling these knots can also be helpful.

Press-Spheres (Ryu), Press-Tack Needles (Empishin), and Intradermal Needles (Hinaishin)

Press-spheres or press-tack needles are usually safe to use for musculoskeletal problems, provided the child is not very run down or overly sensitive. Leaving press-spheres on GV-12 for upper limb problems and around GV-3 to GV-4 for lower limb problems can be helpful. If you leave press-spheres or press-tack needles on other points or areas, make sure to use appropriate dosage levels for the child. Because many children will be kidney vacuity pattern, leaving something on BL-23 bilaterally can be useful, provided you have paid attention to the dose.

For children with mental development problems, the dose needs to be much more carefully controlled. If you leave anything, leave only press-spheres to start with. Only use stronger dose techniques like press-tack needles when you are more certain of how the child responds to treatment. The extra point behind shen men on the ear can be treated with press-spheres. If you find a lot of stiffness or knots on the upper back, especially in the interscapular region, you can apply treatment to those to help reduce the reactions; it is especially helpful to focus on reactions at BL-15 or BL-14 if they are present.

Okyu—Direct Moxa

If the problem includes paralysis or problems of use of the upper limbs it is recommended to apply moxa to GV-12 (Irie 1980; Shiroda 1986), GV-13, or GV-14 (Yoneyama and Mori 1964). If the problem includes paralysis or problems with use of the lower limbs apply moxa to GV-4 (Yoneyama and Mori 1964) or GV-3 (Shiroda 1986). In general, for something like cerebral palsy GV-8 can also be treated with moxa (Irie 1980), especially when there are problems of muscle spasticity. Shiroda (1986) mentions use of okyu on GV-12, BL-18, GV-3, and GB-34 for "childhood polio," which, given the rarity of this today, we can interpret to mean disorders resulting in diminished or lost use of muscles, with difficulty of use of the limbs. If you are thinking of trying the direct moxa treatment, palpate the spine first to see which points are more reactive (exhibit pressure pain, cause the child to flinch or move away), and apply moxa to the more reactive points.

Cupping and Bloodletting

In general these techniques are not often mentioned for treatment of this range of problems. If you use either technique be especially careful of dose, and limit its use for children with locomotor problems rather than mental development problems.

Other Considerations

Home Treatment

As is illustrated in Case 1, giving the parents tools for home treatment can be very helpful as a way of empowering the parents and speeding up treatment progress. It is more difficult when there are mental development problems to give advice for home treatment. You need to spend more time observing the child's responses to your treatments to better understand sensitivity and dose requirements. But for other, more physical, developmental problems, the home treatment can be started as soon as feasible. Again, make sure that you exercise care with the more run down or very sensitive child. For home treatment, using the simple combination of soft stroking mixed with light tapping is usually a good idea.

Further Case Histories

The next case is of a child with a severe disorder due to genetic mutation with physical, neurological, and mental developmental problems.

Case 2
Dianne, Girl Age Almost 4 Years

Main complaints and history: Dianne had Rett syndrome. She had a complex of problems that included the following:

- Significant neuromuscular problems; repeated forceful hand-mouthing, and some biting of hard objects, resulting in irritation of skin of the hands around the thumbs; excessive salivation
- Problems with locomotor coordination; poor gait and instability walking; pronation of feet, especially the right foot, left leg weaker and not as well developed as the right leg; mild scoliosis; some weakness of arms and wrists
- Mental abnormalities and autistic tendencies
- General problems, such as the tendency to have diarrhea and the need to continue wearing diapers because of the inability to self-regulate bowels or urine

Her parents were told that this condition can be progressive and that she needed regular monitoring and possibly strong interventions in the future.[1] She had no history of surgery or hospitalization. She received craniosacral therapy regularly, and her parents were trying a variety of different techniques at home to help with the locomotor problems and mental abnormalities. Although her manifestations were so far quite mild, it was unclear how far the problems might develop. However, she did not appear to be excessively weak. We decided it was worthwhile trying a course of at least eight treatments to see what the treatment did for her.

Examination: She appeared to be quite wary and scared. It was difficult to remove her thumbs from her mouth because of her lack of ease with the new situation. The muscles over the neck, shoulders, back, jaw, and face were very stiff. Left deep pulses were stronger than right deep pulses. Abdominal diagnosis was difficult, but there were indications of a little softness below the navel and depression in the lung reflex area on the right.

Diagnosis: Based on her pulse and other findings, the lung vacuity pattern was chosen. Stomach and/or large intestine channel involvement was suspected because of the jaw tightness and mouthing/biting problems.

Treatment: Using a *herabari*, light tapping was applied over the arms, legs, neck, shoulders, head, and back.

Light stroking was applied down the legs and abdomen using an *enshin*.

Supplementation was applied to right LU-9 and SP-3 using a *teishin*.

Stainless-steel press-spheres were applied to GV-12 and bilateral BL-23.

Second visit—15 days later

At times, the pronation of the right foot was better. She seemed to have greater ease climbing the stairs, and had possibly shown a little more presence with her parents. The press-spheres had caused a minor skin irritation.

Treatment: Using a *herabari,* light tapping was applied over the arms, legs, back, abdomen, neck, shoulders, head, and jaw.

Light stroking with an *enshin* was applied down the back and the neck.

Using a *teishin,* supplementation was applied to right LU-9 and SP-3.

Stainless-steel press-spheres were left around GV-13 and bilateral BL-23.

Third visit—20 days later

She was much more active than usual. She was hand-mouthing a little less, but biting things a little harder (as compensation?). Her hands were warmer. She seemed to be a little more functional and more responsive to parental requests.

Treatment: Using a *herabari*, light tapping was applied over the arms, legs, back, abdomen, neck, shoulders, head, and jaw.

Light stroking with an *enshin* was applied down the arms and legs.

Using a *teishin*, supplementation was applied to right LU-9 and SP-3.

Stainless-steel press-spheres were left around bilateral TB-17 and bilateral BL-52.

---

[1] The scoliosis, for example, is usually progressive so that Rett syndrome sufferers often require surgery.

Fourth visit—6 days later

There were no clear changes to report. Maybe she was hand-mouthing less, but it was not clear.

Treatment: Using a *herabari*, light tapping was applied over the arms, legs, back, abdomen, neck, shoulders, head, and jaw.
 Light stroking with an *enshin* was applied down the arms, legs, and back.
 Using a *teishin*, supplementation was applied to right LU-9 and SP-3.
 Stainless-steel press-spheres were left around bilateral ST-37 and bilateral BL-23.

Fifth visit—2 weeks later

She had had a bad flu the week before but was now recovered. No clear changes in her condition.

Treatment: Tapping over arms, legs, abdomen, chest, back, neck, head, and jaw with the *herabari.* Stroking was applied down the arms, legs, and back with the *enshin.*
 Using a *teishin*, LU-9 and SP-3 were supplemented and left LR-3 was drained.
 Press-spheres were left at bilateral BL-23 and ST-40.

Sixth visit—1 week later

Treatment was very similar to the last visit.

Seventh visit—1 week later

Treatment was again similar to the last visit, with the exception of the insertion of needles (0.12 mm) shallowly for ~30 seconds to GB-20. After this the parents reported a small reduction in the hand-mouthing and more use of the hands for pointing at things.

Eighth visit—1 week later

Treatment was similar to the last visit.

Ninth visit—2 weeks later

The parents reported that her sleep was better, she was walking better, hand-mouthing was better, and that there was more use of her hands. She was more sociable and made more efforts at oral communication. Because of this apparent success, the same treatment as the last were repeated. This produced an immediate adverse reaction. She became very fearful, tired, and unwilling to walk. She needed to sleep a lot after treatment. These symptoms persisted over the next few days. It was obvious that she had been overtreated.

Tenth visit—1 week later

Her locomotor abilities had regressed this week, while her hand-mouthing remained somewhat improved. A lighter variation of the same treatment was given with light needling at ST-36 instead of GB-20. A week later her walking was still not so good, and the same treatment was repeated.
 At this time my teacher, Toshio Yanagishita, was visiting. On consulting him it became clear that a much lighter treatment should be given, eliminating the tapping with the *herabari* and replacing it with extremely light stroking with the *teishin* along the stomach and large intestine channels, down the abdomen and back and neck regions. He also advised that her pattern was a kidney pattern and that she should be treated as such. He also commented that, in cases like hers, the spleen was typically slightly replete, but that this should be treated by supplementing ST-36.

Twelfth visit—2 weeks later

Treatment: Following the recommendations of Mr. Yanagishita, the treatment consisted of applying very light stroking with the *teishin* down the large intestine and stomach channels on the arms and legs, twice each channel, down the abdomen twice, down each side of the back twice, and down the neck twice, with a light rubbing with the *enshin* down the back of each leg. Supplementation was applied to right KI-7, LU-5, and left ST-36.
 This revised treatment worked better for Dianne, with more consistent improvement and no more adverse reactions due to overtreatment. Over the next 8 months, 22 similar treatments were applied with small variations. Her symptoms overall gradually improved. Occasionally draining techniques were added to points like TB-5, GB-37, and BL-58. Press-spheres were left on points like ST-36,

GV-12, and BL-23. At the end of these 8 months of treatments she went to a special clinic for a full evaluation of her condition. The doctors were very surprised that her scoliosis had not progressed at all (usually it progresses in this syndrome) and that her back seemed to be in quite good shape. Her walking was clearly better. Her hand-mouthing was clearly better; she was also more communicative and participatory. The medical team that evaluated her recommended that the parents apply a daily tactile stimulation on her body by using soft brushes and brushing on the torso and limbs. The parents started doing this at home daily.

Fifteen similar treatments were given over the next 6 months. During this time, she became more participatory and started interacting with other children better. Her walking became more stable. However, she showed increasing signs of counterflow *qi,* with stronger and stronger emotional outbursts, especially angry outbursts, and showed repeated flushing of the face, neck, and shoulders. She became extremely ticklish, and showed increasingly difficult resistant behavior. She would show signs of hyperactivity and signs of extreme fatigue as well. While the home treatments that the parents were doing daily seemed to be helping her physical coordination, it seemed that she was being overstimulated and had developed counterflow *qi* reactions as a result. The parents were advised about the possibility that this was happening and that they should cut back on or stop the home brushing. Also, after consulting Mr. Yanagishita again, the side of treatment was changed to the left side and the treatment was made lighter again. At the 50th treatment supplementation was applied to left KI-10 and LU-5[2] with right ST-36.

Following this change in treatment side, she started becoming less irritable, could sleep better, and showed fewer signs of counterflow *qi*. As she became calmer she became more communicative again. But the brushing was continued. Five similar treatments were applied over the next 2 months, then she returned to the special clinic for a further evaluation. They were very pleased with her progress but stated that she seemed to be too sensitive to the tactile stimulation and that it should be cut back to only a very small amount

each day. Over the next 8 months, 21 treatments were given. During this time her concentration and social skills improved. She tried using words more to communicate. She had been assessed by another team and was found to show skills with numbers and counting. She remained calmer, laughing and playing more. She was less scared by change and was more nimble on her feet. Her parents were very pleased with her progress. It is not possible to cure a child of Rett syndrome, but during the 29 months of treatment her condition did not become progressively worse, which is very unusual for Rett syndrome. Her hand-mouthing and biting of hard objects significantly improved, her locomotor coordination improved, her communication skills were better, as were her socializing skills. She showed signs of understanding more things around her and was better able to follow simple instructions in task performance.

The following case illustrates how my colleague Mourad Bihman from Berlin, Germany, treated a boy with severe behavioral problems that had been diagnosed with extreme hyperactivity by one doctor and autism by the next. As Mourad described it, "I wanted to report on this case because of the incredible progress he made during the first treatments. It clearly shows how big the effect of minimum stimulation treatment can be on small children. What I also consider worth mentioning is that after those initially tremendous changes it took time and patience to make further progress." This is often what we see treating children when the treatment works.

Case 3
Bert, Boy Age 4½ Years

When Bert first came for treatment, he did not speak, meaning he did not form any words but made sounds to communicate (sometimes extremely high-pitched screaming). He did not stand still and was running around in the clinic while his mother was answering questions. He had a very short attention span, even if he seemed interested in something. His muscle tonus was very high, and he had well-developed muscles due to his permanent tension and movement. He would tense up his arms and/or legs or the whole body every minute and then relax for a second before starting to

---

[2]   The *he*-sea points were used because of their recommended use for counterflow *qi* in the *Nan Jing (Classic of Difficulties)*, Chapter 68.

run in circles again. He did not have any social contact with his family because he was very difficult to handle. He could hear well and follow instructions, but his restlessness and inability to communicate made social interaction almost impossible.

History: Until the age of 2½ years he developed normally. He had started to speak, but later than others. Then, for no apparent reason, he became increasingly silent and withdrew from the outside world. At the same time he developed this extreme form of activity as described above. He was diagnosed as hyperactive by one doctor and as autistic by another. He was receiving pediatric occupational therapy. He also had gluten intolerance, and after this diagnosis his diet was changed to be gluten-free. He took omega-3 and -6 supplements as prescribed by a doctor. No other therapy was recommended.

Assessment: It was not possible to take his pulse or feel his channels or his abdomen for diagnostic assessment. He could not be persuaded to lie down on the treatment table or to stop moving. So, on this first visit, he was treated underneath the table because that was a place he stopped to rest for a minute.

Diagnosis: The kidney vacuity pattern was chosen with probable weakness of the heart channel.

Treatment: Using a *teishin*, KI-7 and LU-5 were supplemented on the left and HT-7 was supplemented on the right.

While I was treating KI-7 he stared in awe and was completely still and silent so it was possible to go on treating LU-5 and HT-7 with the appropriate low dose. This stillness lasted for ~1 to 2 minutes, during which he looked astonished and relaxed. He was scheduled to come in for treatment twice a week.

Second visit—3 days later

He was calmer than usual on the way home and more perceptive on the evening of the treatment.

Treatment: A *teishin* was used to supplement left KI-7, LU-5, and right HT-7.

Using a *herabari*, light tapping was applied over the neck and head, especially around GV-20.

Third visit—4 days later

The occupational therapist had for the first time been able to work with him in a concentrated manner for 20 minutes. He was more interested in the world around him. He was also calmer, and better communication seemed possible. He came in for treatment in an excited (not overactive) state and was very keen to be treated (knocking on and opening the treatment door several times then immediately jumping on the treatment table).

Treatment: Using a *teishin*, left KI-7, LU-5, and right HT-7 were supplemented.

Gold-plated press-spheres were placed on BL-23.

Fourth visit—3 days later

He was more relaxed again and seemed to be in a good mood.

Treatment: The same treatment as the last visit, with a gold-plated press-sphere that was left on GV-12 instead of BL-23.

Fifth visit—3 days later

He had been less restless.

Treatment: The same treatment was given as on the last visit.

The sixth through eighth treatments were identical to the fifth. After the eighth treatment, stroking of the *yang* channels using an *enshin* was added, and the mother was taught this stroking as homework to be done daily using a spoon. The stroking was applied down the arms and legs (stomach and bladder channels), down the back, and down the abdomen.

Treatment continued for another 30 sessions with slight variations, but all of them included stroking of the *yang* channels and treating the combination of KI-7, LU-5, and HT-7. Usually gold-plated press-spheres were placed on GV-12, but if this irritated him CV-12 was used instead.

He continued to make progress up to a stage where he was much calmer, more concentrated, more perceptive, and much easier to handle for his family. His extreme hyperactive behavior significantly improved.

During the last 10 treatments there were no further signs of improvement so the parents decided to take a break in treatment and continue with the home treatment. It was not possible to obtain follow-up information on how he progressed after stopping treatment.

The following case from my colleague in Seattle, Brenda Loew, is of a girl with facial atrophy from birth. Treatment was helpful to trigger more normal functioning of the facial nerves that had been diagnosed as damaged and non-functioning.

Case 4
Rebecca, Girl Age 3 Years

She and her family were vacationing in Seattle for the summer when treatment began.

Main complaints: Rebecca presented with left-sided facial atrophy since birth. The doctors at that time had diagnosed that three out of five facial nerves functioned normally, while two facial nerves did not function normally, resulting in no upper forehead flexion or downward frown function. She wakened occasionally at night and evidenced occasional irritability. Otherwise she had no other problems.

Examination: There was a U-shaped area of weakness in the lower abdomen involving the entire inguinal area. The rest of the abdomen showed fairly good luster and tone. The left wrist pulse was overall slightly weaker than the right.

Diagnosis: These two signs together indicated a clear liver vacuity pattern.

Treatment: Using a *teishin*, right LR-8 and KI-10 were supplemented.
Light warmth was applied over the affected side of the face using a "Tiger warmer."[3]
Light stroking was applied down the back using an *enshin*.

Second visit—2 days later

The parents had nothing to report.

Treatment: In addition to applying the same treatment as the first session, supplementation to left LU-9 was added, as was light stroking with a needle[4] around the eyes, eyebrows, mouth, face, and entire head, particularly the left posterior skull region.

Third visit—2 weeks later

Since the last treatment she had had nerve conduction exams, which determined that she did have nerve conduction in all five cranial nerves and that the muscles were slightly atrophied in the left forehead and mouth area.

Treatment: The same treatment as on the second visit was repeated.

Fourth visit—1 week later

The parents had nothing to report.

Treatment: The same treatment as on the second visit was repeated.

Fifth visit—5 days later

Her mother had noticed more mobility in Rebecca's left cheek and side of the mouth.

Treatment: The same treatment as on the second visit was repeated.
After this the family returned home where Rebecca continued receiving *shonishin* treatments from a colleague.
Two years later at age 5, Rebecca returned for further treatments. It was clear that she had significantly more mobility in her left mouth, forehead, and cheek. Her parents had recently separated, and the child appeared slightly irritable during the first treatment.

---

3   This is a metal tubular hand-held instrument that holds burning incense within it. As the incense burns, the casing warms up, and one can apply a massage-like technique with the instrument.

4   In Japan the technique is called the *sanshin*, or contact needle technique. There are many different styles of *sanshin* among traditional acupuncture practitioners in Japan. When treating children it is important that the point of the needle is held safely so that as the needle body is stroked lightly over the skin the needle tip cannot prick the child.

Treatment: Using a *teishin*, right KI-7 and LU-5 were supplemented.

Using a *Yoneyama zanshin*, stroking was applied lightly down the leg and arm *yang* channels.

Using the *teishin*, light tapping was applied around the ears and along the occiput. KI-2 was also tapped bilaterally.

Press-spheres were placed on CV-12 and GV-12.

Reflection: Tia came for treatment over a period of a year and a half, sometimes with gaps between sessions as long as 6 weeks, but more generally coming in every 3 weeks or so. The treatments were all as described above, which is to say a fairly routine approach was taken, even though the condition is serious. In that time she experienced only one ear infection, and that was after coming back from a family vacation during which she ate a lot of sweets. I last saw Tia for a treatment 3 years ago. In the final treatment the last thing she said as she left the room was, "I love you, Bob." It was the first time she had said that, and it was a comment worth a million dollars to me, as she had become very dear to me. Her dad followed up with me in an email 6 months ago telling me that Tia is doing very well developmentally. She is happy and exceeding all expectations. Her mother still regularly, though not daily, does the stroking treatment with her special penny.

This case illustrates again how an extremely light and simple *shonishin* treatment coupled with a basic Meridian Therapy treatment can not only stop the problem of recurrent ear infections, it seemingly contributes toward better development for a child genetically predisposed toward having developmental problems. Bob's elegance of treatment is apparent in his ability to stick with such a simple repeatable treatment.

26 Weak Constitution

This is a broad category that refers to the child who has had, from birth, recurrent problems because of a constitutional weakness. In their description of this, Yoneyama and Mori (1964) recommend the basic core treatment and then additionally the use of moxa on BL-18 and BL-20 and possibly GV-12, which would seem to target respiratory and digestive symptoms. Shimizu (1975) differentiates three basic types of weak constitution: (1) the respiratory type with chronic respiratory symptoms, (2) the digestive type with chronic digestive symptoms, and (3) the combined respiratory and digestive type with chronic digestive and respiratory symptoms, and he provides more extensive treatment descriptions. However, as a Meridian Therapist I think that the descriptions of this category are limited. Following the patterns in Meridian Therapy, I identify four distinct weak constitution patterns, based on which I recommend differentiated treatments.[1]

There are some important features associated with these weak constitutions. The problems are usually present from birth, though it is possible that they can be caused by accidents or infections after birth, starting soon after those events. There are often signs apparent in the structure and build of the child, for example, being thinly muscled, being small-boned, having a flat rib cage, having shoulders pulled back (Shimizu 1975). The child is often very sensitive (Shimizu 1975; see discussions of sensitivity in Chapter 4, this volume) and usually has one or more symptoms present all the time.

The child's problems may respond to regular medical therapy, such as drug interventions, but they recur soon after the therapy is discontinued. Some types of constitutional weakness can recover with treatment, other types cannot. For the latter types (e.g., autism, mental retardation, birth defects, severe cerebral palsy), the words of my teacher, Toshio Yanagishita, are very important: you have to be realistic, you cannot fix these problems, but you can help lessen their manifestations, improve the child's quality of life, and help the parents in their continuous efforts to care for their child. There are some cases where you may feel that you really can't do anything because the problems seem so severe. When such feelings occur, you need to deal with the following:

- Put aside your own insecurity in the face of such problems and remember that it is most likely that this child will not improve if left untreated. Therefore, trying a few treatments to see if anything seems to change is a realistic investment for the parent.
- Make a realistic assessment of what is possible and inform the parent of the assessment— for example, informing the parent of an autistic child that you cannot cure the autism, but you will try treatments that you and they can apply to make its manifestations easier to deal with. In this case, you are giving the parents tools for helping with the daily life of their child. You are not only trying to help the child have fewer symptoms, but you are also helping the parents to develop more skills in the child's care and the management of the child's condition; you are not trying to "cure" the child.
- Think about an adjusted cost of treatment for the parents because they will likely need to return over the long term once you have agreed that treatment is worth trying.
- Trust the judgments of the parent with regard to assessing how the child is doing. When you see a child only once a week and do not have to participate in the child's daily

---

[1] I do not follow another idea of Shimizu who describes the broad category of *kanmushi* (see Chapter 21) as a sign of weak constitution and then relates this to evolving 20th century models of developmental stages (Shimizu 1975). I prefer to stay within the framework of traditional acupuncture because it allows both the usual core non-pattern-based root treatment approach and a specific pattern-based treatment approach, which in my experience is usually more rapid acting than either alone. It has not only to do with how I treat patients but practically it allows two different root treatment approaches that can be used together.

General Approach for Patients with Weak Constitution

You must assume from the start that the child is more sensitive than other patients. Thus, trying a softer, milder treatment to begin with is generally important (review Chapter 4 for discussions of this and Chapter 7 for discussions of how to modify the core treatment). Once you have an idea of how the child responds to treatment, you can gradually increase the dose by adding or replacing treatment methods.

Figuring out a simple core non-pattern-based treatment and using that regularly is important, as is teaching the parent to start using this at home. Applying a simple pattern-based treatment according to the pattern type of constitutional weakness is also important. Here it is often useful to focus on the manifestations and symptoms to choose the pattern rather than the usual diagnostic methods of pulse and abdomen. Some patients show combined constitutional weakness, such as the patient with severe atopic dermatitis with airborne, contact, and food allergy triggers (combination of lung and spleen types); the child who both has severe eczema since birth and does not gain weight due to food allergies, poor appetite, chronic diarrhea (combination spleen and lung types); the child with mental development problems as well as severe gastrointestinal disturbance with food allergies (combination kidney and spleen types).

Goals of Treatment

Treat to improve the constitutional weakness. Where feasible, apply treatment to target symptoms. For example, for the child with mental retardation, symptomatic treatment can be difficult, but the root treatments (pattern-based and core non-pattern-based) can start creating change in daily activities and parental care of the child.

Root Treatment for the Lung Weak Constitution Type

Core Non-pattern-based Root Treatment
Apply light stroking down the arms, legs, back, abdomen, and chest (*do not do this if the child has*

skin problems; see Chapter 19 on skin problems). Apply light tapping around GV-12.

If the child has respiratory problems additional tapping can be applied around LU-1 and the area around ST-12 (**Fig. 26.1**).

Lung Vacuity Pattern Treatment
Apply supplementation to LU-9 and SP-3. If the child is very run down and weak, the skin feels too soft or loose, also supplement bilateral TB-4 or ST-36. Generally do not apply draining techniques until the child is stronger. If the child has severe skin symptoms try LU-5 and SP-9 instead of LU-9, SP-3 for the treatment of the primary pattern.[4]

Additional Treatment
Place a press-sphere or new press-tack to GV-12.

If the symptoms in the lungs are very severe or there are recurrent infections, try applying *okyu* instead to GV-12.

If the child has chronic skin problems, tap or apply moxa to the relevant large intestine channel points (see Chapter 19, pp. 135 and 136)

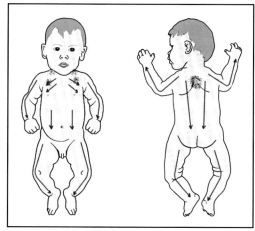

Fig. 26.1   Lightly stroke down:
- Down the back (bladder channel)
- Down the abdomen (stomach channel)
- Down the legs (stomach and bladder channels)
- Down the arms (*yang* channels)
- Across the chest

For a lung pattern add tapping:
- Around GV-12, possibly LU-1 and ST-12 regions

---

[4]   This recommendation comes from my teacher Akihiro Takai (personal communication). According to *Nan Jing* (*Classic of Difficulties*), Chapter 68, *he*-sea points are good for counterflow *qi* manifestations.

instead of applying the core non-pattern-based root treatment with stroking and tapping.

Shimizu's (1975) recommended treatments for the respiratory type are useful to consider. *Okyu*/direct moxa can be applied to BL-12, GV-12, GV-10, LU-5, or LU-6, BL-23 with needling of KI-26, LU-1, BL-11, and BL-17, depending on current symptoms (e.g., easily fatigued, easily catches cold, recurrent fevers, swollen tonsils, bronchitis, chronically swollen lymph nodes in the neck) and reactions in the acupoints. This list of acupoints offers additional options to be added over successive treatments on top of the core root treatment methods.

Root Treatment for the Spleen Weak Constitution Type

Core Non-pattern-based Root Treatment
Apply light stroking down the arms, legs, back, abdomen, and chest. Apply light tapping around GV-12, CV-12, and from GV-3 to GV-4. The area around ST-36 to ST-37 can also be lightly tapped. It can also be helpful to lightly tap around BL-18 and BL-20 (**Fig. 26.2**).

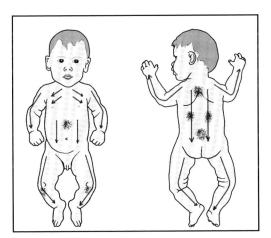

Fig. 26.2 Lightly stroke down:
- Down the back (bladder channel)
- Down the abdomen (stomach channel)
- Down the legs (stomach and bladder channels)
- Down the arms (*yang* channels)
- Across the chest

For a spleen pattern add tapping:
- Around GV-12, CV-12, GV-3, and possibly around ST-36–ST-37, and BL-18–BL-20

Spleen Vacuity Pattern Treatment
Apply supplementation to SP-3 and PC-7. If the child is very run down and weak, and the skin feels too soft or too loose, also supplement KI-3 on the other side and bilateral ST-36. Generally do not apply draining techniques until the child is stronger.

Additional Treatment
Place a press-sphere to GV-12. Also place press-spheres to BL-18 on one side and BL-20 on the other.

If the child is not responding sufficiently to treatment and/or the symptoms are very severe, apply *okyu* instead to BL-18 on one side and BL-20 on the other. The general rule for selecting which side for boys is left BL-18, right BL-20, and for girls, right BL-18, left BL-20. Although some moxa specialists recommend applying the moxa bilaterally (Irie 1980), it is better to use this contralateral treatment because it reduces the number of points you have to treat, reducing by half the amount of irritation and distress the treatment can cause. A press-sphere can be placed at CV-12 as well, if reactive.

If the child has food allergies, apply moxa to the extra point *uranaitei* (below *nei ting*—ST-44) on the bottom of the foot. This is a special point for food allergies (see Chapter 16, p. 105 for the point location).

Shimizu's (1975) recommended treatments for the digestive type of weak constitution are useful to consider. *Okyu*/direct moxa can be applied to GV-12, BL-23, right BL-18, left BL-20 with needling of CV-12, KI-16, or ST-25, LR-13, ST-36, depending on current symptoms (e.g., poor appetite, frequent abdominal pain, diarrhea) and reactions in the acupoints. This list of acupoints offers more options to be added over successive treatments on top of the core root treatment methods.

Root Treatment for the Kidney Weak Constitution Type

Core Non-pattern-based Root Treatment
Apply light stroking down the arms, legs, back, abdomen, and chest and light tapping around GV-12 and GV-3. If the problems are of mental development,

Diagnosis: The kidney, liver, and spleen areas of the abdomen showed signs of reaction. Her pulse was slightly floating, slightly rapid and weak. Weakest pulses: liver and kidney, spleen. Conclusion: liver vacuity pattern with spleen also vacuous.

Treatment: Because she was a more mature girl, the core non-pattern-based root treatment was not used. She was not particularly afraid of the treatment.

Using regular needles,[8] supplementation was applied to left LR-8, KI-10, and right SP-3. Right ST-40 and BL-58 were drained.

Symptomatic treatment: Using the theory of midday–midnight, LU-7 was supplemented to help reduce symptoms in the bladder.

Second visit—1 week later

The hip had felt better for 3 days. The bladder problem was a bit better, not hurting as much

Treatment: Using non-inserted needling method, left LR-8, KI-10, and right LU-9 were supplemented with 0.18 mm silver needles. Draining was applied to right SI-7.

CV-6, BL-18, and BL-23 were supplemented bilaterally to support the root treatment.

Light stroking was applied down the back and the backs of the legs using an *enshin.*

A press-sphere was retained at GV-12 as home therapy.

Light needling was applied to tight areas in the lateral abdomen regions and around the right hip.[9]

A moxa stick was applied over the spine to warm it.

Third visit—1 week later

The hip felt better and she was finding it easier to walk. The bladder did not hurt as much as before starting acupuncture.

Treatment: Using regular needles, left LR-8, KI-10, and right LU-9 were supplemented. Right SI-7 and GB-37 were drained.

CV-6, BL-18, and BL-23 were supplemented bilaterally to support the root treatment.

Press-spheres were retained at GV-12, right BL-18, and left BL-23 to support the root treatment.

Light needling was applied to tight areas in the lateral abdomen regions and around the right hip and the supraclavicular fossa region.[10]

*Chinetsukyu/*warm moxa was applied to CV-3 for the bladder.

LU-7 was also supplemented with a needle to help reduce symptoms in the bladder.

Fourth visit—1 week later

She had found it harder to control her urination this week. She had stumbled and fallen the day before but recovered well. The hip felt all right, though she had been wakened by pain two or three times this week. She was also having problems with nosebleeds (reported by her mother to be due to the diclofenac).

Treatment: Examination showed a kidney vacuity pattern rather than the usual liver pattern.

Using regular needles, left KI-7, LU-5, and right SP-3 were supplemented. Left SI-7 and LI-6 were drained.

BL-13 and BL-23 were supplemented bilaterally to support the root treatment.

Press-spheres were retained at GV-12 and bilateral BL-23.

Light needling was applied to the supraclavicular fossa region.

A moxa stick was applied over the spine to warm it.

Fifth visit—1 week later

She continued having problems with nosebleeds. Sometimes she found it difficult to fall asleep because of the hip pain. However, although the hip had been quite sore she had still been able to get down stairs by herself using the banisters as support. Urination still hurt but seemed overall easier.

Treatment: Examination showed the usual liver vacuity pattern.

---

[8]   In the style and using the methods of the Toyohari system of Meridian Therapy.

[9]   This is called *muno* treatment in Toyohari (Fukushima 1991; Birch and Ida 2001; Yanagishita 2001b).

[10]   This is called *naso* treatment in Toyohari (Fukushima 1991; Birch and Ida 2001; Yanagishita 2001a).

Using regular needles, left LR-8, KI-10, and right LU-9 were supplemented, left GB-37 and BL-58 were drained.

Light stroking was applied down the back and the backs of the legs using an *enshin*.

BL-18 and BL-23 were supplemented bilaterally to support the root treatment.

Press-spheres were retained at GV-12, left BL-18, and right BL-23 to support the root treatment.

Light needling was applied to the lower abdomen and supraclavicular fossa regions.

A moxa stick was applied over the spine to warm it.

Sixth visit—2 weeks later

This week she had found it easier to get down the stairs without help. She had had a problem with alternating diarrhea and constipation. She was able to urinate more freely now with less distress. But she had still had problems with nosebleeds the last two mornings. Because she was feeling better she had tried cutting out the lunchtime tablet of diclofenac.

Treatment: An overall lighter treatment was applied.

Using regular needles left LR-8, KI-10, and right LU-9 were supplemented, left GB-37 and BL-58 were drained.

Light needling was applied to the lower abdomen region.

A mild warm moxa stick technique was applied over the abdomen for the bladder.

Seventh visit—1 week later

She was still having problems with nosebleeds, but had been all right without the lunchtime tablet of diclofenac. Her pain overall was better. Urination was now much better.

Treatment: Treatment was similar to the previous session.

Eighth visit—3 weeks later

She was much better, and some days she did not take the diclofenac. Urination had improved further. Nosebleeds were less frequent and sleep was better, but one day before this visit she had fallen and irritated her back and hip.

Treatment: Using regular needles left LR-8, KI-10, and right SP-3 were supplemented.

BL-18 and BL-23 were supplemented bilaterally to support the root treatment.

Press-spheres were retained at GV-12, left BL-18, and right BL-23 to support the root treatment.

Light needling was applied to the lower abdomen and supraclavicular fossa regions.

A moxa stick was applied over the spine to warm it.

Okyu/direct moxa was applied to *josen* (an extra point below L5; see Chapter 16, p. 105).

Ninth visit—2 weeks later

She reported that she was doing well. She could now go up the stairs on her own. She was walking more, had more stamina, and was coping better. Urination was still a bit uncomfortable but much easier. She was still having some problems with nosebleeds at night. She had only taken diclofenac once or twice a week. Overall sleep was better, and abdominal discomfort was better.

Treatment: Using regular needles, left LR-8, KI-10, and right SP-3 were supplemented.

BL-18 and BL-23 were supplemented bilaterally to support the root treatment.

Press-spheres were retained at GV-12, left BL-18, and right BL-23 to support the root treatment.

Light needling was applied to the lower abdomen and supraclavicular fossa regions.

A moxa stick was applied over the spine to warm it.

Okyu/direct moxa was applied to *josen* and BL-28.

After this, the next four visits were similar as she continued improving.

Fourteenth visit—4 months later

She was doing much better. She had stopped taking diclofenac, occasionally needing paracetamol for pain relief. Her mobility was improving; she was now able to run up and down stairs, the hip and back were much better, and she was walking more easily. She was able to go on longer walks with the dog. Urination was satisfactory.

Treatment: Using regular needles, left LR-8, KI-10, and right SP-3 were supplemented.

BL-18 and BL-23 were supplemented bilaterally to support the root treatment.

Press-spheres were retained at GV-12, left BL-18, and right BL-23 to support the root treatment.

Light needling was applied to the lower abdomen and supraclavicular fossa regions.

A moxa stick was applied over the spine to warm it.

Okyu/direct moxa was applied to josen, BL-28, and GV-12.

Fifteenth visit—6 weeks later

She had had a review at the hospital the previous Friday—everything was fine. She had grown 4 cm in the last 4 months. She had not taken diclofenac for a long time. Her sleep was generally satisfactory. Urination was also much better. The day before the visit she had had a slight setback, playing netball, and had a pain in the left foot—she was worried because the original problem had started with pain in the right foot. She was using lavender heat bags, which she found helpful. She was taking pilates lessons as well.

Treatment: Using regular needles left KI-10, LU-5, and right SP-3 were supplemented.

Light needling was applied to the lower abdomen and supraclavicular fossa regions.

Okyu/direct moxa was applied to GV-12 and BL-23.

Summary: She came for periodic treatment for another 16 months. During this time she had no setbacks and returned to normal activities, including physical education and swimming. She had more stamina, was able to stand for longer, but still had some digestive issues.

The following case is from my colleague Marian Fixier, who practices in London, United Kingdom. Her patient presented with a very severe lung weak constitution condition with severe skin problems, breathing problems, allergies, and tendency to develop infections. He responded well to treatment.

Case 3
Julian, Boy Age 4 Years

Main complaints: He had severe eczema and asthma.

History: Starting around age 8 to 9 months, Julian's skin began to show signs of dryness. At age 1 year, he experienced an allergic reaction after eating baklava (Turkish sweet pastry). The reaction was an instant swelling, though it did not affect his airways. He was given chlorphenamine (Piriton, GlaxoSmithKline) antihistamine for this. He was tested for nut allergy, which was negative. He subsequently also had a reaction to eggs and lemon juice that resulted in instant blistering of the skin. From age 18 months, he developed itchy skin, particularly following a cough or a cold. This was diagnosed as severe eczema, for which he was prescribed steroid and antibiotic creams. These continued to be used as needed. From age 2 years he started having asthma attacks when catching a cold. This would go to his chest and he would develop a wheeze. He had been hospitalized five times for 3 days at a time. The eczema also got worse when he had a cold. The family was trying to manage the asthma better by administering steroids when a cold developed. Eczema flare-ups could last for days or weeks and easily became infected.

Family medical history: His mother had asthma, his mother's sister had eczema, and his father had some allergies. He had had all his vaccinations with no adverse reactions afterward.

General health: He was a lively and animated little boy with a loud voice. His mood was generally good. His sleep was sometimes disturbed by the itching, though he had no problem falling asleep. His parents used silk leggings as a barrier at night. His appetite and bowels were good. He regularly caught cold and developed a cough; this was happening before he started with the asthma attacks. He did consume some milk products.

Appearance: Overall, the skin was rough, dull, and lusterless. It was very itchy at night, worse on the right side. The skin was also red and very dry, and bled when scratched. The eczema was worse on the folds of the knees, hands and arms, and lower abdomen. The eczema was less severe on the legs but more noticeable on the thighs. The eczema had previously appeared on his face, but this cleared up at the age of 3 years.

Treatment: Due to the extensive presentation of eczema over Julian's body, I didn't feel it was appropriate to use the *shonishin* rubbing technique.

Using a *teishin*, supplementation was applied to left LU-8 and SP-5, draining technique to right LR-3.

Using a *zanshin*, light tapping was applied around the patches of eczema; SP-10, LI-11, and BL-40 were also tapped.

Using the *teishin*, supplementation was applied to LU-1, CV-17, and CV-12.

A press-sphere was placed on GV-12.

Second visit—1 week later

He had a bit of a cold, which was a danger sign. He was slightly congested with it but there was no wheezing. An albuterol (Ventolin, GlaxoSmith-Kline) inhaler had been given the night before preventatively. He was happy in himself and, in spite of some itchiness, not irritable with it. The itchiness was still waking him at night. He had had a flare-up of eczema 2 days after the last treatment on the cheek (first time for over a year), and still had a bit on the face around the jaw and eyelids. The steroid cream was used daily. I recommended trying to avoid dairy completely and using soya and rice milk instead. I also suggested goat and sheep products as alternatives to cow products.

Treatment: Using a *teishin*, supplementation was applied to left LU-8 and SP-5, draining technique to right LR-3.

Using a *zanshin*, light tapping was applied around the patches of eczema, and SP-10, LI-4, LI-11, LI-15, BL-40, GV-14, GV-12, and BL-17 were also tapped.

Using the *teishin*, supplementation was applied to LU-1, CV-17, and CV-12.

No press-sphere was left on GV-12 because Julian wasn't happy with these when his mother tried to put them on.

Third visit—1 week later

The cold had continued to progress for 3 to 4 days before abating. The cold triggered asthma with heavy wheezing, worse at night. This was the second time this month. He needed hourly Ventolin given at night when the cold was at its worst to avoid hospitalization. Now only a little bit of a cold remained. He was very itchy at night, but his mother thought it was overall better than previously. It was generally less red and was not weeping. The skin was clearer on the backs of the legs, buttocks, and lower abdomen.

Treatment: Using a *teishin*, supplementation was applied to left KI-7 and LU-8, draining technique to right SP-9.

Using a *zanshin*, light tapping was applied around the patches of eczema, and SP-10, LI-4, LI-11, and GV-23 (for nasal congestion) were also tapped.

Press-tack needles (0.6 mm) were applied to the asthma *shu* points with instructions to the mother to change them if needed.

Fourth visit—1 week later

The cold had cleared and he had not experienced any breathing problems all week. No medication was needed, and he had tolerated the press-tack needles better than the press-spheres. The eczema had flared up for a couple of days after he ate some candy. But overall the quality of the skin appeared improved, less rough, and with better luster. His mother commented that his skin never usually cleared up completely, as it had now on certain parts of his body. His legs had now been clear for 2 weeks. The abdomen and back were completely clear, and the legs improved.

Treatment: Using a *teishin*, supplementation was applied to left KI-7 and LU-8, and a draining technique to right SP-9.

Using a *zanshin*, light tapping was applied around the patches of eczema, SP-10, LI-4, LI-11, BL-40, and GV-23 were also tapped.

Press-tack needles (0.6 mm) were applied to the asthma *shu* points with instructions to the mother to change them if needed.

Fifth visit—1 week later

The family had moved out of their house and were staying with friends while the carpets were being removed at home. This had caused some changes in diet and emotional stability—he had had a huge tantrum during the week. His skin was worse and he had had some loose bowel movements, but no breathing issues at all and no nasal congestion.

Treatment: Using a *teishin*, supplementation was applied to left LU-8 and SP-5, and a draining technique to right LR-3.

Using a *zanshin*, light tapping was applied around the patches of eczema, and SP-10, LI-11, and BL-10 were also tapped.

Light needling was applied to right LI-11 and BL-10.

Because Julian would not allow me to place the press-tack needles at the time, I gave them to his mother to be placed later at the asthma *shu* points. I also gave his mother an article on eczema and the possible effect of chemicals used in the home.

Sixth visit—3 weeks later

He had not experienced any breathing difficulties at all over the 3 weeks. The skin problem was up and down, but overall better now. His mother reported that she felt the skin to be much better than it was 1 year previously. Since having acupuncture, the flare-ups were shorter in duration and less severe. The skin was no longer red and raw "as if on fire," and was not getting infected or weepy. The winter had so far been better than the year before. He had had some problems with loose stools. His mother was also working on making their house more ecofriendly to expose Julian to fewer allergens.

Treatment: Using a *teishin*, supplementation was applied to left LU-9 and SP-3, and a draining technique to right LR-3.

Using a *zanshin*, light tapping was applied around the patches of eczema, and SP-10, LI-4, LI-11, LI-15, and BL-40 were also tapped.

Press-tack needles (0.6 mm) were applied to the asthma *shu* points with instructions to the mother to change them if needed.

A press-sphere was placed on GV-12.

Report 2 weeks later

His asthma was completely quiet, with no breathing difficulties. This was a dramatic change; this

time 1 year before he had been hospitalized twice already and the weather was cold, which was usually an irritant to the asthma. Because the symptoms had disappeared, he had not been using the inhalers, in spite of advice from doctors to use it all the time during the winter. The eczema symptoms were moderate, and he was exposed to many different things and foods in the weeks before Christmas.

Seventh visit—8 weeks since sixth visit

The family had been away in India for a month. He had had no symptoms of asthma, though they used the inhaler preventatively when it got cold. The eczema was better while they were away because he fared better in a hotter, drier climate. He even ate foods he normally reacted to with no reactions. The skin had been itchy at night since they returned.

Treatment: Using a *teishin*, supplementation was applied to left LU-9 and SP-3, and a draining technique to right LR-3.

Using a *zanshin,* light tapping was applied around LI-4, L1-11, and BL-40.

A press-sphere was placed on GV-12.

Eighth visit—2 weeks later

Julian didn't seem himself. He appeared to be out of sorts and fell asleep while waiting in the clinic. He had started with a cold at the beginning of the week, with nasal congestion and a chesty cough on the day of treatment. He was breathing heavily but not wheezing. He was using the inhaler daily. His mother commented that this time 1 year before, they had had several asthma crises. The skin was pretty good overall, a little bit up and down but nothing severe; it looked much less dry and red.

Treatment: Using a *teishin*, supplementation was applied to left LU-8, SP-5, and right LR-4.

Using a *zanshin,* light tapping was applied around LI-4, L1-11, LI-15, BL-40, GV-12, and GV-23 for the nasal congestion.

No press-spheres or press-tacks were placed. I gave some to his mother to place later.

Ninth visit—3 weeks later

While free of asthma symptoms he had been to the hospital for treatment of a skin infection. His skin had deteriorated with the very cold weather and central heating on very high at the nursery. His mother thought they were not moisturizing him enough there and that the heating was having a big effect on his skin. The skin became infected 2 weeks before with red, raised, and angry spots with pus. These spread wherever he scratched. He was placed in an isolation room at the hospital because they didn't know what it was. Julian developed a high fever. He was given intravenous antibiotics and antivirals. He had to spend a couple of days in the hospital. He was also put on oral antibiotics. The dermatologist diagnosed an opportunistic infection (eczema herpeticum) due to the fragility of the skin. At that time his family was strongly advised that, since Julian had chronic asthma, he should be given the steroid inhaler daily despite his condition being stable without it. His mother said Julian was tearful in anticipation of coming for treatment after so much intervention in the hospital. However, he was happy for me to do treatment and was quite playful.

Treatment: Using a *teishin*, supplementation was applied to left LU-9, SP-3, and right LR-3.

Using a *zanshin*, light tapping was applied around LI-4, LI-11, LI-15, SP-10, BL-40, and GV-23 for the nasal congestion.

A press-sphere was placed on GV-14.

His mother called the next day to report that Julian was back in the hospital with a worsening of the skin infection and a replacement diagnosis of a bacterial rather than a viral infection. He had been resistant to the previous antibiotics and new ones were prescribed. His mother called again 2 weeks later; Julian had needed to be hospitalized for a further course of antibiotics. The initial diagnosis of eczema herpeticum had been incorrect. The last update was 25 days later. After the skin infection finally cleared up, his underlying eczema was not too bad, and he still had no asthma symptoms. They had been advised to continue with topical steroids and the steroid inhaler on a daily basis.

Summary: During the time that Julian came for acupuncture his asthma stabilized and he did not have any acute asthma attacks. This was a considerable improvement over the year before when he had had several admissions to hospital. In addition to regular acupuncture treatments, the parents were trying to be more proactive and administer inhalers preventatively as and when he developed a cold. They observed that colds did not lead to asthma symptoms, which had always occurred before. Inhalers were not being used on a daily basis outside of periods of upper respiratory infections.

His skin condition also improved overall during the time that he was coming for treatment. Wintertime was a particularly challenging time for his skin, with the combination of cold and damp weather and central heating on high in his nursery. His mother commented on several occasions that his skin was better than it had been before treatment, though it never fully cleared up.[11] The acute bacterial infection caused a severe worsening of his condition with a severe outbreak of spots on top of the underlying chronic eczema condition.[12] I encouraged his mother to continue to try to exclude certain foods from the diet, particularly damp-producing foods (due to his tendency to develop nasal congestion with the first signs of a cold). This advice was followed sporadically, though more recently, since the acute episode, they were making concerted efforts to exclude cow's milk products from his diet. They also made many changes to the chemicals being used in the home, favoring more ecofriendly products.

---

[11] It is worth noting that in cases such as Julian's, where there is a strong lung weak constitution, it can take considerable treatment to create more change of the condition. Julian was treated over a less than 5-month period, and the severe symptoms showed a significant improvement. Further treatment has a good chance to slowly create more changes. In cases like this the parents need to be patient. You, as therapist, need to convince them that it is worthwhile to continue with treatment. My usual strategy for this is to apply a certain number of treatments, and after demonstrating that symptoms improve, parents can start to appreciate the idea of continued longer-term treatment.

[12] Case 1, Chapter 19, describes a child (Han) with very severe atopic dermatitis, similar to Julian. On occasion he would develop opportunistic skin infections in the skin lesions. We found it helpful to use mild tea tree oil baths to help contain the infections. Of course, if they don't work, appropriate consultation with the doctor should be made because stronger therapy may be needed, but it is good to bear such simple home treatments in mind.

Summary of treatments administered: Due to the extensive presentation of the eczema, it was not appropriate to do the whole body *shonishin* using the stroking technique. The focus instead was on root treatment to strengthen his underlying constitution and to address the chest and skin condition using Toyohari Meridian Therapy diagnosis and treatment. Root treatment points were treated using a small gold *teishin* with non-inserted needling.

Treatment generally focused on a primary lung vacuity pattern, based on findings on the channels and the abdomen. The pulse was more difficult to analyze, though the lung position was weak. Generally, even though the liver pulse felt somewhat weak, draining was applied to the liver given the presentation of red, raised skin (which is interpreted as an excess liver condition). On the occasions when Julian presented with cold signs, usually with nasal congestion, the *jing*-river, metal points were treated instead of the usual treatment points, according to *Nan Jing,* Chapter 68.

For the first two treatments a primary lung vacuity pattern with liver repletion was treated. Because he was not noticeably improved at the second treatment, this was reconsidered, and the pattern was changed to kidney vacuity pattern, with spleen repletion. This pattern also felt appropriate due to the chronicity of the condition and the family medical history, which indicated a hereditary component. Although, this seemed to bring about improvement, after the second treatment using this new pattern the skin seemed to be slightly worse again (though this also coincided with the family having to move out of their home and Julian's diet being affected). It then felt more appropriate to treat the lung vacuity pattern and to drain the liver channel to address the red, raised skin condition. The skin improved after this treatment, so I continued with the lung vacuity pattern.

As treatment progressed, his skin became less angry and less red, so focusing more on supplementing the liver felt more appropriate. On the last treatment, when Julian had already been diagnosed with a bacterial skin infection with red, raised spots, it would, on reflection, have been more appropriate to drain the liver. It seemed that this had a part to play in the condition flaring up again.

Shonishin tapping technique was used on *yang* channel points specifically to address the skin condition, in particular with focus on the typical large intestine channel points that are good for skin problems, and additional points on the legs good for skin problems.

Press-spheres were used and applied at home by Julian's mother on GV-12, a main point to strengthen the constitution and also press-tack needles on the asthma *shu* point on a couple of occasions.[13]

As a result of the recent acute episode, the parents were advised to administer daily topical steroid cream and steroid inhalers, in spite of the improvement in Julian's asthma over the last year.[14]

Treatment recently resumed with Julian. Before he came he had been encouraged to consult with a well-known herbal specialist famous for treating chronic skin disease. However, his skin's appearance was really good, with much more luster and very little eczema. It was decided that it was not necessary to see the herbalist at the time.

The next case from my colleague, Joke Bik-Nowee, who practices near The Hague in the Netherlands, illustrates the importance and power of getting the constitutional treatment right.

Case 4
Jan, Boy Age 3½ Years

Main complaint: Eczema over the whole body (atopic dermatitis), which was very itchy.

---

[13]   The asthma symptoms improved and stayed improved after the asthma shu points were treated for the first time.

[14]   This is a complicated problem. In Chapter 18, p. 119, I discussed our role as therapists when treating a patient on medication for control of a life-threatening disease like asthma. The doctors will insist on the asthma medication even as the symptoms become quieter. This requires ongoing dialogue. It is not our place to make alternative recommendations regarding the steroid asthma medications, but we can encourage the parents to discuss this periodically with their doctor so long as the asthma symptoms remain absent for a prolonged period. My experience has been that the parents and child start forgetting to use the medication because it has been so long since the symptoms appeared, and as this gradually happens more often over time, I then recommend discussing this with the doctor to see if they can move toward using medication on an as-needed basis rather than automatically every day. The decisions lie in the discussions between the parents and the doctor.

History: He had had skin problems since birth. At age 2 months the skin was bad on his chest. Now it was worst on the inside of the elbows and the back of the knees. His skin was itchy and he scratched it until blood was drawn. At the time of the first visit the skin was better than usual and his legs were more affected than the upper part of his body. He had been prescribed many different creams by his doctor, including corticosteroid creams. These did not really help much in the long run, and his mother did not want to use those creams for long periods. This is why she decided to visit an acupuncturist. At age 2 years he had pseudo croup, but he had no breathing problems now. He had no allergic reactions. It was difficult for him to fall asleep, but when he slept he didn't wake till morning. He had had all the usual vaccinations. His mother also had atopic dermatitis and she was an asthma patient. He had a normal appetite, and his bowel movements were daily and without problems.

Examination: He was small for his age, and thin, with pale-white skin. His face was especially white, and his hair was almost white. Under his eyes he had dark circles. He had a good mood and was cheerful, talkative, and unable to sit still for a long time. The skin felt very dry to the touch in many places, especially on the elbows and the back of the knees. His back (upper and lower) had been scratched until small wounds occurred. The skin was thicker at those places. He showed reactions in the lung, kidney, and spleen regions of the abdomen. It was very difficult to feel his pulse because he would not stay still, but perhaps the kidney and lung pulses were weak.

Diagnosis: Kidney vacuity pattern seemed to fit best.

Treatment: Using a *teishin*, left KI-7 and LU-5 were supplemented, right SP-9 and LI-6 were drained.

Using the pointed end of the *teishin,* tapping was applied softly around the eczema spots on the legs and elbows.

Using a *zanshin*, light stroking was applied over the healthy areas on the back, abdomen, chest, legs, and arms.

Second visit—1 week later

His mother reported that the itching had been less for 2 days; thus I gave a similar treatment.

Treatment: Using a *teishin*, left KI-7, LU-5 were supplemented, right SP-3, LI-6, and left SI-7 were drained.

Tapping and stroking similar to the first visit were also applied.

Third visit—1 week later

This week the skin was not good.

Treatment: Using a *teishin,* left KI-7, LU-5 were supplemented, right SP-9, and left GB-37 were drained.

Tapping and stroking similar to the first visit were also applied.

Press-spheres were added to LI-11.

Fourth visit— 1 week later

There was no change in his complaints. Because of this I reflected on my choice of diagnosis and decided to treat the more obvious lung vacuity pattern based on symptoms.

Treatment: Using a *teishin,* left LU-9, SP-3 were supplemented, right LR-3, ST40 were drained.

Tapping was applied a round the areas of skin problems on the elbows and knees.

Using the *teishin,* BL-13 and BL-20 were supplemented to support the root treatment.

Fifth visit—1 week later

The skin was much better this week; the itching had stopped. Many eczema spots had disappeared, and the remaining spots were much smaller.

Treatment: The same treatment was applied as the last except for draining LI-6 instead of ST-40.

A few days later the mother reported that his skin was very good and that she wanted to stop the treatment. About 1 year later the mother came to me for treatment and told me that Jan was still much better, having few problems with the eczema.

Comments: The reason why the skin problems did not change much during the first treatments was probably because the wrong pattern was treated. When the pattern was changed to the lung vacuity pattern the skin became much better. I changed pattern because I was not satisfied with the results of the second and third treatment. I searched for more information in Fukushima (1991) and found that small children with such problems more often have a lung vacuity pattern rather than a kidney vacuity pattern.[15]

Not all cases of constitutional weakness are so difficult. Sometimes the problem appears due, for example, to being born prematurely, but the resulting weakness this can trigger overlays an otherwise relatively well developed infant. The following case of Freddy illustrates how even a child who has chronic recurrent problems and appears to be run down can recover quite quickly with the right treatment.

Case 5
Freddy, Boy Age 20 Months

Main complaints: He has a problem with recurrent colds. No sooner has one finished than another starts. His lungs are usually congested, he has recurrent sore throat, repeated cough, and usually nasal congestion.

History: He was born 5 weeks premature and needed to stay in the hospital for the first week. He breast fed the first 7 months, after which, once he started on bottled milk, he was found to be lactose intolerant and now avoids lactose products. Repeated visits to the doctors have revealed nothing abnormal with no particular treatment offered. In the colder 6 months of the year the colds are almost continuous, one after the other. The colds cause coughing and sore throat, which leaves him almost constantly fussy

---

[15]   We can also suspect that Jan was lung weak constitution pattern, but the protracted use of the corticosteroid creams was slowly weakening his kidneys and changing to a kidney vacuity pattern. In this case Jan was probably still lung vacuity pattern but was showing signs of the weakening kidney, which were accurately identified. Getting the pattern right the first time can be tricky when more complex manifestations start to appear. But at the same time, the changes were quite dramatic once the proper pattern was identified and treated.

and weepy, and with the colds sleep can be disturbed, with waking and crying. He can develop a fever with the cold and often loses his appetite when sick. When the cold does not affect his appetite it is usually good. When he is not sick his mood is generally good. The last several weeks he has had a problem with diarrhea and usually tends to loose stools. His skin is fine. His parents are run ragged since he often has difficulty settling and feeling comfortable and is very weepy a lot of the time.

Assessment: Despite my best efforts he cried very hard on this first visit. Examining pulse and abdomen was impossible. General assessment of his skin condition showed nothing remarkable.

Diagnosis: The history of symptoms indicated a lung vacuity pattern.

Treatment: With a lot of struggle and crying, treatment could be applied very tentatively.
   Using a *herabari,* light tapping was applied to GV-22 and GV-12.
   Using an *enshin,* light stroking was applied (attempted) down the arms, legs, abdomen, and back.
   Using a *teishin,* supplementation was applied to left LU-9 and SP-5.
   A 0.3 mm press-tack was placed on GV-12.
   I finished the treatment as quickly as I could, not sure how he would respond and thinking that the way the symptoms manifested and with his early history treatment might take a lot of time to produce effects and that I might even need to use *okyu* moxa to help fight the repeated infections.

Second visit—6 days later

He has been better the last few days. The cough has improved, his sleep, appetite, and mood have been better. His mother described it as the best he had been for many months.

Treatment: This time he was much more settled and hardly struggled with me about the treatment.
   Using an *enshin,* light stroking was applied down the arms, legs, abdomen, chest, shoulders, and back.

Using a *herabari*, light tapping was applied to GV-22, GV-12, and bilateral LU-1 and around LU-5 (the stop coughing point).

Using a *teishin*, supplementation was applied to left LU-9 and SP-5, with draining applied to right LV-3.

A 0.3 mm press-tack was placed on GV-12.

Press-spheres were applied bilaterally to the stop coughing points in the elbows.

Third visit—6 days later

He has improved further. His mood was a lot better, his energy better, he was happier and he was more open to other people, able to tolerate and enjoy them better. His appetite was good. The stools were firmer but still slightly soft. His mother was really happy and relieved; she described him as almost a different child.

Treatment: Using an *enshin*, light stroking was applied down the arms, legs, abdomen, and back.

Using a *herabari,* light tapping was applied to bilateral LI-4, GV-12, the supraclavicular fossa regions, and left LU-1.

Using a *teishin*, supplementation was applied to left LU-9 and SP-5, with draining applied to right LV-3.

A 0.3 mm press-tack was placed on GV-12.

Press-spheres were applied bilaterally to the stop coughing points in the elbows.

Fourth visit—21 days later

He had had a cold with fever the last 2 days. Before this he had been good, with all symptoms much improved. He still had a fever while at the clinic.

Treatment: Using the more pointed end of a *teishin*, stroking was applied between the fingers and toes for the fever.

Using a *herabari,* light tapping was applied to bilateral LU-1, GV-12, the supraclavicular fossa regions, and GV-20.

Using a *teishin*, supplementation was applied to left LU-10 and SP-2, with draining applied to right LV-2.[16]

---

16 Using the idea described in *Nan Jing*, Chapter 68, the *ying*-spring points were drained because of the presence of the fever.

A 0.3 mm press-tack was placed on GV-12.

Press-spheres were applied bilaterally to the stop coughing points in the elbows.

Fifth visit—15 days later

He improved quickly after the last treatment. But a few days before he had started with some diarrhea, vomiting and poor appetite, and a mild cough. Yesterday he had had a mild fever, but today no fever.

Treatment: Using a *herabari,* light tapping was applied to bilateral LU-1, GV-12, the supraclavicular fossa regions, and GV-20.

Using an *enshin*, light stroking was applied down the arms, legs, abdomen, and back.

Using a *teishin*, supplementation was applied to left LU-9 and SP-3, with draining applied to right LV-3.

Press-tacks (0.3 mm) were placed on GV-12 and the stop coughing points in the elbows.

I taught the mother to do home treatment with light tapping and stroking.

Sixth visit—7 days later

The gastrointestinal symptoms improved. He has been doing much better, though there remains a slight congestion in the lungs. His mood is good, and he really likes the home treatment and has become excited about coming to the clinic for treatment.

Treatment: Using a *herabari,* light tapping was applied to bilateral LU-1, GV-12, and the supraclavicular fossa regions.

Using an *enshin*, light stroking was applied down the arms, legs, abdomen, and back.

Using a *teishin*, supplementation was applied to left LU-9 and SP-3, with draining applied to right LV-3.

Press-tacks (0.3 mm) were placed on GV-12 and the stop coughing points in the elbows.

Seventh visit—35 days later

He has been doing really well. No colds, no cough, no gastrointestinal problems. He likes to have the home treatment daily.

Treatment: Using a *herabari,* light tapping was applied to bilateral LU-1, GV-12, and GV-20.

Using an *enshin*, light stroking was applied down the arms, legs, abdomen, chest, and back.

Using a *teishin*, supplementation was applied to left LU-9 and SP-3.

A 0.3 mm press-tack was placed on GV-12.

Press-spheres were placed to bilateral LU-1.

Treatment stopped here. We agreed to do occasional follow-up visits, or, if symptoms recurred, he could come in as needed. I had expected when I heard his history that treatment would take a long time to create clear change. But in retrospect I can see that his bodily constitution and vitality were good, but that probably being born 5 weeks premature left his lungs susceptible and hence he had the recurrent infections.

For examples of treatment of the kidney weak constitution see the cases in Chapter 25, in particular Case 2 (Dianne, who has Rett syndrome).

27 Recurrent Infections

Recurrent Respiratory Tract Infections

Case 1
Mary, Girl Age 3 Years

Main complaints: Multiple recurrent colds over the last year. On several occasions the colds worsened and developed into bronchitis. On two occasions the bronchitis progressed into pneumonia, one episode of which led to her being hospitalized. She had to take many rounds of antibiotics over the last year because of the episodes of bronchitis and pneumonia. Along with the colds she had some problems with ear infections as well, but this was less of a problem than the continuous cycle of catching colds. At the time she presented, Mary was recovering from a cold that had started several days before; she had a congested nose and mild cough.

History: Until 1 year previously she did not have too many health problems. But over the last year she had been more tired and showing signs of emotional distress. Her appetite, sleep, and bowel movements were regular and all right. Her mother was a student of mine and had recently learned *shonishin* from me, which made her think to bring her daughter for treatment. While discussing her daughter's problems the following history emerged: Mary's mother worked and studied full time. Two years before, while a student and working she was found to have breast cancer. After starting treatment for the breast cancer her husband could not cope and left her. Now she was a single working mother who also was finishing her studies, and in remission from cancer. It seemed to me that probably Mary's problems were related to the difficulties that her mother had been having. Her mother was struggling a lot with her own problems, and when Mary started becoming sick, her mother was increasingly frustrated

about being unable to do anything to help her. This probably created a cycle feeding the downward spiral in Mary's health.

Treatment strategy: Apply the basic non-pattern-based root treatment and teach the mother to do the treatment daily at home.

Treatment: Tapping was applied with a *herabari* on the GV-12 area, GV-22, and occipital areas.
    Stroking was applied with an *enshin* down the back, arms, legs, and abdomen.
    Press-spheres were placed and retained on GV-12 and left BL-13 (hard knot).
    The mother was taught to carefully apply the treatment daily at home.

Second visit—7 week later

Mary had fully recovered from the cold and had nothing else to report. The mother was applying treatment daily in the evening before putting Mary to bed, which Mary enjoyed.

Treatment: Tapping was applied with a *herabari* on the GV-12, GV-22, and occipital areas.
    Stroking was applied with an *enshin* down the back, arms, legs, and abdomen.
    A press-sphere was retained on GV-12.
    After a further discussion about the home treatment the mother agreed to come back with Mary if symptoms started returning.

Follow-up: Five and a half months later Mary had not had a single episode of catching cold. At 1 year, she had had one episode of a mild cold, from which she recovered quickly. She was doing well and was full of energy and very happy.

Reflection: I felt application of the principle of *Nan Jing (Classic of Difficulties)*, Chapter 69, was very important: "For vacuity supplement the mother." It was highly likely that the psychosocial circumstances of Mary's home life contributed to and probably triggered the problems she was having: the illness of her mother, her and her mother's abandonment by the father, her mother's hard-working habits and determination to keep going no matter what. Treating Mary alone would be helpful. But more helpful was to have the treatment given daily by her mother. Not only would treatment be more frequent, it would give mother and child more close contact together, it would help the mother relieve her own feelings regarding her health, her husband's departure, and her inability to help her child stay well. As the mother felt better this would be picked up by Mary and help Mary feel more secure in herself too. It worked well, I think.

Case 1 illustrates how a healthy child under stressful circumstances can respond with developing an illness. The next case shows how those illness patterns are part of a longer-standing issue to do with constitutional tendencies. When the constitutional tendency underlies the illness, it may be necessary to give attention specifically to trying to affect the constitution. This is discussed in Chapter 26, Weak Constitution. In the following case we can see that, despite a history of chronic problems that easily recurred, a little focused treatment was able to trigger big changes. The additional measures that can be needed to address weak constitution problems were unnecessary, as were treatment approaches (such as *okyu*/direct moxa) to help stimulate the immune system to deal with the recurrent infections.

Case 2
Tom, Boy Age 4½ Years

Main complaints: He caught cold easily and had recurrent colds and ear infections, with continuously swollen lymph nodes in the neck.

History: He had taken many rounds of antibiotics in the past. He was hospitalized 16 months before with a *Streptococcus* infection in the lymph nodes of the neck accompanying a bad ear infection, and has had swollen lymph nodes in the neck since then. He had problems with chronic loose stools, diarrhea, and vomiting. These symptoms improved after elimination of wheat gluten from the diet following identifica-

tion of a gluten allergy. His mother had many problems as a child, with chronic swollen lymph nodes in the neck. At age 19 she was diagnosed with sarcoidosis of the lungs. The mother was thus worried that her son may have the same problem or similar tendencies. His mood was good, his sleep was good, and all other systems were unremarkable.

Diagnosis: Based on the symptoms and findings on the abdomen and pulses, he had lung vacuity with a liver repletion pattern.

Treatment: Tapping was applied with a *herabari* over the head, occipital, and neck regions, the GV-12 area, around the ears, and on the abdomen.

Stroking with an *enshin* was applied on the abdomen, down the back, arms, and legs.

Using a *teishin*, left LU-9 and SP-3 were supplemented and right LR-3, left BL-58 drained.

Press-spheres were left on GV-12 and CV-12.

Second visit—7 days later

The week was unremarkable, with not much to report.

Treatment: Tapping was applied using a *herabari* on the head, occipital and neck regions, GV-12 area, around the ears, and on the abdomen, back, arms, and legs.

Stroking with an *enshin* was applied on the abdomen, down the back, arms, and legs.

Using a *teishin*, left LU-9 and SP-3 were supplemented and right LR-3, left BL-58 drained.

Press-spheres were left on GV-12 and CV-12.

I taught the mother how to do home treatment, with light tapping (around the ears, neck, and GV-12 regions) and light stroking down the back, abdomen, arms, and legs.

Third visit—6 days later

He was doing well. The home treatment went well with nothing much to report.

Treatment: Tapping was applied using a *herabari* on the head, occipital, and neck regions, GV-12 area, around the ears, and on the abdomen, back, arms, and legs.

Stroking with an *enshin* was applied on the abdomen, down the back, arms, and legs.

Using a *teishin*, left LU-9 and SP-3 were supplemented and right LR-3, left BL-58 drained.

Press-spheres were left on GV-12 and CV-6.

Fourth visit—8 days later

He had had a slight cold, from which he recovered quickly, and he was generally doing well.

Treatment: Tapping was applied using a *herabari* on the head, occipital, and neck regions, GV-12 area, around the ears, and on the abdomen, back, arms, and legs.

Stroking with an *enshin* was applied on the abdomen, down the back, arms, and legs.

Using a *teishin*, left LU-9 and SP-3 were supplemented and right LR-3, LI-6 drained.

Press-spheres were left on GV-12 and TB-17.

Fifth visit—3 weeks later

Over the last few days the lymph nodes had been a little larger (but without ear infection). He had had some problems with cough and mild headache symptoms. Otherwise he was quite well.

Treatment: Tapping was applied using a *herabari* on the head, occipital, and neck regions, GV-12 area, around the ears, and on the abdomen, back, arms, and legs.

Stroking with an *enshin* was applied on the abdomen, down the back, arms, and legs.

Using a *teishin*, left LU-9 and SP-3 were supplemented and right LR-3 drained.

Press-spheres were left on GV-12, bilateral TB-17.

Sixth visit—19 days later

He had had some mild digestive symptoms (loose stools, abdominal pain) over the previous week. He had started with an ear infection, but it cleared up without developing much, and he was still coughing a little.

Treatment: Tapping was applied using a *herabari* on the head, occipital, and neck regions, GV-12

area, around the ears, and on the abdomen, back, arms, and legs.

Stroking with an *enshin* was applied on the abdomen, down the back, arms, and legs.

Using a *teishin*, left LU-9 and SP-3 were supplemented and left TB-5, SI-7 drained.

Press-spheres were left on GV-12, bilateral TB-17.

Seventh visit—23 days later

The lymph nodes were smaller, but they were still a little swollen below the left ear; he had some problems with headaches.

Treatment: Tapping was applied using a *herabari* on the head, occipital, and neck regions, GV-12 area, around the ears, and on the abdomen, back, arms, and legs.

Stroking with an *enshin* was applied on the abdomen, down the back, arms, and legs.

Using a *teishin,* left LU-9 and SP-3 were supplemented and right LR-3, left TB-5, SI-7 drained.

Press-spheres were left on GV-12, and behind the neck point on the back of the right ear.

Eighth visit—19 days later

He was doing generally better; the cough was very mild and occasional, the lymph nodes less swollen.

Treatment: Tapping was applied using a *herabari* on the head, occipital, and neck regions, ST-12, GV-12 areas, around the ears, and on the abdomen, back, arms, and legs.

Stroking with an *enshin* was applied on the abdomen, down the back, arms, and legs.

Using a *teishin*, left LU-9 and SP-3 were supplemented and right LR-3, left BL-58 drained.

Press-spheres were left on GV-12, behind TB-17 bilaterally.

Ninth visit—15 days later

He was doing well and the lymph nodes were much less swollen.

Treatment: Tapping was applied using a *herabari* on the head, occipital, and neck regions, GV-12

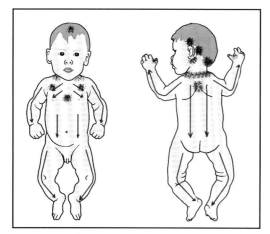

Fig. 27.1 Stroking:
- Down the arms (*yang* channels)
- Down the legs (stomach and bladder channels)
- Down the back (bladder channel)
- Down the abdomen (stomach channel)
- Across the chest

Tapping:
- Occipital area: 10 times
- Behind the ear: 10 times each
- Above the ear: 10 times each
- Below the ear: 10 times each
- CV-12 area: 10 to 20 times
- LI-4: 5 to 10 times each
- ST-12 area: 5 times each
- GV-20 area: 10 times
- Across the shoulders: 10 to 20 times

problem proves stubborn or resistant, *okyu*/direct moxa is probably the best method for stimulating the immune system of the child. However, it is, as discussed elsewhere, not always easy to apply this method, thus we tend to apply other techniques first in addition to the root treatment and use the moxa if still not working.

Press-Spheres *(Ryu)*, Press-Tack Needles *(Emp-ishin)*, and Intradermal Needles *(Hinaishin)*

It is common to leave press-spheres on points like GV-12 and BL-13. If there is a lot of lymphatic congestion below the ears (usually seen when the ears also become infected after catching cold), it can be helpful to leave press-spheres at the harder, more painful points, often around or below TB-17. For children with cough, palpate and treat the stop coughing points on the elbows near LU-5. On some children when the lungs are congested, a strong reaction will show around the

asthma *shu* point; it is good to treat this point for the lungs.

If the symptoms prove stubborn or resistant, increase the dose by using the new Pyonex press-tack needles (Seirin-America). The intradermal needles are used if the symptoms persist after increasing the dose of treatment with press-tack needles.

Additionally, for the child who has a tendency toward lung weak constitution and has a problem of recurrent infections, it can be helpful to treat related back *shu* points, such as treating BL-13 on one side and BL-20 on the other. Press-spheres can be used, but if the child is older or symptoms are more stubborn, the 0.6 mm Pyonex press-tack needles can be used.

If the child has secondary liver-related symptoms, such as sleep or behavioral problems, it can be helpful to leave a press-sphere on the point on the ear behind *shen men.*

Needling

If the child has very stiff shoulders, which is a symptom of the lung vacuity pattern, and the stiffness does not change much with the pattern-based root treatment and the non-pattern-based root treatment that includes light tapping of the shoulders, needling may be required. It can be helpful to lightly insert needles to one or two of the most reactive acupoints on the stiff shoulders, such as GB-21, TB-15, and SI-14. The needling should be shallow (2–3 mm) and the needles not retained for very long.

Palpate the area around GB-20 for the child with recurrent infections, chronically congested nose, or nasal infection if these symptoms have not responded to treatment. If it is stiff here use either the retained needling or in and out needling method to treat the stiff reactions. On the older child (3 years and older) for the same stubborn symptoms of the nose, palpate around GV-22 to GV-23 for a spongy, painful reaction. If present, apply retained needling on the reactive point, angled toward the nose. For the child with additional problems of ear infections, if there are strong reactions in the region below the affected ear(s) around TB-17, and the problems have not been resistant so far to treatment, you can apply light needling to this reaction to speed up the process of change. Sometimes a reaction is found around GB-12 rather than TB-17, in which case needle this.

If the child with the problem of recurrent infections, which is a typical lung vacuity sign, also has concurrent liver symptoms, such as behavioral problems or sleep disturbance, treat related acupoints. If tapping LI-4 and the stiff region around GB-20 has not yet helped, use in and out needling to LI-4 and either in and out or retained needling to the reaction around GB-20.

Okyu—Direct Moxa

If the responses are too slow in developing, or the child requires a more urgent treatment, *okyu*/direct moxa can be applied at GV-12. But, as explained in Chapter 13, this can be difficult to do, both for the parent and for the child. It is not usual to do this immediately, but rather, later in the treatment series. Because of the effects of this moxibustion technique, the desired biological changes will start regardless of where you apply the moxa. We choose GV-12 first because it has a reputation as being good for all pediatric conditions, second because there is a history of applying moxa to this point to prevent infections, and third because it is easier to do moxa on as few points as possible. Choosing a midline point on the back is much easier than bilateral points elsewhere. When you start applying moxa to this acupoint, use the "80%" method at first (see Chapter 13)—let it get hot then take it off. When the child is more used to the technique you can let it burn down more. In more severe or acute cases you may choose to let the moxa burn down further to get the stronger treatment effects.

Chinetsukyu—Warm Moxa

This is a technique we do not use often on children and only on older children who you are confident will stay still long enough. The technique is used as a soft supplementation method (see Chapter 13) for children who show weakness of all the *yang* channels. In such a case use a cone of moxa on GV-14. Make sure that the cone is removed *before* the child feels any heat. The stronger supplementation effect comes just before the patient starts to become aware of some vague feeling of warmth. Thus use this for the child who shows softness and loss of springiness of the skin with overall weak deep pulses (see earlier discussion).

Cupping

If there is chronic congestion in the lungs it is often helpful to apply cupping over the interscapular region to help break up the congestion. It depends on the age, strength, and dose requirements of the child as to how to apply the cupping—see Chapter 14 for ideas about these dose adjustments.

Bloodletting

On some children there is a lot of lymphatic congestion in the neck. One finds chronically swollen lymph nodes in the neck, below the ears. If other treatment methods have proved insufficient to help with this, one can try light bloodletting of either LI-1 or LU-11; both are helpful for this kind of problem. LI-1 is better selected in more acute circumstances.

Some children with the lung constitutional weakness and recurrent infections show vascular spiders on the upper back in the space between the scapulae and from the levels of GV-14 down to GV-11. If you see this, first try applying light (usually brief) cupping to help improve the blood stasis. Light cupping is recommended because one will often notice that the skin in this area is thin, a sign of lung vacuity, and lesser dosage of treatment is indicated. If the improvements are not satisfactory, then one can start to carefully apply vascular spider bloodletting on the area. Because the skin is usually thin here, apply only the stabbing and squeezing method, rather than the cupping method. See Chapter 15 and also *Japanese Acupuncture: A Clinical Guide,* Chapter 10 (Birch and Ida 1998, pp. 218–229).

■ Other Considerations

Dietary

It can be important to test for, and eliminate as needed, cow's milk products. The cow's milk products (milk, cheese, cream, yoghurt) may need to be eliminated while the child recovers, but they can be consumed again later when the child is stronger and has broken the cycle of recurrent infections. Sugar intake can also contribute to the problem; thus it can also be important to control this.

Home Treatment

To strengthen the body and give parents tools for treatment, teach a simple form of the core non-pattern-based root treatment as soon as you can (usually not on the first visit). This most often includes light stroking (especially with a silver spoon rather than a stainless-steel spoon) and some minimal targeted tapping, such as GV-12 (almost all cases) and LU-1, in the area below the ears, and so on. For ear involvement, the tapping is done above, behind, and below the ears. For nasal involvement the tapping is done on LI-4 and over the occipital region. For coughing, tap over the interscapular region, maybe LU-1.

■ Further Case Histories

Case 3
Eric, Boy Age 18 Months

Main complaints: He caught cold easily, seven times in the last 6 months. Often he had high fevers with each cold. His nose was chronically stuffy, and his lungs were congested most of this time.

History: The last week he had had a bad cold with high fever for 2 days. He seemed to slowly recover from each cold and then quickly start another. His nose was stuffy so that he had to breathe with his mouth open all the time, which at night caused dryness and irritation of the mouth and throat. He was delivered by suction method, resulting in a mild head trauma, affecting his left side, which is slightly less well developed than the right. Despite this, he was a relatively well-developed and full-bodied (slightly replete type) child. He tended to have loose stools and some abdominal bloating. All other systems were unremarkable. His parents were very busy, and the family lived a distance from the clinic, making regular weekly treatments difficult.

Diagnosis: The lung and spleen areas on the abdomen showed a reaction, the lung and spleen pulses were weak, and the liver pulse was hard. The diagnosis was lung vacuity pattern with probable repletion of the liver.

Treatment: Tapping was applied using a *herabari* on the abdomen, back, arms, and legs, GV-22, GV-20, GV-12, and occipital area.

Using a *teishin*, left LU-9 and SP-3 were supplemented, right LR-3 drained.

Press-spheres were retained on GV-12 and left BL-13 (a palpable knot was found here).

The parents were instructed to test for sensitivity to cow's milk products.

Second visit—8 days later

He was doing well, no cold and no fever, and there was not much to report.

Treatment: Tapping was applied using a *herabari* on the abdomen, chest, arms, and legs, GV-22, GV-20, GV-12, around the ears, and over the occipital area.

Using an *enshin*, stroking was applied down the back.

Using a *teishin,* left LU-9 and SP-3 were supplemented, right LR-3 drained.

Press-spheres were retained on GV-12 and bilateral BL-15.

The parents were instructed to do home therapy daily, stroking down the back, tapping arms, legs, chest, GV-22, GV-12, and the occipital area.

Third visit—6 weeks later

Home treatment had been pretty consistent and had gone well. He was clearly better without cow's milk and was using a soy-based replacement. Other than an infection of the left eye, he had generally been OK, without any colds, was able to breathe through his nose more, and had fewer problems with loose stools and abdominal bloating. But a recent test showed he had a slightly low white blood cell count, which the parents were quite concerned about.

Treatment: Tapping was applied using a *herabari* on GV-22, GV-12, LI-4, around the ears and over the occipital area.

Using a *teishin,* very light stroking was applied down the back, abdomen, arms (large intestine channel), legs (stomach and bladder channels), chest, neck, and shoulders.

Using a *teishin,* left LU-9, SP-3, and right ST-36 were supplemented.

Press-spheres were retained on GV-12 and CV-12.

The parents were instructed to continue daily home treatment.

Fourth visit—6 weeks later

He started kindergarten and immediately had some digestive problems (loose stools and bloating). Generally he was better, with no colds, and the nasal congestion was better. He had a mild rash while traveling but had recovered. On this visit he had a mild runny nose and some congestion in the lungs.

Treatment: Tapping was applied using a *herabari* on GV-22, GV-12, LI-4, ST-36, around ST-12, and over the occipital area.

Using an *enshin,* stroking was applied down the back, abdomen, arms, and legs.

Using a *teishin,* left LU-9 and SP-3 were supplemented, right LR-3 drained, and left TB-4 supplemented.

Press-spheres were retained on GV-12 and bilateral asthma *shu* points.

Fifth visit—13 days later

He had caught cold 4 days earlier. He had nasal congestion, mild fever, coughing, congestion in the lungs, and a mild skin rash on the right cheek.

Treatment: Tapping was applied using a *herabari* on GV-22, GV-12, over the occipital area, arms, legs, back, and abdomen.

Using a *teishin,* left LU-9, SP-3, and right LR-3 were supplemented.

Cupping was applied over the interscapular region.

Press-spheres were retained on bilateral asthma *shu* points and nasal *bi tong* points.

Sixth visit—22 days later

His nose and lungs were generally better, but he was having some problems with abdominal pain and gas. The night before, he had had a mild fever with cough and had evidenced some congestion in the lungs. He was very slightly warm to the touch but had no fever.

Treatment: Tapping was applied using a *herabari* on GV-22, abdomen, back, arms, legs, chest, around the ears, and over the occipital area.

Using an *enshin,* stroking was applied down the back, abdomen, arms, and legs.

Using a *teishin,* left LU-9 and SP-3 were supplemented, right LR-3 drained.

Pyonex press-tack needles (0.6 mm) were applied to bilateral asthma *shu* points.

A press-sphere was placed on the left stop coughing elbow point.

Seventh visit—13 days later

He was good for 2 days after the last visit, then he developed a cold, which turned into bronchitis, and an ear infection. He had fully recovered from these and was generally doing well.

Treatment: Tapping was applied using a *herabari* on GV-22, GV-12, abdomen, back, arms, legs, chest, around ST-12, and over the occipital area.

Using an *enshin,* stroking was applied down the back, abdomen, arms, and legs.

Using a *teishin,* left LU-9 and SP-3 were supplemented, right LR-3 drained.

Small press-tack needles (0.6 mm) were applied to bilateral asthma *shu* points.

Eighth visit—6 weeks later

He had been good since the last visit, but a few days previously he had had a bad cold with strong coughing. He was still coughing.

Treatment: Tapping was applied using a *herabari* on the head, abdomen, back, arms, legs, and chest.

Using a *teishin,* left LU-9 and SP-3 were supplemented, right LR-3 drained.

Cupping was applied over the interscapular region.

Pyonex press-tack needles (0.6 mm) were retained on bilateral BL-13.

Press-spheres were placed on the left stop coughing elbow point and bilateral LU-1.

Ninth visit—22 days later

He had generally been good, but with some sleep disturbance the last few nights, crying at night, waking around 2 a.m., and not falling asleep easily. He had also had some irregularity of bowel movements over these few days.

Treatment: Needles were inserted and retained at bilateral GB-20.

Tapping was applied using a *herabari* on the head, abdomen, back, arms, legs, and chest.

Using a *teishin,* left LU-9 and SP-3 were supplemented, right LR-3 drained.

Cupping was applied over the interscapular region and around the navel.

Press-spheres were retained on GV-12 and bilateral ST-25.

Tenth visit—20 days later

He had been good, no lung and nasal symptoms, but some irritability and waking at night.

Treatment: Needles were inserted and retained at bilateral GB-20.

Tapping was applied using a *herabari* on the head, occipital area, abdomen, back, arms, and legs.

Using an *enshin,* stroking was applied down the back, arms, legs, and abdomen.

Using a *teishin,* left LU-9 and SP-3 were supplemented, right LR-3 drained.

Cupping was applied over the interscapular region.

Press-spheres were retained on GV-12 and bilateral ST-25.

Eleventh visit—27 days later

He had been pretty good this last month. He had some signs of irritability, a little coughing, and some loose stools over the last few days.

Treatment: Needles were inserted and retained at bilateral GB-20.

Tapping was applied using a *herabari* on the head, abdomen, back, arms, legs, chest, around ST-12, and over the occipital area.

Using an *enshin,* stroking was applied down the arms, legs, and back.

Using a *teishin,* left LU-9 and SP-3 were supplemented, right LR-3 drained.

Cupping was applied over the interscapular region.

Press-spheres were retained on GV-12 and bilateral ST-25.

Twelfth visit—22 days later

He had been doing well, no complaints. It was decided to stop treatment at this time because the main reasons for coming, the repeated infections, had clearly stopped and his digestive problems were much better. The parents agreed to continue applying some home treatment and call for an appointment if Eric had any recurrence of these problems.

Treatment: Needles were inserted and retained at bilateral GB-20.

Tapping was applied using a *herabari* on the head, abdomen, back, arms, legs, chest, around ST-12, and over the occipital area.

Using an *enshin,* stroking was applied down the arms, legs, and back.

Using a *teishin,* left LU-9 and SP-3 were supplemented, right LR-3 drained.

Cupping was applied over the interscapular region and around the navel.

Approximately 1 year later I was in contact with his parents who reported that he no longer had any problem with catching colds or with lung or nasal congestion. These problems had not recurred since the treatment.

Reflection: I had worried that we might need to apply *okyu* to try to kick-start his immune system, especially after we heard about the low white blood cell count, but without the moxa and with regular home treatment, Eric did very well. He had a clear lung weak type constitutional tendency (see Chapter 26, Weak Constitution), which presents with allergic sensitivities and the tendency toward repeated infections. It would probably have been useful to apply cupping earlier than I did. It is also interesting that as his lung weak tendency improved he showed less of the symptoms associated with the pattern (lung, nose, and digestive). The associated repletion of the liver showed up as sleep disturbance, irritability, and more crying *kanmushisho*-type symptoms (see

Chapter 21). I changed the treatment approach once I recognized this, hence the needling of GB-20 and the refocusing of the core treatment pattern. Such a change is usually a good sign, though the parents do not always see it as such. Changing a chronically weak constitutional tendency so that it triggers fewer of the associated symptoms can take time; not only do those gradually improve, but secondary problems emerge as being of more concern. We see this tendency in many adult patients when they stop talking about the symptoms that brought them for treatment and instead talk a lot about other problems that they had before, but which they had barely mentioned in passing.

The following case from my colleague Dan Zizza, who lives and works in Seattle, illustrates very succinctly how the basic *shonishin* root treatment coupled with a Meridian Therapy pattern-based root treatment and hardly any symptomatic interventions can very successfully treat a child with recurrent infections of the respiratory tract.

Case 4
Olivia, Girl Age 19 Months

Main complaints and history: Olivia was brought to see me by her mother for recurring and unresolved upper respiratory tract infections over the last 6 months. Her main symptoms were continual nasal congestion and thick white/clear nasal discharge. She also had a frequent wet, phlegmy cough, low-grade fever, and lethargy. She mouth breathes and produces gurgling sounds with breathing. Her sleep is disturbed because she wakes frequently through the night with coughing. Her mother has been keeping her off dairy products and giving her an elderberry syrup. She took her to a naturopathic doctor (ND), but not an allopathic physician (MD).

Appearance: Olivia looked pale, drawn, and tired. She was timid, clinging to her mother, and she would not look directly at me. Her skin showed both white and dark areas with poor luster. She didn't speak, but she would whimper occasionally. She had a thin build.

Examination: On palpation of Olivia's channels I found that the lung channel felt dry and sunken, and the spleen channel felt damp. On her abdomen I found the spleen reflex area to be puffy, and the lung area to feel rough and depressed. Her pulses were floating, rapid, and vacuous. The lung and spleen positions on the pulse felt the weakest.

Diagnosis: Her examination revealed lung vacuity pattern.

Treatment: Using the *teishin*, supplementation was applied to right LU-9 and SP-3.
  Using an *enshin*, light stroking was applied down the lung, large intestine, spleen, and stomach channels.
  Using the *Yoneyama* instrument, light tapping was applied to the occipital area, upper back, GV-14, and GV-12, GV-24, and *yintang*.
  Light stroking was then applied with the *enshin* along the sides of the nose and down the bladder channel on the back.
  A press-sphere was retained on GV-12 for 24 hours.

Second visit—3 days later

Olivia's nose stopped running after her first treatment, and her energy improved a lot. She still had some coughing and was still making gurgling sounds with breathing, and she continued to mouth breathe.

Treatment: Using the *teishin,* supplementation was applied to right LU-9 and SP-3.
  Using an *enshin,* light stroking was applied down the lung, large intestine, spleen, and stomach channels and down the back and legs, and along the sides of the nose and down the chest.
  Using the *Yoneyama* instrument, light tapping was applied to the upper back area.
  The *teishin* was used at GV-24, GB-20, *yintang* point, LU-1 and KI-25, GV-12, and right BL-13 and right BL-20.
  A press-sphere was retained on GV-12 for 24 hours.

Third visit—6 days later

Olivia improved more after the second treatment. She no longer had any nasal drainage, had good energy, and was able to sleep through the night.

She was coughing only occasionally, and it was now a dry cough, no longer wet and productive.

Treatment: Using the *teishin,* supplementation was applied to right LU-9 and SP-3.

Using an *enshin*, light stroking was applied down the lung, large intestine, spleen, and stomach channels and down the back and legs, and along the sides of the nose and across the scalp.

The *teishin* was used at CV-12, GV-14, and GV-12.

A press-sphere was retained on GV-12 for 24 hours.

Fourth visit—5 days later

All respiratory symptoms, including the cough, had completely resolved following the third treatment. However, two episodes of vomiting occurred 2 days prior to the fourth visit. Olivia's mother said that she was a little more whiny but otherwise had had no additional symptoms, and she was still eating normally. Given the acute symptoms I switched the root treatment to a spleen vacuity pattern.

Treatment: Using the *teishin,* supplementation was applied to right SP-3 and PC-7.

Using an *enshin,* light stroking was applied down the pericardium, large intestine, spleen, and stomach channels and down the back and abdomen.

Using the Yoneyama *zanshin* light scraping was applied to the stomach channel, and tapping was used on the upper back and BL-21 area.

The *teishin* was used at CV-12, CV-4, and GV-12.

Fifth visit—9 days later

No vomiting or any other digestive disorder symptoms occurred after the fourth visit, and no respiratory symptoms returned. Olivia's mother reported that Olivia is happy, playful, with good energy, a strong appetite, and good quality sleep.

Treatment: Using the *teishin*, supplementation was applied to right LU-9 and SP-3.

Using an *enshin,* light stroking was applied down the lung, large intestine, spleen, and stomach channels and down the back and abdomen.

Using the Yoneyama *enshin*, light scraping was applied on the upper back area.

I did not see Olivia again for nearly 1 year, and her mother reported that she stayed well until 2 weeks prior to her next visit.

Sixth visit—12 months later

Olivia had been diagnosed with an ear infection. The illness began with viral-like symptoms of a runny nose, a fever up to 39.4°C, and a phlegmy cough. She appeared pale and run down, and she developed ear pain. Visual inspection of the ear drums revealed blistering. She was put on antibiotics but remained on them for only 48 hours because she began displaying behavioral problems. It was at this point that her mother brought her in for treatment.

I again diagnosed a lung vacuity pattern, finding the lung and spleen channels sunken and vacuous upon palpation as well as the lung and spleen areas of the abdomen, and the lung and spleen positions of the pulse. The pulse quality was floating, rapid, thin, and vacuous.

Treatment: Using the *teishin,* supplementation was applied to right LU-9 and SP-3.

The *teishin* was also used to treat GB-20, TW-16 and TW-17, GV-14, right BL-13, and right BL-20.

Using the Yoneyama *zanshin*, light tapping was applied over the mastoid/occipital area behind the ears and down to the upper back, GV-14, and GV-12 areas.

Using an *enshin*, light stroking was applied on the lung, large intestine, triple warmer, spleen, stomach, and bladder channels on the arms and legs.

The treatment was finished with the use of a copper disk on right TW-5 and a zinc disk on left GB-41 to treat the ears,[3] retaining the disks on the points for ~ 20 seconds.

Seventh visit—3 days later

Olivia was feeling a lot better. She no longer had any ear pain, her energy was good, she was happy

---

3   Dan is a Toyohari practitioner and teacher; this use of TB-5 and GB-41 is a typical Toyohari extraordinary vessel treatment.

and playful. She still had some nasal congestion, clear nasal discharge, and a wet-sounding cough.

Treatment: Using the *teishin,* supplementation was applied to right LU-9, SP-3, and bilateral ST-36.

Using an *enshin,* light stroking was applied on the lung, large intestine, spleen, and stomach channels on the arms and legs, down the back, chest, and abdomen.

The *teishin* was also used to treat GV-24, *yintang,* LI-20, and GV-12.

Using the Yoneyama *zanshin,* light tapping was applied over the occipital and upper back areas.

A copper disk was placed on left LI-4 and a zinc disk on right ST-43. They were retained for around 20 seconds.

Eighth visit—6 months later

Olivia's mother reported that all of Olivia's respiratory symptoms had resolved in the days immediately following her seventh visit. She was brought to see me again following the onset of cold-like symptoms, which began 3 weeks earlier. She presented with coughing and a runny nose, clear nasal secretions, no fever, and lethargy. Based on the abdominal and pulse findings, a lung vacuity with liver vacuity pattern was chosen for the root pattern.

Treatment: Using the *teishin,* supplementation was applied to right LU-9, SP-5, and left LV-4.[4]

Using an *enshin,* light stroking was applied on the lung, large intestine, spleen, and stomach channels on the arms and legs, down the back, chest, and abdomen, and from GV-24 to *yintang* and over the LI-20 and GB-20 areas.

The *teishin* was also used to treat GV-14, GV-12, right BL-13 and right BL-20, and CV-12.

Using the Yoneyama *zanshin,* light tapping was applied over the occipital and upper back areas.

A copper disk was placed on right LI-4 and a zinc disk on left ST-43. They were retained for around 30 seconds.

---

[4] Please note that I chose to use the metal phase points on the spleen and liver channels this time because they brought about a better change in the pulse and felt like the more active location for supplementing the *qi* on palpation, and theoretically strongly supported the lung channel vacuity.

Treatment ended with a press-sphere at GV-12.

Olivia's mother left open the possibility of a return visit in another 3 days if Olivia was still displaying symptoms, but she didn't make that visit because all of Olivia's respiratory symptoms resolved over the next few days.

Candida albicans Infection

I report here two cases of successful treatment of *Candida albicans* infection. Although I have not much experience treating this condition (I think parents do not usually think of acupuncture treatment for a condition like this in their children), I report the cases as a guide for how to proceed should you have a patient come to you for treatment of this problem. The general treatment principles should by now be obvious, and in the absence of more experience treating this particular problem and the dearth of written literature on it I do not add much other detail afterward. In both cases I applied a simple form of the core non-pattern-based treatment, a simple pattern-based root treatment, and minimal symptomatic treatment with good success. In both cases improvement in symptoms was immediate and lasting, thus I did not need to try any stronger tactics nor did I need to teach simple home treatment.

Case 1
Carol, Girl Age 4½ Years

Main complaints: Vaginal yeast infection causing itching and pain.

History: She had had this problem for several months. The general practitioner diagnosed it as *Candida albicans* and prescribed no treatment. She was somewhat distressed by the symptoms. Her mother had placed her on a lactose-free and yeast-free diet and had been using tea tree oil in the bathwater but none of these had made any real change in symptoms.

Additional complaints: She had frequent abdominal pain with bad-smelling gas. She also had stiff shoulders, which she had difficulty relaxing. She tired easily. All other systems were unremarkable, and she had no other complaints.

Diagnosis: Weak spleen and heart pulses and her digestive symptoms and tiredness suggested a spleen vacuity pattern.

Treatment: Tapping was applied using a *herabari* on the GV-12 area, GV-20, GV-3, bilateral LI-4, and lower abdomen.

Light stroking with an *enshin* was applied on the abdomen and down the back, arms, and legs.

Using a *teishin*, supplementation was applied to right SP-3, PC-7, left GB-37,[5] draining to left ST-40.

Press-spheres were placed on GV-12, GV-3, and left BL-20.

Second visit—6 days later

She had had no itchiness or pain from the *Candida albicans* since the previous treatment. The abdominal pain had decreased, and she had fewer problems with gas.

Treatment: Tapping was applied using a *herabari* on the GV-12 area, GV-20, GV-3, bilateral LI-4, and lower abdomen.

Light stroking with an *enshin* was applied on the abdomen and down the back, arms, and legs.

Using a *teishin*, supplementation was applied to right SP-3, PC-7, and left GB-37.

Press-spheres were placed on GV-12, GV-3, and left BL-20.

Third visit—7 days later

She had no *Candida albicans* symptoms at all. This was the longest stretch of time with no symptoms since their onset. She also had no abdominal pain or bad gas. However, she had caught cold during the week and still had a stuffy nose and slight cough.

Treatment: Tapping was applied using a *herabari* on the GV-12 area, GV-20, GV-3, bilateral LI-4, arms, and lower abdomen.

---

5   GB-37 was supplemented to counterbalance the relative repletion of the liver, rather than draining the liver channel.

Light stroking was applied with an *enshin* on the abdomen and down the back, arms, and legs.

Using a *teishin*, supplementation was applied to right SP-3, draining to left LR-3.

Press-spheres were applied on GV-12, GV-3, and right BL-20.

The next visit was canceled. At follow-up 2 weeks later, she had no *Candida* or abdominal symptoms at all. The mother was very satisfied and chose to stop treatment, partly because of the improvement and partly because of heavy work commitments. She agreed to reschedule if any symptoms returned.

Case 2
Mary, Girl Age 20 Months

Main complaints: She had a vaginal yeast infection causing itching and pain with white grainy discharge.

History: She was Carol's sister and had the problem for the same period of time, for several months. The general practitioner diagnosed it as *Candida albicans* and prescribed no treatment. She was somewhat distressed by the symptoms. Her mother had been using tea tree oil in the bathwater, but this did not improve the symptoms

Additional complaints: She had a bad nasal infection with green phlegm and a continuous bad smell from the nose—the doctor suspected a problem of the adenoids but offered no clear treatment. She also had problems of frequent diarrhea (several times daily). Mary was fairly small and just below the normal growth curve; she also had some irritation of the skin around the nose. All other systems were unremarkable and she had no other complaints.

Diagnosis: Weak lung and spleen pulses, skin problems, and diarrhea indicated a lung vacuity pattern.

Treatment: Tapping was applied using a *herabari* to the GV-12 area, GV-20, GV-22, and GV-3.

Light stroking with an *enshin* was applied on the abdomen and down the back, arms and legs, chest, and neck.

Using a *teishin*, supplementation was applied to right LU-9, SP-3, draining to left LR-3.

Press-spheres were applied to GV-12 and bilateral BL-23.

Second visit—6 days later

She had had no symptoms of the *Candida albicans* since the previous treatment. She had also had no diarrhea this week. The nasal symptoms were unchanged.

Treatment: Tapping was applied using a *herabari* to the GV-12 area, GV-20, GV-22, LI-4 bilaterally, and on the arms, legs, back, and neck.

Light stroking with an *enshin*, was applied on the abdomen and down the back, arms, and legs.

Using a *teishin*, supplementation was applied to right LU-9, SP-3, draining to left LR-3.

Press-spheres were applied to GV-12 and *yintang*.

Third visit—7 days later

No *Candida albicans* symptoms at all. Also no diarrhea. Both problems had remained absent since the first treatment, but she had caught cold during the week. Although her sleep was poor, she had no green phlegm, just a small amount of thin nasal discharge, and no bad smell from the nose!

Treatment: Tapping was applied using a *herabari* to the GV-12 area, GV-20, GV-22, bilateral LI-4, and on the arms, legs, abdomen, and back.

Light stroking with an *enshin* was applied on the abdomen and down the back, arms, and legs.

Using a *teishin*, right LU-9, SP-3 were supplemented and left LR-3 drained.

Press-spheres were applied on GV-12 and *yintang*.

The next visit was canceled. At follow-up 2 weeks later there were no *Candida* symptoms and no diarrhea. The nasal symptoms were much better, with no smell and no green phlegm, only a little thin, clear nasal discharge. The mother was very satisfied and chose to stop treatment, partly because of the improvement and partly because of heavy work commitments. She agreed to reschedule if any symptoms returned.

■ Further Considerations

It could be useful to consider the following if your results are slow to appear or the effects of treatment are only short-lasting.

If the parent is not already using something like tea tree oil in the bath it could be helpful to recommend it. You may need to help the parent figure out if there is an irritant in what the child eats or drinks, and help identify and eliminate that. Of course, with slower-responding patients, figuring out and teaching a simple home treatment using tapping, stroking, and so on can be strongly indicated.

If the symptoms are more severe or nonresponsive I would consider trying *okyu*/direct moxa to points like GV-3 or GV-4. I would also consider applying light cupping over the lower back and lower abdominal regions.

I suspect that, if the condition is more chronic or severe, the kidney or liver pattern may show. In the two cases presented here, additional symptoms helped me identify the spleen and lung patterns. I thought about whether Mary might not be a spleen pattern rather than a lung pattern. I decided to try lung (thinking the issue could be weak lung, making lower resistance to infection) and change to spleen pattern later if there was insufficient progress.

28 Improving Vitality

There are two classes of patients for whom the primary focus of treatment is to "improve vitality." In the first there are no symptoms for you to treat, since you are providing auxiliary therapy to help the patient receive strong Western medical therapy, such as surgery, chemotherapy, and so on. Here you are trying to strengthen and balance the overall condition of the patient before or during those therapies to improve resilience and the ability to recover. In the second, you are faced with a patient who is in such a poor condition, usually with multiple chronic debilitating problems, that it makes no sense to focus on treating symptoms. Instead, the best approach is to provide general support by strengthening and balancing the overall condition of the patient, which can allow the patient to start improving more naturally from some of the problems.

At the beginning of Chapter 17, I described the three-, four- and five-level models for understanding and thinking about what you are trying to do. Taking the basic five-level model, you are primarily trying to strengthen the third level (vitality) rather than focus on techniques to trigger symptom improvements in level 1 (functional-structural systems level). As is discussed there, it is usually advantageous to target both the overall *qi* (*yuan qi/zheng qi/sheng qi*) with the core non-pattern-based root treatment and to balance the channel system using the pattern-based Meridian Therapy treatments. Chapter 26, Weak Constitution, further discusses the treatment of the weak constitution. What is described there is often helpful when thinking about how one applies this general treatment approach to improve vitality. Your treatment approaches will overlap. If we don't obtain satisfactory results in the treatment of a constitutionally weak patient, we can increase the dose of treatment to try to stimulate more of the desired changes, with, for example, use of direct moxa at specific acupoints. Treatment for improving vitality employs the general treatments of the non-pattern-based and pattern-based approaches but not the stronger stimulation methods. I have found that, for both

children and adults who need this approach, we obtain the best results by avoiding more stimulating, symptom-targeting approaches and instead focusing on only the channels and vitality. This is reinforced by the teachings of my Toyohari Meridian Therapy teachers, such as Toshio Yanagishita.

The following case is of a very ill little boy who, without surgical and other drastic medical interventions, would have died long before. I was called in to help him recover from the next major surgery that was planned.

Case 1
John, Boy Age 5 Years

Main complaints: He had been hospitalized for the last 3 months with severe gastrointestinal (GI) disturbance. He had chaotic peristalsis in the GI tract causing fecal matter to pass back up through the intestine to the stomach and out through the nose and mouth. This is life-threatening. To deal with this problem he had a tube placed through his abdominal wall around left ST-26 to drain his small intestine. He had a tube placed down his throat to drain his stomach. He had enemas twice daily to clear out his colon. The name of the diagnosis of this problem is chronic intestinal pseudo-obstruction syndrome. It is very rare. Life expectancy is very poor. He was not able to eat solid food and was fed through a tube (a portacath) in the right thoracic region.

History: By the age of 1 year his parents figured out that his gastrointestinal system was abnormal, and the problem was first diagnosed. Since that time he had spent about half his life in hospital. He had multiple abdominal surgeries to investigate and try to remedy the problem, including surgeries for obstructed bowel. He had continuous medical interventions with multiple tests for over 4 years. He could not eat normally. His teeth were abnormal and in poor condition. At this stage, eating solid matter only increased the amount of material drained out into the stomach and small intestine drainage bags. One measure of how well he was doing was the amount of fecal matter drained out of the stomach. He spent most of his time sitting in bed. As a result, he had developed problems of hip dysplasia and could not walk normally or well. He also had very stiff and, at times, painful back muscles.

It was decided that probably the best thing to try next was a colostomy surgery to disconnect the small and large intestine and to install an external drainage bag. He was on the waiting list for this surgery. It was decided to try acupuncture before he had the surgery to help prepare him for it. His mother was staying with him at the hospital, which was very disruptive to family life. He had had so many medical interventions that he reacted with fear in the presence of a new therapist. This is normal in a small child with his medical history. For the first visit, a case worker from the hospital assisted with explaining and helping through the various stages and methods of the diagnosis and treatment. He showed an especially strong fear reaction when hands approached the region of his mouth, again considered normal given the number of times that he had been orally intubated.

Assessment: Besides being fearful as described, he was in a generally good mood. He had a strong clear voice. His face was slightly swollen and round, probably as a result of medications that he was taking, such as prednisone. Sitting on the bed he had no problem playing and moving around, except to make sure that he did not pull on any of the tubes to which he was attached. He sat with very splayed legs as a result of the hip problems. His skin was a slightly dull white. Once the case worker had explained what was going on it was possible to get him to strip down to his underwear.

Abdominal diagnosis was not possible because of the numerous tubes and scars on the abdominal and thoracic walls. The muscles of his arms were very stiff, the muscles on his back were stiff and jumpy on palpation, and the shoulders and neck regions were also very stiff. The pulses were difficult to take as he would not stay still for very long, but the quality was overall slightly sinking and weak. The pulse rate was difficult to assess because of his repeated movements. The heart (first left deep) pulse, the spleen (second right deep) pulse, and the *ming men*/pericardium (third right deep) pulse were weak.

Diagnosis: In Japanese Meridian Therapy, he had a spleen vacuity pattern. He was not, as one might expect, in an advanced state of vacuity. The *yang* channels were probably all slightly weak. It was decided to target the treatment to apply supplementation techniques for the spleen vacuity pattern and possibly the *yang* channels, and to apply techniques to try to release some of the tightness of the muscles. As it was the first visit and it was possible to schedule the next visit the next day at the hospital, it was decided to apply a simple low dose of treatment.

Treatment: Using a *teishin*, supplementation was applied to left SP-3 and then left PC-7. The pulses were rechecked, and it was noted that the kidney (third left deep) pulse was relatively weak.

Supplementation was then applied to right KI-3 using the *teishin*. The pulses were then rechecked. It was not clear whether or how to select any draining techniques on the *yang* channels, and there remained a slight weakness of the *yang* channels. Thus supplementation was applied to bilateral TB-4 and then ST-36 using the *teishin*.

Using a *herabari*, light, rhythmic tapping was applied over the back of the neck and over the tops of the shoulders.

Press-spheres were placed at GV-12 and bilateral ST-36.

Next visit—1 week later

There was no significant change. There had been no word yet about when the surgery might take place, and since it would be almost a week before the third treatment, it was decided to try to increase the dose of treatment.

Diagnosis: He showed the same spleen vacuity pattern but was obviously more relaxed with the treatment.

Treatment: Using the *teishin,* supplementation techniques were applied to left SP-3, left PC-7, right KI-3, and bilateral TB4.

Using the *herabari*, light, rhythmic tapping was applied over the neck, *naso* regions, arms, and back.

An *enshin* was lightly stroked down the back.

Intradermal needles were placed at bilateral ST-36 with instructions to replace them the next day with press-spheres.

John's mother was also given appropriate tools to use and was taught how to apply the light, rhythmic tapping over the back, arms, legs, and neck, with recommendations to do this daily for a few minutes.

Next visit—5 days later

He had had a lot of intestinal gas and pain the day of the treatment with increased counterflow of food and draining of matter from the stomach bag. This improved the next day. It was discussed further and was decided that, although it could happen at any time, there was a high suspicion that the intradermal needles were possibly the cause. It was decided not to use them again. He was also scheduled for the surgery the next day, thus the treatment was principally to help him prepare for and recover from the surgery.

Diagnosis: Spleen vacuity pattern. It was decided that the counterflow symptoms recommended the use of the *he*-sea points for the root treatment. It was also decided to use the extraordinary vessels to affect the abdomen.

Treatment: A small copper disk was placed on left KI-6 with a small zinc disk on left LU-7.[1] These were retained for ~2 minutes. The pulse filled out and John became visibly relaxed.

Supplementation was applied using the *teishin* to left SP-9, PC-3, then to right KI-3 and TB-4 on both sides.

Light, rhythmic tapping was applied on the arms, legs, neck, and back using the *herabari*.

An *enshin* was stroked lightly down the arms, legs, and back.

Press-spheres were applied to left and right ST-36.

The parents agreed to call to set up the next appointment. John usually spent 2 or more weeks recovering in bed following any abdom-

---

[1]   This treatment method comes from the Toyohari tradition. See Fukushima (1991, pp. 243–251).

inal surgery, during which time he was quieter and not very active.

Next visit—9 days later

John had recovered remarkably well and quickly from the surgery. Instead of lying in bed quietly for 2 weeks, he was up playing after only 2 days! He was quite active at this visit. Since the surgery, the stomach drainage had decreased slightly, but not significantly. The parents had been trying to postpone this surgery for years. Now that they had decided to go ahead with the surgery they found themselves torn about what to do with the acupuncture. On the one hand, they could see that it had done something for John. On the other hand, it was very important to see what the surgery could do for him. As a result of this they decided to discontinue the acupuncture, so that this would be the last visit. Since it was obvious from the outset that John's parents were confronted with life-and-death situations not infrequently, and that they were under enormous personal strain, it was decided at that time to agree with their wishes without debate, and to ask them only to call if it may ever be appropriate in the future.

Treatment: The spleen vacuity pattern showed. Supplementation was applied using the *teishin* to left SP-3, left PC-7, right KI-3.

Draining technique was applied to left BL-58 and supplementation to right TB-4 and ST-36.

Light, rhythmic tapping was applied over the arms, legs, neck, back, and shoulders using the *herabari*.

Press-spheres were applied to ST-36 on both sides.

Next visit—17 months later

John's parents called out of the blue asking for more acupuncture treatments. John, who was now 7, had recovered well from the surgery and had been able to go home for a while. But 4 months before the parents called me he had to be readmitted with acute abdominal pain resulting from an obstructed small intestine. He required emergency surgery, from which he spent over 2 weeks recovering. Ten weeks later he required further emergency surgery for a similar problem, from which he also spent weeks recovering. The professor in charge of his case had found during the last surgery that John's colon was completely abnormal and after consultation with international experts had decided that the best course of action was to completely remove the colon. Since John also had a tube down his throat to the stomach and a tube through the abdominal wall into the jejunum, it was decided to replace these at the same time. John was also on parenteral feeding with a tube directly into the small intestine. These surgeries were planned for 10 days later and John's parents remembered that he had recovered well after the acupuncture the previous year; thus they called to see if acupuncture could be used to prepare him for surgery and help with the postsurgical recovery. Two more appointments were scheduled before the surgery.

Diagnosis: Despite having been in the hospital for the last 4 months and having major surgeries during that time he looked quite well. His voice was strong, he had grown, and he was both more active and more mature. He had daily schooling at the hospital. His flesh was full and strong, but the muscles were still very tight. When I inquired about his walking, the parents discussed how John was also scheduled for a brain computed tomographic (CT) scan to see if there was any abnormality of the brain that might be causing the muscle spasticity. Abdominal diagnosis was not possible. Using a *teishin*, supplementation was applied to left LI-4 as a method of confirming the pulse diagnosis. The pulse diagnosis showed a spleen vacuity pattern.

Treatment: Supplementation was applied to left SP-3, left PC-7, and right KI-3 using the *teishin*.

Draining technique was then applied to left SI-7, right LI-6, and supplementation to ST-36 on both sides.

Using the *teishin*, super light stroking (*sanshin*) was applied down the large intestine and stomach channels on the arms.

Using an *enshin*, very light stroking was also applied down the backs of the arms and legs and down the back.

Light, rhythmic tapping was applied on the head and over the areas ST-36 to ST-37.

Next visit—1 week later

Two days before, his portacath feeding tube mechanism had mechanically failed. This required that he have emergency minor surgery to replace the tube. Following such minor surgeries with general anesthetic John would spend at least a couple of days recovering. This time he was out of bed playing 2 hours after the surgery!

Treatment: Supplementation was applied using the *teishin* on left SP-3, left PC-7, right KI-3, ST-36 on both sides, with draining technique on left SI-7.

The *sanshin*-style super light stroking was applied down the large intestine and stomach channels.

Light stroking down the back was applied using an *enshin*.

Light, rhythmic tapping was applied over the head, neck, and shoulders using the *herabari*.

Press-spheres were applied to ST-36 on both sides.

Next visit—2 days later, 7 days before the surgery

John was doing well and was ready for the surgery.

Treatment: Identical to the previous session, except that SI-7 was not drained and a press-sphere was also added to GV-12.

Next visit—15 days later, and just before I was to leave for Japan to study

John had recovered amazingly well from the surgery. The surgery had gone well so that he now had no colon left. It was expected that he would be in intensive care after the surgery for 3 to 4 days. He was out in 20 hours! It was expected that he would be laid flat on his back in bed for 2 weeks. He was sitting and playing in 3 days! This was the first time that even the surgeon was wondering about the acupuncture. John was still on pain medication and still had postsurgical pain, but he was doing very well. He was quite active and had no difficulties getting around. The CT scans of his brain had come back negative. It had been decided to start pediatric physical therapy (often for digestively disrupted/spleen vacuity patients), and BL-23 for patients with strong kidney vacuity signs. If the child is having difficulty sleeping, try leaving the press-spheres at BL-17 and, if not reactive, around GV-9. If the child is in a very run-down state the extra points, lateral *pigen*, can be used (see Chapter 16 for location).

Chinetsukyu, warm moxa, is very useful for a simple general supplementation. The technique is not used often on children if they will not stay still or have respiratory problems that could be irritated by the smoke. The "supplementing" form of *chinetsukyu* can be used for the very run-down child as a direct treatment of the vitality by applying it to GV-14, GV-3, and the lateral *pigen* points. I have been using this extensively on adults with very good results. The difficulty of using this technique on very sick children, such as those for whom you have chosen the improving vitality treatment approach, is that either (1) they are hospitalized and you can't burn this kind of moxa or (2) they are too fearful, move too much, or have difficulty dealing with the smoke. But if you are in a position to use this *chinetsukyu*, it can be very helpful.

Other Considerations

Home treatment can be applied in a soft, light manner to help support what you are trying to do, and it gives the parents a simple approach for dealing with their very ill child. It is strongly recommended to try this wherever feasible.

Further Case History

The following remarkable case from my Barcelona-based colleague Rayén Antón is of the treatment of a 7-year-old girl with severe heart disease for whom the prognosis was poor. Rayén was on a field trip to Gaza with the UK-based organization World Medicine in October 2009. This case shows the power of the core non-pattern-based root treatment and its regular application by the parents at home.

Case 2
Malek, Girl Age 7 Years

Main complaints: She experienced sudden extreme tiredness, fatigue, lack of vitality, difficulty breathing. The parents stated that "her heart pumps more blood from one side than the other."

History: At the age of 5 years, Malek was diagnosed by the specialists at the hospital as having severe pulmonary hypertension. She underwent cardiac catheterization; the procedure was successful, but the condition remained and her parents were told that she would need to continue on medication for the rest of her life. She had developed increasing exercise intolerance and was generally quite limited in her activities.

Examination: Malek had a fearful expression, sad eyes, and timid behavior. She had a cyanotic complexion and big dark bags under her eyes. Her skin looked a bit rough and lackluster. Her abdomen was noticeably bloated (she was taking diuretics for her heart condition), and she was very thin and small for her age. The pulse was deep, of normal speed, and weak. It disappeared easily with pressure.

Diagnosis: The pulse and abdominal findings showed a lung vacuity pattern. This pattern was gradually introduced during the course of treatment rather than applied from the first visit, so that dose responses could be more carefully gauged using only a very light core non-pattern based treatment, which was applied as the main focus of treatment in this clinical context.

Treatment: Light stroking was applied with an *enshin* down the arms, the lower part of the legs, and along the back.

Tapping was applied on the GV-12 and GV-4 areas, around ST-36, and in the supraclavicular fossa region.

Remarks: During the treatment the pulse improved a lot, becoming fuller. Malek's general look was brighter by the end of the treatment. The mother was taught the basic core non-pattern-based root treatment using a spoon to apply the stroking. She was instructed to do this daily.

Second visit—2 days later

Malek's mother reported: "After the treatment she started running, at night she was tired." Home treatment had been applied daily. Malek had a better complexion and was less lackluster. The pulse was much better.

Treatment: Light stroking was applied with an *en-shin* down the arms, the lower part of the legs, and along the back. Special attention was paid to "opening" the chest (stroking from the sternum to the sides).
Tapping was applied around GV-12, the inter-scapular region, and ST-36 bilaterally.
Using a *teishin*, supplementation was applied to right SP-6.

Third visit—2 days later

Her mother reported, "Before I could never take her to weddings, because she was always so tired. Yesterday I took her to one and she was playing with the rest of the kids with no problem." Home daily treatment continued. During the previous visit it was clear that the mother's eyes had changed, and on this visit they were bright and strong (very different from the first day, when they were not bright and were carrying an evident amount of sorrow and exhaustion). The pulse was strong in all positions, and balanced. The abdomen was less bloated.

Treatment: Light stroking was applied with an *en-shin* down the arms, the lower part of the legs, and along the back. Special attention was applied to "opening" the chest (stroking from the sternum to the sides).
Tapping was applied to the GV-12 and GV-4 areas.
Using a *teishin,* supplementation was applied to GV-12, right LU-9, and SP-6.

Fourth visit—1 day later

Malek continued to improve. Her face was shiny, the abdomen less bloated, and her mother continued with the daily treatment at home. The pulse was healthy and full.

Treatment: Light stroking was applied with an *en-shin* down the arms, the lower part of the legs, and along the back. Special attention was applied to "opening" the chest (stroking from the sternum to the sides).
Tapping was applied around GV-12, the inter-scapular region, and ST-36.
Supplementation was applied using a *teishin* to GV-12 and bilateral SP-6.

Fifth visit—7 days later

She had improved further. She was able to climb onto the treatment table by herself, with an agile movement. Daily treatment was ongoing. The pulse was good.

Treatment: Light stroking was applied with an *en-shin* down the arms, the lower part of the legs, and along the back. Special attention was applied to "opening" the chest (stroking from the sternum to the sides).
Tapping was applied around GV-12, the inter-scapular region, and ST-36.
Using a *teishin*, supplementation was applied to GV-12, right LU-9, and SP-6.

Sixth visit—2 days later

Malek remained improved. Her mother applied treatment daily at home. The pulse was good, and the abdomen was less bloated.

Treatment: Light stroking was applied with an *en-shin* down the arms, the lower part of the legs, and along the back. Special attention was applied to "opening" the chest (stroking from the sternum to the sides).
Tapping was applied around GV-12, interscapular region, and GV-4.
Using a *teishin*, right LU-9 and SP-6 were supplemented.

Seventh visit—1 day later

She remained improved. She entered the room smiling, with gifts (it was the last treatment before Rayén returned to Barcelona). Malek and her mother both had a distinctly improved appearance. The pulse was good.

cated in a child who has a fever of over 37.8°C and one has to think about whether one should apply this core treatment on a child who has a raised body temperature up to 37.8°C. If the parent has made the effort to come and see you with the child, it behooves you to treat the child. You may, however, have a child present who has strong symptoms and a high fever. As an acupuncturist, I always feel sorry to send someone away without treatment, and I can always find something to try to help. I will first recommend that the parent take the child to their usual doctor for a consultation and then apply a treatment. I further instruct the parent to either go immediately to the doctor or, if the symptoms progress at all, to go to the doctor at that point. There will be some variations in how you might express yourself, depending on the parent and the condition of the child, but the message should be simple: it is better to have the child checked by the doctor in this case. If the child presents with only a mild fever (say around 37.8°C) I will proceed with treatment, albeit carefully. At the end I instruct the parent if the condition worsens, and especially if the fever increases, to please consult the doctor.

Although the core non-pattern-based root treatment can be contraindicated, there are a few aspects of it that can be applied and which can be helpful for a child with fever. Tapping lightly around the head can help encourage release of heat by sweating. Mr. Yanagishita recommended use of a very light stroking over the webs of the fingers (Yanagishita 2007, personal communication). Here the technique is applied by holding the needle or instrument between the index finger and thumb so that a small part of the instrument (*teishin, herabari,* etc.) protrudes. One strokes on the dorsal surface of the hand from near the wrist moving toward the web between the digits, moving your fingers between the fingers as you come over the web, angling slightly toward the palmar surface of the hand. Apply one to two light strokes over each area on both hands. This treatment is applied very quickly and does not take much time.

The pattern-based root treatment can also be modified to target the symptom of fever. Following the ideas from *Nan Jing (Classic of Difficulties)*, Chapter 68, we can use the *ying*-spring (fire) points for fever and the *jing*-river (metal) points for alternating fever and chills. The first time my

son was sick with a fever (around age 1 year) and we were figuring out what to do, we had just taken his temperature, which was 38.2°C. I applied supplementation with a *teishin* to LU-10 (the *ying*-spring point) instead of LU-9 to try to target the fever. We both felt some immediate difference, we rechecked the temperature and it was now 37.2°C and he looked less feverish! It was very curious. I continued treatment by supplementing SP-2. He recovered quite quickly and the fever did not (on that occasion) return. Of course, we do not always see such rapid changes, but we can get a hint from this experience. For the child who has the liver vacuity pattern and who today has a mild fever that alternates with chills, recovering from a cold that started several days ago, instead of using LR-8 and KI-10 you can try using LR-4, KI-7, and the *jing*-river points.

The symptomatic aspects of treatment offer several opportunities to target the fever. The most common approaches we might use on an adult patient with fever are moxa and bloodletting. Both of these can be difficult to apply on the pediatric patient, especially the younger child.

Studies in China found that applying a moxa pole to GV-14 on patients with a fever reduces the fever.[1] This matches clinical experience. We might use *okyu*/direct moxa to achieve this or a more hot but indirect form of moxa, such as a moxa pole. Probably the easiest technique on the typical child with fever is the use of the moxa pole at GV-14. I have not described the use of the moxa pole in this book because we do not usually use moxa poles in the treatment of children, and, in general, in the Japanese acupuncture approaches I practice I do not use them. However, unless one's *okyu* techniques are very good, you are not likely to use that technique on the feverish child; hence I will describe the use of the moxa pole here. First, do not apply this technique on the child with the higher fever (very rarely seen in our clinics).

Children usually do not stay still, especially the small child who makes unpredictable movements and on whom, if you try to constrain the child's movements, you create opposite reactions, struggling and more movements, or crying. We prefer

---

[1]   See, for example, the studies by Tian and Wang (1987) and Wang, Tian, and Li (1987).

not to do this. When we use something like a moxa pole, the danger for children is that they will not stay still and will move, bumping into the burning end of the pole, which would be disastrous. We thus need a simple way of maintaining safety if we are to use the moxa pole. There are two simple methods. First it may be better to use a lighted incense stick on the baby or small child rather than the moxa pole, which burns much hotter. Second, you need to fix the lighted end of the pole at a set distance from the skin and in such a way that the child cannot bump into the lighted end. One way to do this is to hold the pole close to the lighted end with the index finger and thumb, holding both bent, while extending the other fingers of that hand so that they touch the child. As the child moves he or she presses against the extended fingers, which are kept straight, thus allowing the lighted pole to be kept at the same distance from the skin. With your other hand you also need to touch the child to feel his or her responses. The child may move upon feeling the heat of the pole, or the child may move simply because he or she won't stay still. When the child feels the heat, move the lighted end away and then a little while later bring the lighted end back, moving away again as the child feels the heat. This approaching and moving away from the point GV-14 will allow the point to gradually warm up. Once it starts to appear a little red around GV-14, stop the technique.

On children, it is sometimes indicated to apply bloodletting, especially of *jing*-well points. Shimizu (1975) recommends bleeding of LI-1 and/or SI-1 for early-stage mild fever in children who also have a sore throat. On adults we can apply bloodletting to *jing*-well points for fever; thus we have a similar idea here. However, *jing* point bloodletting can be difficult on children and requires a good technique that is painless for a child. Chapter 15 describes how to do this technique, but you definitely need to practice on other people before you try it on a child with fever. If you choose to use the technique on a child with fever make sure of the following:

- Select the point for treatment by visual signs— the point and surrounding area are slightly reddish, maybe slightly swollen.
- Make sure to apply the technique not only painlessly but also so that when you want the blood to stop oozing, it does so (i.e., don't stab at all deeply).

- Remove a few drops of blood from each point, do not remove too much from each (i.e., do not stab too deeply and do not wait till the blood flow changes color or consistency).
- Have small plasters or bandages on hand to place over the treated point to be removed a short while later when the child arrives home.

Teething Problems

For teething problems *shonishin* can be very helpful. If the child is crying a lot and is very irritable, ask about general moodiness and sleep. If not so good, treat the baby child as the *kanmushisho* pattern. In addition to the core non-pattern-based root treatment, add extra tapping around the occipital region, LI-4, GV-20, GV-12, on the jaw, and below the ears. For the Meridian Therapy treatment, if the pulse and other findings are not clear, treat the liver vacuity pattern (supplement either LR-8, KI-10 or LR-3, KI-3); otherwise follow the pattern that you find.

If the teething problems are triggering nasal congestion problems, or problems of catching cold easily, apply the core non-pattern-based root treatment and apply additional tapping to the GV-22 to GV-23 area, LI-4, GV-12, and LU-1 regions. For the Meridian Therapy treatment, if the pulse and other findings are not clear, treat the lung vacuity pattern (supplement LU-9 and SP-3); otherwise follow the pattern that you find.

Applying press-spheres to GV-12 can be helpful, if there are hard, reactive points either on the jaw or behind the jaw around TB-17, applying a press-sphere to this can also be helpful.

If the symptoms are stronger and resistant to the foregoing treatment, insert needles with the in and out method to LI-4.

In more severe cases bloodletting can be applied to the thumbnail corner, especially LU-11 or LI-1 (Maruyama and Kudo 1982).

Infectious Diseases

Today, especially in the West, when a child develops an infectious disease such as mumps or tonsillitis, it is common that the parents seek the help of their pediatrician. Some parents may also seek help from, for example, a homeopath, but in general parents do not tend to think that acupuncture might be useful for such conditions and thus tend not to consult acupuncturists in these cases. In the past, in Japan, especially before the current health care system had developed, parents were much more likely to go to the acupuncturist for treatment. Thus, some of the older practitioners describe treatment of these conditions. It is possible that we as acupuncturists in modern Western countries may be called upon to see children with such infections; thus it is useful to know what to do to help, because the *shonishin* treatment approach can be quite effective.

Yoneyama and Mori (1964) caution for such conditions that if the child has a fever of 37.8°C or higher not to apply treatment. It is better that the conversation about whether treatment should be applied or not is best done over the phone so as to prevent unnecessary clinic visits and associated travel. In the case of tonsillitis, Yoneyama and Mori say if the fever is mild treatment can be applied.

Tonsillitis

Tonsillitis causes symptoms of sore throat, pain on swallowing, and, when very enlarged, mouth breathing due to obstructed nasal airways. The tonsils can start to become enlarged around age 2 to 3 years with significant swelling around age 6 years.

Several authors have different recommendations for the treatment of tonsillitis. I present them all here so that one has choices in the approach one wants to take.

Yoneyama and Mori (1964) recommend a two-stage treatment for tonsillitis: (1) needle around LI-18 to ST-9, angling toward and almost to the depth of the tonsils; (2) look for a swollen vein around KI-6 and let blood from it (they comment that the bloodletting is especially effective).

For chronic tonsillitis Hyodo (1986) recommends needling of LI-18 and ST-9 or placement of press-spheres to these acupoints.

Shimizu (1975) comments that we can view tonsillitis as lung and/or kidney related. As well as applying the core non-pattern-based root

treatment he recommends treatment of acupoints such as KI-27, KI-16, KI-6, BL-23, LU-5, LI-4, and BL-13 to help regulate the lungs and kidneys. Additionally, needle over the area of the tonsils to acupoints such as TB-17, BL-11, and ~ 0.5 *cun* lateral to C6/7. Finally *okyu*/direct moxa can be applied to acupoints such as GV-12, BL-12, BL-23, LU-5, and KI-6 (half rice grain size, three to five cones per point). If you use moxa reduce the number of acupoints needled and do not needle and moxa the same acupoints.

From the perspective of Meridian Therapy, if the condition is acute and has not occurred before, it is more likely to be a lung vacuity pattern (but we will rarely see children in such an acute stage). If the condition is chronic, with recurrent symptoms, it could be a kidney vacuity pattern. One needs to differentiate from the pulse and various findings. Supplementing KI-7 and LU-8 can be helpful, but if there are signs of fever at all, use of KI-2, LU-10 (*ying*-spring points for fever) may be better.

Writing in general about the use of moxa treatment, Shiroda (1986) recommends the following acupoints be palpated and reactive points be treated with moxa for tonsillitis: LU-5, BL-11, GV-14, BL-12, LU-6, LU-7, and KI-3. Maruyama and Kudo (1982) mention that bloodletting can be applied to the thumbnail corner, especially LU-11.

Mumps

Yoneyama and Mori (1964) recommend that, for mumps, it is better to avoid treatment when there is a fever. Treatment can be applied when the fever has subsided. For treatment: insert thin needles shallowly or place intradermal needles over the area so as to surround the swollen region.

Shimizu (1975) has a more detailed description. This is mostly seen in 5- to 15-year-old children. The child presents with early signs of headache, fever, a strange feeling over the swollen area, and a poor appetite. As the condition progresses the glands become swollen and painful, with difficulty chewing and opening the mouth. It can manifest on one or both sides. For treatment, quick relief of the pain can be obtained by placing an intradermal needle at the center of the swollen region (below the ear and toward the lower jaw). If there is no fever, then one can also apply the core non-pattern-based root treatment, focusing especially on the shoulders, upper back, upper abdomen, and lumbar region. Needles can be inserted to acupoints such as BL-14, BL-22, TB-9, and TB-15. Bloodletting can be applied to the thumbnail corner, especially LU-11 (Maruyama and Kudo 1982).

From a Meridian Therapy perspective you are likely to see a problem with stomach and triple burner channels, which point toward a spleen vacuity pattern. Because the child is older you should be able to perform pulse and abdominal diagnosis to select the pattern for treatment. It is also possible that the pattern is lung vacuity, perhaps with a disturbance of the heart pulse or kidney vacuity pattern, perhaps with a disturbance of the heart or spleen pulses. Treat according to what you find.

Rheumatologic Conditions

The following case from my colleague Bhavito Jansch in Switzerland illustrates the surprisingly quick changes that can happen in cases of arthritis. Following the case I outline general principles for treatment of rheumatologic problems.

Case 1
Maria, Girl Age 5 Years

Main complaints: She has joint and muscle pain over the whole body, especially in both legs. She could hardly walk and her parents needed to drive her to kindergarten and carry her up and down any stairs. She is always tired during the day, especially in the morning.

History: The pediatrician at the hospital had diagnosed juvenile arthritis. Maria has been taking the COX-2 selective nonsteroidal anti-inflammatory drug (NSAID) Celebrex (Pfizer) for the pain. The doctors have discussed their desire to start prescribing glucocorticoids, which her mother wants to try to avoid her taking; hence she brought Maria to my clinic for treatment.

Maria also has problems falling asleep and tends to have vivid dreams. She easily sweats at night, and her feet are always hot and sweaty. Her appetite is generally poor, and she sometimes has pain and abdominal bloating after eating. She also has dry eyes.

Assessment: She and her mother are very close. Even on the treatment bed during diagnosis they hold hands together.

The abdomen around the navel was slightly raised and tense. The liver area was also tense. The pulse was slightly fast, weak, and deep with some hardness. The right pulse was weaker than the left side except for the floating hard stomach pulse. Palpation of the left and right spleen channels showed a difference between them. Her knees were swollen and warm to the touch.

Diagnosis: The abdominal symptoms and pulse findings suggest a spleen vacuity pattern[2] with probable repletion of the liver as a secondary pattern.

Treatment: From the beginning we had a good connection, and we could send the mother back to her seat.

Using a *teishin*, right SP-3 and PC-7 were supplemented. Then a gentle draining was applied to left LV-3.

Using a *Yoneyama* instrument, light tapping was applied over the four limbs. Tapping was applied around the knees and the bladder channel.

Using the *teishin*, light stroking was applied over BL-40 and GB-34 on both sides.

Treatment finished with a cone of *chinetsukyu* to CV-6.

Second visit—5 days later

Her appetite and the bloated abdomen had been clearly better these few days. The pain was okay, but as expected there was no clear improvement. Energy seemed to have been a bit better.

Treatment: Using a *teishin*, right SP-3 and PC-7 were supplemented. Then gentle draining was applied to left LV-3. The whole upper back was

---

[2] In Toyohari Meridian Therapy joint problems are seen as a spleen channel sign (Fukushima 1991). This, coupled with the imbalance of the spleen and stomach pulses and the reaction in the spleen area, is sufficient to choose the spleen pattern.

sweating, so BL-20 and BL-18 were also supplemented.

Using a *Yoneyama* instrument, light tapping was applied over the four limbs. Tapping was applied around the knees and the bladder channel.

A press-sphere was applied to GV-12, and treatment finished with a cone of *chinetsukyu* at CV-6.

Third visit—7 days later

Her energy seemed to be improved and she had less pain. She was running around in my clinic, and she had been able to walk stairs this week. Her night sweats had not changed.

Treatment: Using a *teishin*, right SP-3 and PC-7 were supplemented. Then gentle draining was applied to left LV-3.

Using a *Yoneyama* instrument, light tapping was applied over the four limbs. Tapping was applied around the knees and the bladder channel.

A press-sphere was applied to GV-12, and treatment finished with a cone of *chinetsukyu* at CV-6.

Fourth visit—8 days later

She had had almost no pain this week. She was in good condition and running and jumping around like a normal child. The parents had not needed to give her any Celebrex during the whole week. Still, bending her knees for crouching remained difficult. Her energy was good. The night sweats had stopped.

Her mother reported that she was still anxious when Maria was jumping up and down on her bed.

Treatment: Using a *teishin*, right SP-3, PC-7, and then left LV-3 were supplemented.

Using a *Yoneyama* instrument, light tapping was applied over the four limbs. Tapping was applied around the knees and on the back.

Treatment finished with a cone of *chinetsukyu* at CV-6.

Fifth visit—10 days later

Maria's left knee was pain free. She still had a bit of pain in the right knee when crouching.

Treatment: Since the pain remained in the right knee I changed the sides of treatment.

Using a *teishin*, left SP-3, PC-7 and then right LV-3 were supplemented.

Using *okyu* moxa I applied mild *okyu* to BL-40 and some points around the right knee.

I noticed that she did not relax the same way during this treatment and speculated that it might have been due to changing the side of treatment.

Unfortunately the mother wanted to stop the treatments at this point, even though Maria insisted to come back for more treatments. I tried to make the mother clear that she should come back if the pain gets worse and tried to convince her to continue treatments for a while. She did not reschedule and I did not hear back from her.[3]

Comments: Bhavito performed a very good treatment on this girl. How many practitioners would have the courage to apply such a simple treatment on a child with these kinds of pains? We can suspect that, although Maria has juvenile arthritis, there are probably no changes inside the joints, which was why the simple and limited treatment was enough to produce such clear changes. When irreversible changes have occurred inside an arthritic joint, pain management requires much more and sometimes we have to add stronger techniques.

■ Summary of Treatment Ideas for Rheumatologic Conditions

Pattern-based Root Treatment

As mentioned earlier joint problems are seen to be spleen related; thus if the pulse and abdominal findings are not clear enough for you to choose the pattern, assume a spleen pattern. Also in *Nan Jing*, Chapter 68, the *shu*-stream points are said to be good for pain of the limbs; thus, in general, for treatment we tend to use the *shu*-stream/source points on the *yin* channels for the root treatment. If, however, the joints are really inflamed, red, swollen, and hot to the touch, we can try to

---

3   In clinical practice this is all too familiar. Not wanting to be intrusive or appear to be insistent we usually don't call to see how the patient is doing, and when we don't hear anything we don't know for sure how it has gone. But it is surprising how often the patient remains better when they quit early in treatment like this.

use the *ying*-spring points because they are indicated for signs of body heat (usually understood to be fever but can include conditions like this).

Non-pattern-based Root Treatment

In general this should be applied carefully, with caution when one is working around the joints. Light tapping around the affected joints can provide a comfortable local treatment.

Symptomatic Treatment Approaches

If one is needling, use of thin needles painlessly around the affected joints at stiff, uncomfortable points can be applied. A child who is in pain may exhibit sleep problems and generally appear more stressed out. Application of needling to points such as BL-17 for sleep and upper limb problems can be recommended. Generally, needling on the neck/shoulder region to help relax the area can be recommended, commonly around GB-20/BL-10 and around GB-21 are reactive areas and are treated.

But for local treatment in rheumatic conditions such as rheumatoid arthritis it is better to use *okyu* direct moxa. It is thought that the moxa has stronger local anti-inflammatory effects and can help modulate the immune system.[4] As we have discussed in this book, this form of direct moxa is difficult to apply on children; thus you will usually not apply it until after you have tried other approaches, the child is already familiar and comfortable with you, and everyone agrees that it is all right to try the technique. At first use the 70% style (i.e., not letting it burn down all the way to the skin).

For knee arthritis, paired points, such as ST-34–SP-10 and GB-34–SP-9, are recommended. For the wrist, TB-5–PC-6 can be used. For the ankles SP-6–GB-39 or KI-6–BL-62 can be used. Moxa treatments on adults with arthritis are described elsewhere, and in more severe cases it is also helpful to apply moxa to certain back *shu* points (Manaka, Itaya, and Birch 1995, p. 216; Shudo 2003).

Retaining press-spheres, press-tack needles, or intradermal needles can be very helpful for joint problems. For the knees, around the head of the greater trochanter and either SP-10 or ST-34 are recommended; for pain in the feet, palpating along the anterior line between the ankles and treating the most painful point can be helpful; for wrist and hand pain, around TB-4 can be helpful (Akabane 1986). Application of these methods on adults can be found elsewhere (Manaka et al 1995; Birch and Ida 1998).

Nervous Conditions

■   Stuttering and Stammering

This is not a condition for which many parents have brought their child for treatment. Usually parents seek help from specialized speech therapists. If the parents bring their child to you, and the child is receiving treatment from such a therapist, this is ideal. If they come to you and have not sought help from a speech therapist, it is useful to advise such therapy. Sometimes the parents have taken their child for psychological therapy to help with this problem. This can also be a useful therapy to help the child learn to relax and cope better with stress, and it may also be a good referral for the parents. If you want to try your treatment first and then refer after you have seen the response this can also be useful to help you understand whether your treatment is helping and how it is helping. A main target of your treatment will be to help the child feel more relaxed and help change the way that the child's body responds to what the child perceives as stressful situations.

Yoneyama and Mori (1964) describe treatment of this condition and report that this problem generally responds well to the *shonishin* treatment. Conditions that developed more recently are more easily cured. Severe, chronic conditions can be corrected with continuous treatments by the age of 5 to 6 years (if the treatment is started early enough).

Treatment

Use the core non-pattern-based whole body treatment with stroking and tapping needle (especially of the neck, shoulder, and upper back regions), as is used in the treatment of *kanmushisho*. You may find abnormal tension patterns in

---

4   In Chapter 13 I summarize ideas about how moxa that causes small local tissue damage might affect the immune system and inflammatory processes. This is an explanation for why moxa is a recommended treatment in Japan for rheumatoid arthritis.

the muscles of the jaw, around ST-7 and ST-6, so apply tapping to these. You may also find abnormal tension patterns around TB-17; target treatment to this area as well. On some children there can be abnormal tension on the sternocleidomastoid muscle; apply a little extra tapping to this region as well. Once you have established a pattern of treatment that seems to fit the child well, it is strongly advised to teach the parents a simple form of home therapy to be applied regularly at home.

I think for the pattern-based root treatment, this condition will show either a liver vacuity pattern or a lung vacuity pattern. Look to the pulse and other signs to differentiate which. In terms of point selection, this condition is usually associated with nervousness or worsened by stress causing nervousness. Look to see if there are any signs of counterflow *qi* in such cases (flushing of the face, neck) and try the *he*-sea points instead of the usual points.

In severe conditions one will usually find a lot of stiffness on the neck, shoulders, and upper back. One can apply light needling to the stiff points around GB-20 and BL-10. If there are knots around BL-14 or BL-15, one can apply press-spheres or press-tack needles to these knots, being careful about doses. One can also leave press-spheres at GV-12 and/or the point on the back of the ear behind *shen men.*[5] On older children one can palpate the thoracic vertebrae between T2 and T9. For the reactive point(s) apply *okyu.* This is Fukaya's "psychosomatic" moxa treatment (Irie 1980; Fukaya 1982). This is used a lot on adult patients within the Fukaya moxa tradition and is helpful whenever the patient shows a physical symptom due to psychological or emotional issues or stress. Stuttering and stammering usually manifest as such a "psychosomatic" problem. It is difficult to do this treatment on smaller children because it involves the use of more direct moxa. If there is a single intervertebral space that shows a clear reaction, apply around nine cones of moxa (the reaction should diminish with the treatment). If there are two or more intervertebral spaces that show reaction apply three cones of moxa to each space. For example, if below T4

is distinctly reactive, apply nine cones of moxa. If below T4, T5, and T7 are reactive, apply three cones to each.

Neurological Conditions

■ Convulsions—Including Epilepsy

Yoneyama and Mori (1964) describe the treatment of children with convulsions. This includes both the condition "epilepsy" and children who have febrile convulsions. Today it is not very common for children to come for acupuncture for treatment of these conditions. The epileptic patient is usually on medication, and if this does not work sufficiently, appropriate medical specialists are visited rather than the local acupuncturist. However, because children do occasionally come with the problem of convulsions, I include treatment recommendations as a guide to treatment.

Yoneyama and Mori indicate that children prone to convulsions (or epilepsy) can show slow, steady improvement with regular application of the whole body general treatment. The core non-pattern-based root treatment is good for the constitutional tendency, helping prevent the tendency to convulse. To deal with acute episodes, more aggressive and stronger treatments are necessary. *As a rule, great caution is advised in the treatment of epileptic or seizure-prone children. Proper referral and consultation with the child's pediatrician are very important. Treatment of the acute episode should be embarked upon with even greater caution.*

Treatment

For the emergency or acute treatment, insert needles to the *jing* points, or needle GV-26 and apply bloodletting to LI-2. Also add strong touching/tapping needle methods to the temporal regions. However, it is much more likely that, if a child has a seizure in your clinic, you will wait for the parent(s) to manage the seizure before you continue.

For the constitutional treatment, apply the core non-pattern-based root treatment with stroking and tapping, and moxa GV-12.

Root treatment using Meridian Therapy will be possible based on a full assessment of the

---

[5]   This is recommended by Mike Smith of the Bronx as useful for children with attention deficit hyperactivity disorder, and I have found it useful for children who have difficulty expressing themselves.

patient. On the older child you will be able to access the pulse and abdomen and choose the pattern accordingly. The most likely pattern will be liver vacuity pattern, in which case supplement LR-8 and KI-10. It is also possible that the liver may be replete (showing with a clear hardness of the liver pulse). In this case the child will either be lung vacuity pattern or spleen vacuity pattern. Examine the pulse and abdomen and other findings to select which of these patterns to treat. For the lung vacuity pattern supplement LU-9 and SP-3 on one side and drain LR-3 on the other. For the spleen vacuity pattern supplement SP-3 and PC-7 on one side and drain LR-3 on the other.

For symptomatic treatment, moxibustion is described by several authors. Irie (1980) describes the application of moxa to GV-8, GV-12, and GB-8 (three moxa each). Manaka, Itaya, and Birch (1995) indicate the use of moxa on GV-20 and CV-4 for infantile seizures.

■ Facial Paralysis

Occasionally in practice a child presents with paralysis of the facial nerves. Shimizu (1975) describes treatment of this condition, indicating that treatment of this problem on children is more effective than on adults, and one sees changes usually within 3 to 4 weeks.

Treatment

Apply the core non-pattern-based root treatment. After this apply in and out needling techniques to some of the following acupoints: BL-18, GV-8, CV-14, and LR-14 (to help regulate the liver); GV-20, GB-20, GV-12, and GB-21 (to help regulate the state of the nervous system). Then select and needle up to four acupoints from among the following on the affected region: for example, GB-1, ST-7, ST-5, TB-17; then needle up to two acupoints on the limbs at, for example, TB-9, GB-34. Finally, place intradermal needles to distinctive pressure pain points on the affected region, such as at GB-1 or more posterior to it, SI-18, ST-5, TB-17, GB-3, and ST-7. Also place some intradermal needles at distinctive pressure pain points on the limbs, choosing from among TB-9, LI-10, GB-34, and ST-36. Retain the intradermal needles for 3 to 5 days, then change them to other reactive points, rotating among the various reactive points continuously.

As Shimizu indicates, this can be treated also as a liver-related problem. The most likely pattern will be liver vacuity pattern, in which case supplement LR-8 and KI-10 on the unaffected side. It is also possible that the liver may be replete (showing with a clear hardness of the liver pulse). In this case the child will either be lung vacuity pattern or spleen vacuity pattern, so examine the pulse and abdomen and other findings to select which of these patterns to treat. For the lung vacuity pattern supplement LU-9 and SP-3 on the unaffected side and drain LR-3 on the affected side. For the spleen vacuity pattern supplement SP-3 and PC-7 on the unaffected side and drain LR-3 on the affected side.

■ Facial Pain following Brain Tumor Surgery

Case 2
Charlie, Boy Age 5 Years

Main complaints: He had nerve pain in the face on the right side.

History: At 18 months Charlie was found to have a brain tumor on the brain stem, which was monitored by the hospital specialists. At age 4 it had grown sufficiently that surgery was performed. They found it was a benign astrocytoma and were able to remove almost all of it, but due to the location they could not remove everything. The surgery caused some damage to the nerve controlling the windpipe so that breathing was initially disturbed but is now all right. There was also some minor locomotor control problem of the head and neck muscles so that his head easily leans to one side a bit, but while the head still leans a little, this is now not considered a problem. Following the surgery he also had facial nerve pain, which improved to the point that it only started when he had a fever from, for example, a cold. But recently the nerve pain started without fever and occurs almost daily. Also since the surgery, he easily develops mouth and nose sores due to herpes simplex and a lowered immune system. When the nerve pain is bad he takes pediatric ibuprofen or paracetamol, which offers some relief.

As a baby he had eczema and often caught cold. He is a surprisingly happy and emotionally stable boy.

Assessment: The history of eczema and repeated colds as a baby suggests a lung vacuity pattern.

Abdomen: The kidney and lung regions of the abdomen feel slightly soft and weak.

Pulse: the kidney and lung pulses are weak with a very slight hardness in the spleen/stomach position.

Given his medical history the first treatment should be very light, and he should be carefully watched to see how he responds.[6]

Diagnosis: The pulse, abdominal findings, and symptoms indicate kidney vacuity.

Treatment: Using an *enshin*, light stroking was applied down the arms, legs, abdomen, and back.

Using a *teishin*, left KI-7 and LU-5 were supplemented. Rechecking the pulse revealed a repletion of the spleen pulse; thus right SP-9 was drained.

A 0.3 mm press-tack was placed and retained on GV-12.

Second visit—6 days later

For the first few days he had no facial pain, and for the last couple of days he has had some intermittent pain, but at a lower intensity. He just came from a routine visit to the neurologist who declared that he is doing very well.

Treatment: Using an *enshin*, light stroking was applied down the arms, legs, abdomen, and back.

Using a *teishin*, left KI-7 and LU-5 were supplemented. Rechecking the pulse revealed a repletion of the spleen pulse; thus right SP-9 was drained.

A 0.3 mm press-tack was left on GV-12.

His mother was taught to apply home treatment by stroking gently down the arms, legs, abdomen, and back.

Third visit—7 days later

He has had no pain for the last 4 days. Home treatment is going well.

---

6   My experience treating patients who have had brain problems due to trauma, tumor, and surgery or developmental issues is that one sometimes sees a lowering of normal adaptive mechanisms such that an overdose of treatment or application of inappropriate techniques can trigger extended problems, which it is definitely better to avoid if at all possible. Hence apply minimal treatment.

Treatment: Using an *enshin*, light stroking was applied down the arms, legs, abdomen, and back.

Using a *teishin*, left KI-7 and LU-5 were supplemented. Rechecking the pulse revealed a repletion of the spleen pulse; thus right SP-9 was drained.

A 0.3 mm press-tack was left on GV-12.

Fourth visit—8 days later

He is overall better. He still has some pain, but much less.

Treatment: Using an *enshin*, light stroking was applied down the arms, legs, abdomen, and back.

Using a *teishin*, left KI-7 and LU-5 were supplemented. Rechecking the pulse revealed a repletion of the spleen pulse; thus right SP-9 was drained. Bilateral BL-13 and BL-23 were supplemented.

Press-tacks (0.3 mm) were left on right BL-13 and left BL-23 to support the kidneys.

Fifth visit—35 days later

He had no pain before and during the holidays. Upon returning he caught a cold, which triggered some facial pain.

Treatment: Using an *enshin*, light stroking was applied down the arms, legs, abdomen, and back.

Using a *teishin*, left KI-7 and LU-5 were supplemented. Rechecking the pulse revealed a repletion of the spleen pulse; thus right SP-9 was drained.

Press-tacks (0.3 mm) were left on GV-12 and right BL-20.

Sixth visit—21 days later

The facial pain was almost completely gone; he had had a few episodes of short-lived mild pain.

He just had a full checkup. They found some scar tissue on the brain and have scheduled a meeting with the specialist to discuss this.

Treatment: Using an *enshin*, light stroking was applied down the arms, legs, abdomen, and back.

Using a *teishin*, left KI-7 and LU-5 were supplemented. Rechecking the pulse revealed a repletion of the spleen pulse; thus right SP-9 was drained.

Palpation revealed a hard knot around right ST-6; using a *teishin*, supplementation was applied next to the hard knot on a somewhat softer region.

Press-tacks (0.3 mm) were left on GV-12 and right BL-23.

Seventh visit—21 days later

Although overall there is still less pain, he has had some pain on and off. His mother noticed that it seemed to coincide with episodes of nasal irritation/soreness that were possibly due to the herpes simplex. She had not noticed if the pain had coincided with these possible herpes irritations before.

Treatment: Using an *enshin*, light stroking was applied down the arms, legs, abdomen, and back.

Using a *herabari*, gentle tapping was applied over the shoulders and regions above the clavicles.

Using a *teishin*, left KI-7 and LU-5 were supplemented. Rechecking the pulse revealed a repletion of the spleen pulse; thus right SP-9 was drained. After this the stomach pulse was also found to be replete; hence right ST-40 was also drained.

Press-tacks (0.3 mm) were left on GV-12 and right BL-23.

His mother had been advised to think about a different treatment approach to the nasal irritation and was recommended to try a simple over-the-counter homeopathic approach, such as arnica.

Eighth visit—14 days later

He has had no pain for the last 7 days. He has been taking the homeopathic remedy, which his mother thought was possibly also helping. The mother also noted that there had been some short-lived complaints of pain when he had eaten ice cream or exposed his face to very cold air. This was also a new observation.

Treatment: Needles (0.12 mm) were inserted but not retained to bilateral LI-4 and GB-20.

Using an *enshin*, light stroking was applied down the arms, legs, abdomen, and back.

Using a *herabari*, gentle tapping was applied over the shoulders and regions above the clavicles.

Using a *teishin*, left KI-3 and LU-9 were supplemented. Rechecking the pulse revealed a repletion of the spleen pulse; thus right SP-3 was drained.

Press-tacks (0.3 mm) were left on GV-12 and right BL-23.

Ninth visit—21 days later

The whole family had bad colds, including Charlie. When sick with the cold and a fever he had facial pain for 2 days, but otherwise he had had almost no facial pain.

Treatment: Needles (0.12 mm) were inserted but not retained to bilateral LI-4 and GB-20.

Using an *enshin*, light stroking was applied down the arms, legs, abdomen, and back.

Using a *herabari*, gentle tapping was applied over the shoulders and regions above the clavicles and around GV-12.

Using a *teishin*, left KI-3, LU-9, and SP-3 were supplemented.

Press-tacks (0.3 mm) were left on GV-12 and right BL-23.

The next visit 4 weeks later was canceled. When his mother called in the day before the appointment, she reported that he had been doing very well. The specialist at the hospital had not expressed any need to do anything about the scar tissue except monitor it. She also reported that, with their insurance situation, they would prefer to hold off on having further treatments at this time and would call for further appointments if the facial pain were to return. They were very happy with how helpful the treatment had been.

Kidney Diseases

■ Glomerulonephritis and Nephrosis

Occasionally we see patients who come for acupuncture because of kidney disease problems. This is not so common with adult patients and is even less common with children. In the past in Japan this was more commonly treated by acupuncture. Today, if we see such a patient, the patient is usually undergoing Western medical therapy, such as steroids, and is often being treated over the long term. We tend not to see patients with this condition until they have already been treated over a long period with steroid therapy and concern begins to be expressed about the consequences of such long-term therapy,[7] and/or the fact that the condition is being maintained by the drug therapy but is not improving. Thus, when we see patients with such problems we are not only addressing the kidney disease itself and its manifestations but also secondary issues due to prolonged use of drugs. This can be quite complicated and can require extended courses of treatment to be helpful. Many patients do not have the patience or resources for such extended therapy, and so it is useful when treating children to focus on finding ways to demonstrate to the parents in a sufficiently short period of time that what you are doing does in fact help, and then working out a home treatment regimen so that the parents can continue therapy daily at home, reducing the number of visits to you. As described in the introduction to Chapter 26, p. 263, it is also helpful to find a way of reducing costs for the parents using, for example, reduced treatment rates.

Yoneyama and Mori (1964) report that infantile nephritis can respond very well to *shonishin* therapy. Rest, keeping the child warm, and altering the child's diet are, of course, important, but the *shonishin* treatment is quite effective.

Treatment

Apply the core non-pattern-based root treatment with the stroking and tapping regularly. Apply additional tapping to the area around GV-3/GV-4 and around the navel. As soon as you have established a pattern of treatment that fits the child, teach the parents to apply a simplified form of the treatment daily at home.

On babies and small children this is best treated as a kidney vacuity pattern. On older children where you are able to differentiate more clearly from the pulse and abdominal findings, you may

find a lung or liver vacuity pattern is present. In particular, supplementing the *he*-sea water points may be useful rather than the usual treatment points. If there are signs of inflammation with warmth or fever the *jing*-river points may be better for treatment.

Okyu/direct moxa can be applied to KI-1 (three cones) to reduce edema and increase urine output. One can also try treating the extra point *shitsumin* with direct moxa for the same purposes (Katsuyoshi 2006). Shiroda recommends several points to be treated with *okyu*/direct moxa on adults, especially CV-9, CV-7, and KI-16 (Manaka et al 1995, p. 214). It can be useful in stubborn cases to direct treatment to these points in older children.

Hyodo (1986) recommends light needling or placing press-spheres to BL-23 and KI-1 for this condition. Needling KI-1 is probably more difficult than moxa on this point; thus it could be helpful to apply moxa to KI-1 with needling followed by press-spheres to BL-23.

As additional home treatment on an older child it can be helpful to target heat stimulation to points such as KI-1 and KI-16. At first you can have the parents either use a small moxa pole or thick incense stick held above KI-1, moving the lighted end away when heat is felt and bringing it back again until heat is felt again. Start with KI-1, making sure that the heat is felt at least nine times. Later you can add KI-16 with this mild heat stimulation, making sure that the heat is felt at this point at least five times.

Postnatal Lethargy with Lack of Sucking Reflex

The following case from my Spanish colleague, Manuel Rodriguez, probably helped remove the need for the parents to take their newborn baby to the hospital. Incredibly little treatment was done to produce these immediate effects.

Case 1
Anna, Girl Age 3 Days

Main complaints: Since birth she had not sucked from her mother's nipples. She had been able to

---

[7]   The long-term use of, for example, prednisone, can include the following side effects: facial swelling, blood sugar problems, weight gain, eye problems, and sleep problems, among others.

get minimal nourishment when placed at the nipples as milk spontaneously dripped out, but she had no sucking reflex. She had also only defecated twice since birth. Her urine was very scanty. Her parents reported that she was sleeping most of the time, and they were both distressed and confused about what to do.

Examination: The baby looked small and with a marked tendency to flaccidity and lethargy. When carefully examined she did not wake up. Her muscles and skin felt loose, and the abdomen also looked and felt flaccid.

Treatment: Bearing in mind the baby's young age, a very light core non-pattern-based root treatment was applied using a silver *enshin* with one stroke over each area, followed by supplementation at CV-12 using a *teishin.*

The parents were then instructed in how to apply the core non-pattern-based treatment daily using a spoon. However, ~15 minutes after the treatment the baby awoke and started suckling, which she did continuously for ~2 hours, interrupted once because of the passage of a large amount of stools, requiring that her diaper be changed.

Anna returned 5 weeks later. She had continued with normal feeding, digesting, and defecation. Her length, weight, mobility, abdominal tonus, and activity were all normal.

Surgical Conditions

Sometimes parents present with their child after they have been told that the child needs surgery for conditions, such as inguinal hernia or undescended testicles. The parents come for treatment because they are afraid for their child or afraid of the surgery. If the condition is stable and not urgent, you can try treatment to see if the condition can be improved by preventing the surgery or to at least help prepare the child and parents for the surgery. It used to be relatively common in Japan for parents to bring their child with inguinal hernia for treatment by *shonishin*, and there are clearly described treatments. Today it is not so common for parents to seek acupuncture therapy for such a problem, but according to the published literature, the hernia can respond

very well to treatment. For other surgical conditions, such as an undescended testicle, if the treatment does not help the testicle to descend, it can at least help the child to recover more easily from the surgery (see Chapter 28).

■ Inguinal Hernia

Yoneyama and Mori (1964) and Shimizu (1975) report that inguinal hernias generally respond very well to acupuncture, especially if the treatment can be applied within a short time of the onset of the problem. These authors state that, if the treatment can be begun within 1 week of the onset, the effectiveness rate is as high as 90%. Shimizu states that treatment can still be effective up to 1 month after appearance of the hernia.

Treatment

Yoneyama and Mori have simpler recommendations for treatment: first apply thin shallowly inserted needles so as to surround the area of the hernia. Then thoroughly apply *shonishin*, either rubbing or touching/tapping methods, on the lower abdominal region and on the internal aspect of the thigh. Done regularly this treatment can cure the condition within a short period.

Shimizu has more detailed descriptions: apply in and out shallow needling techniques at two or three sites on the area of the hernia. Apply in and out needling techniques to around BL-54 or SP-11 on the affected side. On older children also needle BL-23 and BL-25. Apply the core non-pattern-based root treatment to help strengthen the body (Shimizu mentions that children with this problem are often a little weaker). On babies apply the tapping/stroking techniques on the head, neck, shoulders, back, and abdomen. On older children add in and out needling to acupoints such as CV-12, ST-25, GV-12, BL-13, and LU-6. On school-age children, as well as applying the latter treatment, add moxa to GV-20, GV-12, LU-6, and BL-23 (half rice grain size, three to five cones), making sure not to moxa the same points that have been needled (Shimizu 1975).

From a Meridian Therapy perspective, hernias can be seen as liver vacuity pattern in babies and small children. Apply supplementation to LR-8 and KI-10 or LR-3 and KI-3.

30 Combining Treatment Methods

This chapter discusses and provides examples of how to integrate the treatment methods described in this book with other treatment systems. Many people reading this book and practicing *shonishin* will have studied other forms of acupuncture. Two cases presented here, one from Diana Pinheiro, a colleague in Lisbon, Portugal, and one from Paul Movsessian, a colleague in Australia, serve as examples of how the systems can be integrated. With the help of Manuel Rodriguez, my colleague in Barcelona, I will also outline ideas about how to combine the treatment methods described in this book with Chinese herbal medicine. I am not an herbal practitioner and make no attempt to describe the practice of herbal medicine. Manuel is an herbal medicine practitioner; thus, with his help, I outline ideas and principles to guide the process of combination and give a couple of case examples from Manuel of when the combination was applied. Manuel has also contributed to the discussion on combining the treatment methods in this book with Bach flower remedies. He and I both use Bach flower remedies. My training was somewhat informal in Boston, whereas Manuel took a course on the method in the UK. I will outline ideas about when and how to combine Bach flowers with *shonishin* and present two cases to illustrate what the results can be.

Shonishin and Other Acupuncture Methods

Diana Pinheiro is a traditional Chinese medicine (TCM) practitioner and teacher who has performed pediatric treatment studies in five pediatric departments/hospitals in China. She studied *shonishin* in Amsterdam several years ago and has been using it in combination with her usual treatment of children. In the following remarkable case she reports on the treatment of Nillian, who, at the start of December in 2005 was a 5-year-old girl with trisomy, a very severe disease, which, from birth, usually leaves children crippled and nonfunctional. Many do not survive. Diana used *shonishin* as one of several tools to treat Nillian. In China, if acupuncture is used for a child with such problems, the tendency is to use very strong techniques because it can work when no other treatments are available. Some of the methods Diana used are from this tradition in China. We include the case here not only to show how *shonishin* can be successfully integrated into other styles of practice but also to demonstrate how this child has progressed far beyond what any doctor would have said was possible. Diana, Nillian, and her parents have done a remarkable job.

Case 1[1]
Nillian, Girl Age 5 Years

Main complaints:
- Gastrostomy (with a gastric button); she could be fed only by the gastric button, she was unable to eat through the mouth
- Hypotonia of the body (all muscles)
- Hypertonia of the Achilles tendon
- Vomiting
- Renal failure, with cysts in the kidneys
- Tendency to become hypoglycemic easily
- Tendency to catch cold easily

History: Nillian was born with a genetic mutation. She had a genetic translocation of chromosomes, monosomy of the ninth chromosome, associated with the 11th chromosome, resulting in the very severe disorder called trisomy. There was no family history of such problems. She was born 2 months premature (at 2.62 kg, 50 cm tall) and required hospitalization after birth. At birth she had edema and required ventilation for 2 months. At age 2½ years she needed heart surgery to correct a heart defect. The Western medical prognosis was dire: she would never eat through her mouth, and she would not easily gain strength in her legs, which meant that she would be unable to walk, with or without help.

---

[1]   From Diana Pinheiro.

Assessment:
- Red face all over, not only on the cheeks
- Hot face, throat, and chest
- Legs and feet were very cold, with cyanotic feet
- Runny nose with yellow mucus; cough with yellow, greasy sputum; mucus in the stools
- Yellow mucus coming out of both ears
- Constant asthenia and apathy
- Vocalizations only with sounds
- The legs were the weakest part of the body during movement, after motor stimulation
- Tongue: red body with thin white coating; coating more greasy and yellow on the sides, the tongue marked by the teeth; the tongue without tonus and slightly pale in the area of the lung
- Vein of the finger, purple, up to the middle phalanx

Diagnosis:
- Gallbladder damp-heat
- Liver *qi* stagnation
- Spleen and lung *qi* vacuity

Treatment:
- Clear the heat, remove the dampness
- Promote the free liver *qi* circulation
- Reinforce the spleen and lung *qi* to reinforce the kidneys

Methods and techniques: Shonishin was applied on the four limbs, the face, behind the ears, chest, and on the back, to regulate the *yang qi* circulation in the body,[2] to expel the excessive and toxic heat; stroking was applied downward.

Ear candles were used to clean the ears, to remove the mucus-dampness directly from the inside of the ears, and release the sinuses and throat.

Acupuncture with semi-insertion was applied[3] along the lung, spleen, stomach channel, and locally on *ding chuan,* ST-36, ST-40, CV-12, SP-6, SP-9, LR-2, GB-34, LR-14.

Flash cupping was applied[4] on LU-1 and LU-2, CV-12, and BL-13.

Tui na massage was performed on the chest to open it and alleviate cough, on the legs and feet to promote blood circulation.

Mustard seeds were left on ST-36, CV-12, SP-6, SP-9, BL-13, BL-23; on the ear points; and liver, lung, spleen, and stomach.

The parents were instructed to perform *shonishin* treatment with a stainless-steel spoon, and press on the mustard seeds, every day. It was recommended that the *shonishin* be done in the evening/night, just before bedtime.

These treatments were repeated weekly in the clinic.

After two treatments, the runny nose, the cough, and the mucus coming from the ears stopped completely, and the face was not so red and hot anymore.

After 1 month the legs became less cold; the muscles of the legs started to become stronger.

Two months from the first treatment, Nillian started to eat through her mouth, and the gastric feeding button was removed!

These treatments were given over an extended period. At the time of writing, almost 4 years since treatments began, Nillian is 10 years old. She has shown the following changes and responses:

She continues to eat through her mouth. She does not easily catch cold anymore. She has real strength in her legs to the extent that she started to stand and walk with assistance. At about the age of 6½ she started to stand up with help. By her eighth birthday she was walking with assistance. Now she walks on her own, using a "wanderer," a support with four legs, provided someone walks behind her for security.

Her body temperature is uniformly distributed throughout her body.

She now comes for treatment just when the seasons change, to strengthen the *wei qi* (immune system), and the organ *qi*, or occasionally, when she gets cold at school. If she is in a weakened state the treatment dose is reduced and, for example, seeds are left only on the ear points, ST-36, and CV-6.

---

2   As a TCM practitioner this is how Diana has understood and translated the basic *shonishin* treatment protocol; it is not the language of *shonishin*, but is an interesting perspective.

3   The semi-insertion technique involves the following: using needles (in this case 0.22 mm gauge) inserted rapidly to a depth of only 1 to 2 mm without retention. There is often a soft and comfortable itching or soft heat sensation, and the skin reddens slightly. The child finds the technique comfortable.

4   Flash cupping involves the application and immediate removal of the cup, so that it remains for only a few seconds.

The *shonishin* is still applied regularly before sleeping; I feel it is helpful to regulate Nillian's *yang qi* circulation, and to reinforce her *wei qi* system.[5] It seems to me to be a wonderful method to help to maintain Nillian's vitality, with more energy and strength.

It was possible to help this child so effectively with all the team's effort and collaboration: Nillian, her parents, myself, and all the knowledge that my teachers, here in Portugal, China, and in Amsterdam shared with me, for which I am very grateful.

Comments: We do not often have the chance to treat children with such severe disorders. How we each approach a child like this, and what we do, will naturally vary depending on our background. This is a remarkable case because it is clear that she would never have walked but for these treatments, nor was it ever expected that she could be free of the gastric feeding button and be able to eat more normally. Although I have cautioned to use very low doses to be able to regulate the effects, in such severe cases stronger, more stimulating methods with much higher doses can also be helpful. But records of cases like this are so few that it is hard to develop concrete guidelines. We try the best we can with the tools that come to hand and based on our own and our teachers' experiences. Special thanks to Nillian, her parents, and Diana for sharing this remarkable story with us.

The following account from my colleague Paul Movsessian from Sydney, Australia, is of a complicated case of a profound reaction to vaccination. Given the time pressures placed on him to try to prevent surgical procedures that were being discussed, Paul elected to combine *shonishin* treatment with Meridian Therapy root treatment (as outlined in this book) together with several treatment methods from the treatment system of Yoshio Manaka, "*Yin-Yang* Channel Balancing Therapy" (in Manaka, Itaya, and Birch 1995); thus this case is another good example of how to combine the treatment methods discussed in this book with other treatment methods. The results of treatment are quite impressive.

Case 2[6]
Sofie, Girl Age 3 Years

Main complaints: Following the measles/mumps/rubella (MMR) vaccination, Sofie had developed profound deafness and behavioral problems as a suspected reaction to the vaccine. The deafness was progressively worsening. Over the last year she had lost the capacity to hear with a hearing aid in the lower frequencies. Her speech was greatly affected. She was seeing a speech therapist but not making any progress. The doctors advised surgical implants to help with the hearing, but her mother wanted to avoid these and asked if I could work quickly to try and get improvements to avoid the implants. For this reason, I chose to perform a lot more treatments and a broader selection of approaches than would normally be done with a child, watching to see if Sofie could cope with the treatment dosage. This was an unusual and exceptional circumstance. Sofie had had various tests to investigate her problems, such as electrocochleography and a brain computed tomographic scan.

Additional problems: Her digestion was not very good, and the doctors suspected that she may have been suffering from leaky gut syndrome. Sofie also caught colds easily and showed signs that her immunity was weak. She became energetic as the night approached and did not fall asleep easily. She disliked waking in the morning and was always tired. As a result of all these problems her mother was emotionally exhausted, very concerned, and upset.

Additional history: In the last year she had had a strep throat, a parasitic infection of the gut, and anemia. She was taking nonprescribed zinc and homeopathic supplements.

Assessment: She showed frustration and irritability in her behavior with emotional lability. Her behavior was lively, and her eyes looked clear, with sparkle. Her breathing seemed even and normal. There was no detectable odor, and her voice had a slight groaning quality with low pitch. Her skin had rough patches but overall good luster. Her limbs and abdomen felt cool to the touch.

---

[5]   This is Diana's TCM conceptual translation of *shonishin* treatment effects.

[6]   From Paul Movsessian.

Diagnosis: Her symptoms and abdominal diagnosis indicated kidney vacuity pattern with secondary vacuity of the spleen.

Treatment: The initial visit was needed to gain her trust, so the treatment was kept short and light to assess her response. Using a copper *Yoneyama* instrument the core non-pattern-based root treatment with a combination of light tapping and stroking was applied down the arms, legs, abdomen, back, and neck for a total time of ~2 minutes.

Using a *teishin* needle, supplementation was applied to right KI-7, LU-5, and left SP-3.

The *teishin* was also used to supplement CV-12, ST-25, CV-6, and then BL-22 and BL-23.

We ended the treatment here, Sofie was happy that the treatment was painless.

Second visit—1 week later

Nothing to report from treatment except that there were no adverse reactions.

Treatment: The same treatment as on the previous visit was applied.

Treatment using the polarity agent methods of the ion-pumping cords (IPCs) was applied bilaterally to TB-5 and GB-41 without using needles.[7] The clips of the cords were pressed to the pair of acupoints on each side for between 5 and 10 seconds.

Sofie was clearly enjoying the treatment and was very comfortable from the beginning of this session.

A press-sphere was left on GV-14.

The mother was asked to study how to do a simple form of the stroking and tapping treatment at home.

Third visit—next day

Her mother reported that Sofie had been calmer and had really enjoyed treatment. She was look-

ing forward to returning for the treatment. Her mother noticed that Sofie seemed to have heard a car alarm that day.

Treatment: The same treatment was applied as on the day before.

Light tapping along the small intestine channel was added using the "Manaka wooden hammer and needle" timed to a metronome at 120 beats per minute.[8]

A gold-plated press-sphere was applied to GV-14.

The mother was taught and asked to apply a simple form of the tapping and stroking treatment daily at home.

Fourth visit—6 days later

Sofie had undergone hearing tests this week. She had scored much higher than usual but the doctors did not feel it was a real improvement. They gave her mother several more months before a decision was made on implants. The naturopath did a live blood cell analysis and found marked improvements.

Treatment: The same as the last visit, with the addition of draining with the *teishin* at left GB-38 and right LI-6.

Additionally *okyu*/direct moxa was applied one grain each to GV-14 and GV-12.

Fifth visit—6 days later

The mother reported that everything was continuing to improve. Sofie was feeling very comfortable with the treatments.

Treatment: The same treatment as the previous visit was applied except that the IPCs were replaced by the ion beam device (IBD), which applies polarized weak fields to the skin at a frequency of 100 Hz for 5 seconds on each side.[9]

Additionally, light tapping with the Manaka wooden hammer and needle was applied using the metronome frequencies to try and stimulate channels around the ears. TB-17 and TB-20 were tapped at a frequency of 152 beats per minute,

---

[7] Ion-pumping cords (IPCs) were developed by Yoshio Manaka and are described in detail in Manaka, Itaya, and Birch (1995) and also in Matsumoto and Birch (1988). The IPCs are simply a wire with a diode placed in them to create tiny electrical effects between the points to which the red (+ve) and black (−ve) clips are attached.

[8] The Manaka wooden hammer and needle is described in detail in Birch and Ida (1998) and Manaka et al (1995).

[9] The ion beam device was developed by Manaka; it is described briefly in Manaka et al (1995).

followed by tapping of KI-2 and KI-3 at 120 beats per minute.

Treatment ended with *okyu* on GV-14.

Sixth visit—next day

Remarkably, Sofie started forming words to speak today.

Treatment: The same as the day before except that the IBD treatment was changed to TB-5 (black) and GB-2 (red) for 10 seconds each side.

Seventh visit—6 days later

Sofie was still improving, but she had a slight cough.

Treatment: The same as the last treatment, except that tapping was applied to GB-21 instead of KI-3 and moxa to GV-12 instead of GV-14.

Eighth visit—next day

Sofie still had a slight cough but overall immunity seemed to have strengthened since treatments began.

Treatment: Same treatment as the day before with the exception that the IBD treatment was changed to black on TB-3 and red on GB-21 for 5 seconds each side at 7,000 Hz, and tapping with the Manaka wooden needle at only KI-2, TB-17, and TB-20.

Ninth visit—1 week later

The cough cleared after the last treatment. More importantly though, the speech therapist found that Sofie had undergone significant improvement in distinguishing letters and words in the higher frequency range. She was also starting to vocalize words and letters. The speech therapist was impressed by this, given the lack of any improvement previously.

Treatment: Same as last visit.

Tenth visit—1 week later

Sofie had shown an overall improvement in her speech, with a marked improvement in her pronunciation of words as well as use of new words.

The whole family had come down with colds; Sofie had surprisingly managed to avoid the cold.

Treatment: Same treatment as last visit except that LU-8 was used instead of LU-5, and the IBD was applied to GB-41 and TB-5.

Additionally, tapping with the Manaka wooden needle was applied lightly around the occiput to BL-10, GB-20, and GB-12.

Sotai (Japanese form of muscular or movement therapy) exercises were added to address tightness of the neck/shoulder region to improve circulation to the head region.[10]

Eleventh visit—5 days later

Sofie had continued improving. She was using more words. Her speech therapist was amazed that she was able to pronounce words outside her estimated range of hearing. At this visit, Sofie was a little more fussy and irritable, so a lighter treatment was applied.

Treatment: The core non-pattern-based root treatment using the *Yoneyama* instrument was applied with tapping and stroking as before.

Using a *teishin*, right KI-7, LU-5, CV-12, ST-25, and CV-4 were supplemented.

IPCs were touched for around 5 seconds to TB-5 and GB-41.

Using the Manaka wooden needle, light tapping was applied to TB-17, TB-20, and KI-2.

Twelfth visit—1 week later

Sofie had had a very good week. She was able to discern tones in her hearing, and the hearing test showed clear overall improvements.

Treatment: Same as previous treatment with the addition of supplementation to BL-22 and BL-23.

Thirteenth visit—2 days later

Nothing new to report.

---

10   *Sotai* exercises, a Japanese form of muscular or movement therapy, are described in Manaka et al (1995) and especially in the text by Hashimoto and Kawakami (1983).

Treatment: Same as last visit with the addition of press-spheres to the auricular points of the auditory nerve, to be placed at night while sleeping and removed during the day—repeated nightly.

Fourteenth visit—6 days later

Overall, Sofie showed marked improvements all around. Digestion, sleep, and tendency to catch colds were all markedly improved. There had been significant improvements in hearing, and she continued to make progress with her speech. It was decided to make this the last visit for now, with an agreement to reschedule as needed.

Treatment: The core non-pattern-based root treatment using the *Yoneyama* instrument was applied with tapping and stroking as before.

Using a *teishin,* right KI-7, LU-5, left SP-3, CV-12, ST-25, CV-4, BL-22, and BL-23 were supplemented.

The IBD was applied for 5 seconds or so to TB-5 and GB-41.

Using the Manaka wooden needle, light tapping was applied to the gallbladder and large intestine channels.

Sofie kept improving with no need for the surgical implants. At the last follow-up 5 months later, the hearing tests showed a marked improvement, and she did not need the implants.

Shonishin and Chinese Herbal Medicine

Chinese natural medicine is a powerful form of therapy. Although in China the materia medica of Chinese medicine includes the use of some mineral and animal products, the vast majority of remedies are of plant origin. Many of the animal products and minerals are difficult to use in Western countries where their use may be restricted or frowned upon. Thus, for all intents and purposes, in Western countries by far the most commonly used materia medica products from China are herbal, of plant origin. It is common outside of China to thus call this medicine Chinese herbal medicine.

Chinese medicine has a long history of use dating back to the time of the earliest medical literatures out of which acupuncture also emerged (Rodriguez 2014). There is a huge body of literature on Chinese medicine documenting extensive use over the centuries. Many traditions of practice have emerged during this long history, with several key figures contributing texts and theories describing its use (Unschuld 1985, 1986a). Among these was Sun Simiao (seventh century), who contributed not only the first specialized treatises on gynecology but also some of the first more extensive descriptions of pediatrics. From the 10th century up to modern times,[11] the vast majority of literature about pediatrics in China describes the almost exclusive use of Chinese medicine products.

In each of these different schools of practice, plants are prepared and prescribed in different forms. The plants, or parts of them, can be taken as they are, ingested raw, powdered, or decocted, but very often the raw plant, or part of it, is prepared by different means, such as being dried, cooked in oil or honey, and so forth, to constitute what the pharmacist will use as materia medica.[12] Sometimes single products are used, but more commonly several prepared products are used together to compose a formula where the components are thought to work synergistically. A thorough diagnosis is performed so that the formula that is composed for the patient matches the specific patterns, disturbances, and symptoms identified through that diagnosis.

This extensive body of literature and documented use over many centuries provides a background for a safe and effective use of Chinese herbal medicine. However, since this medicine is highly active in the way it acts directly on the metabolism of the patient, it is very important that the person prescribing the herbal medicine be adequately trained. In general, the body of

---

[11] Gu 1989 and see Chapter 2 above.

[12] There are many good texts on Chinese medicine available in English, including Bensky, Clavey, and Stoger 2004; Brand and Wiseman 2008; Jiao 2003, 2005; Scheid, Bensky, Ellis, and Barolet 2009. For pediatric TCM herbal medicine texts see, for example, Cao, Su, and Cao 1990; Flaws 2002; Rodriguez 2008; Scott and Barlow 2003.

knowledge required to safely and effectively practice this herbal medicine is quite considerable, probably even greater than that required to practice acupuncture.

Even if the therapist has some familiarity with the use of herbs, we must remember we are dealing with toddlers or children, who are highly reactive. Thinking about the prescribing of Chinese medicine, Sun Simiao said, "Only one in ten treating men dare to treat women; only one in ten treating women dare to treat children" (Rodriguez 2008). This informs us that, according to Sun Simiao, treating children is a hundred times more difficult than treating adult men, at least at the time he was writing. Of course with publication of specialized literatures the situation has improved, and we should thus not take this literally, but it does give us an important perspective: the person who prescribes Chinese herbal medicine for children should be properly trained. Simply being trained in Chinese herbal medicine and practicing it on adults is not enough. The practitioner should also be trained specifically in pediatric herbal medicine prescribing and preferably should have sufficient practical experience as well. If you are a practitioner of Chinese herbal medicine already and wish to start using herbal prescriptions for your pediatric patients, it is important to find a good teacher and training program first. If you are an acupuncturist who does not practice Chinese herbal medicine, as is typically the case in Japan, for example, if you wish to refer patients to an herbal medicine practitioner you need to ensure that the person is adequately trained. This specialized training will involve not only the details of how to make proper diagnosis of children and the corpus of literature on specific pediatric formulae, but also understanding the issue of greatly increased sensitivity to treatment in children.

Criteria for judging the qualifications of a pediatric Chinese herbal medicine practitioner are a matter of common sense and pretty much what you would expect. How do you choose a doctor or dentist? You want to know that they are properly trained, but can pretty much take that for granted since doctors and dentists must have completed extensive training to advertise themselves as such and be able to practice. There are government rules and regulations strictly controlling this. But as with many complementary

therapies, in the case of herbal medicine there is no government certified degree, at least in many countries.[13] Thus the nature and extent of the herbal practitioner's training are important, especially related to the specialty of pediatrics. You also want to know how much experience they have as a practitioner. Again doctors and dentists have quite extensive training before they are allowed to advertise themselves, but for an herbal medicine practitioner there are no obvious requirements in many countries before they start practicing. Finally, you will probably want some evidence that they are good practitioners: Have people you know seen the doctor or dentist? What was their experience? Do they recommend the practitioner? The same for the herbal medicine practitioner and, especially, do you know children that have been treated by this person?

Since you will be referring patients to this person you are indirectly responsible for what happens; thus it is normal for you to find out as many details as possible to help you make your choice of referral.

Training

Has the practitioner completed a full course of Chinese herbal medicine training? How long was that training? Has the practitioner completed a course of training on diagnosis and treatment of children using Chinese herbal medicine? If so, with whom? You can find out from practitioner associations or government agencies if there are government regulation or professional standards for what is normal in relation to these questions. If the practitioner in question belongs to an established professional organization that has good minimum training entry requirements, then you can be sure that person has good basic training in herbal medicine.

Experience

How many years has the practitioner practiced Chinese herbal medicine? How many years has

---

[13] Obviously, in China there are regulations, but outside Asia few countries have specified the required training. In the United States the national exam and state licensing provide extensive coverage. Australia recently enacted legislation, but Europe has as yet no clear government oversight and no requirements, except those developing in Switzerland.

the practitioner treated children with Chinese herbal medicine? And what is the practitioner's normal success rate with children? Getting answers to these questions will probably require you to be flexible as you assess the data and form your judgments.

Do you know of any children that have seen the practitioner? If so, what were the treatment outcomes and how was the experience? It is helpful to know more than one child that has seen the practitioner, but this can often be difficult information to find.

Preparations

Regarding the manner of preparation and administration, most formulas are prepared as a decoction; the raw herbs are mixed and then cooked or boiled according to certain methods. This is usually the best way to take advantage of all the properties of the formula, but the preparation takes time, and often the strained liquid is not very well accepted by the patient, though this is quite variable.[14] There is also a long tradition of using pre-prepared formulas that are available in other forms, such as patent medicines. These can be available in pill form or syrups. In recent decades freeze-dried preparations of the formula or single herbs are also available as concentrated powders, which are usually dissolved in water. Together these forms can be easier for the patient to accept and take because they are easier to consume and require very short or no preparation at all. In addition to tailor-made formulas based on TCM diagnosis, the Chinese Pharmacopoeia has many ready-made, off-the-shelf formulas, usually effective enough to solve many of the most common problems, such as general cough, fever, constipation, and the like. Many herbalists in the West will use such preparations rather than prescribe the raw herbs.

------

14 Manuel Rodriguez notes that, in his experience, from the standpoint of acceptance, he often has less difficulty with children than with adults. Children tend to refuse the decoction the first time, which is only logical, because the taste is unknown to them, but then they usually come to accept it a lot better than most adults.

■ Combining Chinese Herbal Medicine with Japanese Acupuncture and *Shonishin* Treatment

We tend to use Chinese herbal medicine or refer for its use only when the usual external treatments (*shonishin*, acupuncture and moxibustion, *tunia* massage) are too slow acting or aren't producing the desired effects. In these cases, and always taking into account the rules of pediatrics, herbs can be the definitive factor in producing therapeutic change.

Of course it is also natural to think that herbal medicine may be more effective for more internal problems, and in general this can be correct. That said, the case histories in this book demonstrate clearly that the "external" treatments of *shonishin* and Meridian Therapy with simple symptom control interventions can produce profound effects, even for complex internal problems. Thus, as a rule, if *shonishin* is not having the desired effects or if improvement comes too slowly, one might consider turning to herbal medicine.

The following cases from Manuel Rodriguez illustrate the combined use of *shonishin*-acupuncture and Chinese herbal medicine where the combination of external (*shonishin*, Meridian Therapy) and internal (herbal medicine) treatment produced some very positive results.

Case 1
Pablo, Boy Aged 12 Years

Main complaints and history: About 2 years prior he had come back from the countryside with some subcutaneous bleeding related to two insect bites. The reaction was thought to be allergic. Two months after the subcutaneous bleeding had been reabsorbed, the boy started showing petechiae on his legs. His doctor referred him to a specialist pediatrician whose medical diagnosis was Schönlein–Henoch purpura. The pediatrician stated that it should recover on its own in 2 to 3 months. This prognosis was incorrect. Since that time, Pablo has suffered repeated bouts of subcutaneous bleeding, for which he has been repeatedly hospitalized. He also started to have episodes of hematuria. The episodes were usually accompanied by fever, provoked by any infection (respiratory or urinary), which he is very prone to. They are even provoked by any body heating, such as physical exercise. Eventually he was additionally diagnosed as having essential hypertension and kidney insufficiency.

Assessment: Pablo is big for his age, a bit overweight with slightly loose skin. He has poor digestion with a tendency to soft stools. He has a red tongue and a very weak and slightly rapid pulse. Although he is not currently in crisis, he shows petechiae on his legs, and his urine is a bit dark. He says that he is calm, but his nails are bitten quite far down. His mother reports that he is very affected by his inability to live a normal life. He can be irritable and can have a crisis—petechiae and hematuria—if he becomes very angry. He feels cold, but he doesn't like heat, and he feels very tired, especially in the morning. He doesn't eat much. He has pain in the joints, especially in the knees, and he has high blood pressure.

Treatment principles: There were many different factors to consider: blood heat, toxic fire, blood stasis, low defensive system, spleen and kidney vacuity, even liver stagnation and vacuity. Due to the complexity the treatment was divided into two phases: crisis-related and between-crises. I began by treating in the crisis mode, because he showed active petechiae (bright red) and some hematuria.

Taking into account both the complexity of the illness and Pablo's age, I began by combining some *shonishin* with semiadult acupuncture (Meridian Therapy style) and herbal medicine. The first formula was based on *Dao Chi San*,[15] to address the small intestine fire, cool the blood, and promote urination. I also recommended that they keep on hand *Yin Qiao San* so they could give it to Pablo at the slightest sign of fever. Pablo continued taking herbs throughout the course of treatment, although the specific formulas were modified as needed according to his specific state and reactions.

Treatment: I applied the basic *shonishin* stroking and tapping treatment and supplemented KI-7, LU-8 on the left. I applied *okyu* to bilateral BL-17 and LI-11.

---

[15] I do not usually work with off-the-shelf formulas; my preference is for the most traditional herb-by-herb personalized formulas, many times starting with a well-known proven formula but tailored to better match the personal needs of the patient. This is why I say "based on" a particular classical formula.

Second visit—1 week later

The petechiae were improved, and the urine was normal.

I repeated the treatment and instructed him to continue with the herbs.

Third visit—1 month later

Treatment had been interrupted because Pablo had had the flu, which caused the petechiae to return almost to their initial state.

Treatment: I applied the basic *shonishin* stroking and tapping. I changed the Meridian Therapy treatment to the liver pattern, supplementing LV-8, KI-10 on the left and draining ST-40. I additionally supplemented KI-3. *Okyu* was applied on BL-17, BL-23, and LI-11.

Fourth visit—2 weeks later

Pablo was well, but he had become angry about something, which caused a flaring of petechiae.

Treatment: The usual *shonishin* treatment, followed by supplementation of KI-7 and LU-8. Needles were inserted and retained at BL-17 and BL-23 while *okyu* was applied to LI-11. Additionally, somewhat deeper needling was applied on SP-10 and SP-6 for the petechiae on the legs.

Fifth visit—2 weeks later

The petechiae were almost gone. His mother reported that Pablo had started playing as a normal boy of his age, with no bad reactions.

Treatment: Treatment was the same as the previous visit.

After the fifth treatment, Pablo came regularly every 2 weeks and drank his herbs daily. The basic acupuncture treatment remained the same, with the Meridian Therapy pattern varying between kidney and liver vacuity pattern. The purpose of the herbal formulas evolved from solving the crisis to reinforcing the spleen and kidney vacuities (with *Dong Chong Xia Cao*, plus a variation of *Gui Pi Tang*) and to help prevent fevers from infections (with *Yin Qiao San*). He no longer had petechiae or hematuria, but he continued being a bit fragile, producing dark urine almost every time he had a fever, although the hematuria didn't progress, and he didn't produce any petechiae. I recommended *Dong Chong Xia Cao* to help with the kidney insufficiency. He continued under Western medical follow-up.

By the ninth treatment he had been camping for 3 days without problems. After this we agreed to cut back acupuncture treatment to once a month.

Tenth visit—1 month later

He had a fever, but for the first time without petechiae or hematuria.

Eleventh visit—1 month later

He is now living a completely normal life. He plays, he participates in sports, he even has his angry bouts, but he doesn't show any of the previous symptoms. He continues coming to treatment roughly once a month.

Fifteenth visit—4 months later (after ~10 months of treatment)

He no longer has any heat symptoms, and he hasn't been ill at all. Blood analysis shows normal creatinine levels. His doctor says he can now be considered as being free from disease. The family agreed to continue our treatment, coming to see me about once a month, and Paulo continued to drink his herbs but in a much lower concentration.

Comments: As stated earlier, because of both the complexity of the case and the age of the boy, together with the need to get rid of the blood heat and stasis as soon as possible, I used both acupuncture and herbs right from the beginning. Also I think that the two-staged approach (crisis and intercrisis) has been key to the effectiveness of the treatment. Having in mind the severity of this boy's basic diagnosis—kidney insufficiency— and the rarity of its first manifestations, I consider the success of this case as a good example of developing a treatment strategy combining several therapeutic methods.

Case 2
Carla, Girl Age 13 Years

Main complaints and history: She is nervous, irritable, and has had difficulty with concentration since early childhood. She was treated by a psychologist at age 11 but with no improvement. She has had many small obsessions and manias since she was 12.

Problems at school have caused her to become behind in her studies, and the school authorities (including a psychologist) recommended Ritalin (Novartis), a treatment the parents would prefer to avoid.

Other than the behavior problems, she had recurrent respiratory infections from birth up through age 3, treated by her doctor with a mix of antibiotics, bronchodilators, and corticoids. Around the age of 3 the respiratory problems receded, but skin problems started. She was diagnosed as having atopic dermatitis, treated with corticoid creams and an antihistamine medication, Polaramine (Schering-Plough Pty Ltd).

She has allergy reactions, both airborne and contact. While not well identified yet, there appear to be many such irritants.

Additionally she has bed-wetting problems and appears never to have fully mastered control of her bladder. She still uses diapers to go to bed and her family appears not to think much of this.

She began her menstruation at age 12 and has no obvious problems with it.

In addition to her concentration difficulties, which affect her studies, she tends to be irritable and easily frustrated. She is eager to please and always wants to be well appreciated by her peers.

She consumes a lot of cow's milk products and likes sweet confection products, such as cakes, eating them to the point that she can sometimes complain of indigestion and abdominal pain.

Assessment: She has small facial tics and difficulty keeping still. She appears to have low self-esteem; her family ties may need to be explored.

She has dry skin. The skin lesions are ongoing with permanent pruritus; at night this often disturbs her sleep. There are visible scratches. She uses Polaramine to help control the worst periods.

Her weight appears almost normal. She sighs often and reports intermittent feelings of thoracic oppression.

Tongue: The body is red, rough, big, and with dental imprints. The coat is dry and very thin.

Pulse: Her pulse is deep, weak, and tense, threadlike. It is fast, and weaker in spleen and heart.

Treatment principles: Behavior troubles seem to point to several systems, at least spleen (pulse, compulsive behavior, and digestive problems), heart (pulse, concentration problems—together with the spleen), liver (irritability, moodiness). The skin and history of respiratory problems show a strong lung connection, and the early onset of the pathologies together with the urinary troubles also shows kidney. The complexity of the case points to a probable *yin*-fire syndrome.

The complex presentation, the relatively older age, and the presence of regular menstruation put this patient somewhere in the middle between being a child and an adult. So I introduced dietary suggestions (control pastries, avoid cow's milk and dairy products, etc.) and used both *shonishin*, regular acupuncture (Manaka style[16]), and Chinese herbs in a step by step approach, focusing on the behavior problems.

Treatment details: For *shonishin*, I performed and then instructed the mother to do a daily general body tapping treatment with strict explanations about how to avoid the most affected skin lesions, with a special focus on treatment of the head, nape of the neck, shoulders, and around ST-36, GV-12, and GV-4 areas.

Using Manaka style treatment with the ion-pumping cords (IPCs), the patterns changed with the progression of the treatment. I started with a pattern associated with liver–kidney disturbance (according to Stephen Birch "K3L"),[17] and then evolved to treatment of the *yin qiao renmai* pattern.[18] Because the girl was aversive to the use of needles I instead taped small metallic disks to the treatment points and attached the IPCs to them.

I had her come in twice a week for treatment.

---

[16] This refers to the treatment methods of Yoshio Manaka; see *Chasing the Dragon's Tail* for details (Manaka et al 1995).

[17] This treatment is right LI-4 (black) – left LV-3 (red) + right KI-6 (black) – left LU-7 red.

[18] Bilateral KI-6 (black) – LU-7 (red).

She started taking herbal formulas the second week; they are primarily related to helping deal with the *yin*-fire syndrome and helping control the symptoms. They were first a variation of *Xiao Chai Hu Tang*, and then a variation of *Zuo Gui Yin*, alternated with a variation of *Xiao Yao San*.

She already started to improve in the second week. On the third week we decided to make clinic visits once a week because she was already improving. After 4 more weeks of these treatments there were greater improvements such that even the school had commented on them. Carla appeared to be much happier, she was much calmer and able to be still and focused. I continued treating her for a further 6 weeks, after which, because her main complaints were much better and she felt much better, I terminated treatment. At that time I made further recommendations to the family to try to maintain the dietary guidelines and to perform the *shonishin* tapping from time to time, perhaps once a week.

Remarks: All the involved factors, the age, the menstruation, and the complexity, called for a treatment combining pediatric with adult medicines. I thought it good to use the *shonishin* mainly to introduce a psychologically positive input into the family relationships and also to help relieve both the patient and the parents of the idea that "nothing can be done," empowering them with a tool they could use themselves. Carla's response to the whole treatment was unusually rapid. I was surprised and delighted at how fast her behavior changed. The skin also improved, and with it the sleep was better, which in my understanding, was a critical factor in her ability to recover to a normal and more stable neurological and mental state.

Shonishin and Bach Flowers

Bach flowers are a kind of herbal remedy produced in a manner reminiscent of that used for homeopathic products. They were developed by the English physician Dr. Edward Bach in the 1930s and have been used as a form of natural treatment since. There are 38 remedies produced as tinctures of each flower essence. Probably most readers have heard of the rescue remedy, which is one of the Bach flower remedies, specific for shock and trauma.

They are administered by putting a few drops of the selected remedies into some water. They are taken by placing the water essence mix under the tongue. Each remedy is selected not for its effects on physical problems but for its effects on specific emotional manifestations. When you purchase a Bach flower set it will include a list of the remedies with a short list of specific emotional states that are associated with each.[19] If you read Bach's book it gives much more detail and examples of the ways that these emotional states can manifest. The Bach Centre in the UK provides courses that teach in much greater detail how to diagnose and apply the remedies. There are thus very simple and straightforward ways to apply them and, with more in-depth training, more extended ways of applying them. Dr. Bach designed this system for ease of use.

I studied them in a short course in Boston more than 30 years ago. I have used them with some patients over this time, but they have not been a major part of my treatment approach for treatment of adults or children. I am not an expert, and I tend to use the very simple method of selecting them for patients. In some cases I have had good results that I attributed to their use. Thus I am not teaching here how to use them; this information is available in books[20] and courses, where their application can be studied in much greater detail.[21]

The biggest clue that it might be good to try some Bach flower remedies for your pediatric patient will be the emotional states and manifestations of the patient. For example, the child that seems unusually fearful, is having nightmares or disturbing dreams, or has very poor self-confidence, or is very irritable—these are typical indications for thinking about the use of the Bach flowers. You may have treated children with these emotions before and seen them improve with your regular *shonishin* treatments. But in the cases where these emotions do not seem to change with the usual treatments I have tended to use the Bach flowers. Or you may have an insight that, because the emotional states and expressions are so strong, it might be more effective to work more directly at that level and not to wait to try the Bach flower remedies. In the model of treatment I outlined in earlier chapters, Bach flower remedies have the potential to improve the emotional and mental state of the child and thus work at level four in that model.

My method of selecting which remedies to use is very simple. I look over the list and keep in mind an impression of likely remedies that might be appropriate. But since I often have very short periods of time with the child and often little or no discussion with the child, I have the parents instead read through the short list and make a selection. I quickly review their choices, and for those that seem odd I question them and maybe delete them from the list based on our conversation. For remedies that I had thought of but that are not included I ask the parent. I may then add that remedy to the selection based on the response of the parent. Thus I primarily have the parent make the selection and then refine the choice based on my own insights and thoughts. Older children who have followed the discussion may then demand that their parent show them the list and then critique some of the selections. This can also help play an additional role in refining the selection. But I do not ask for this; this happens only if the child chooses to participate by demanding to know what their parent has selected. My colleague Manuel Rodriguez completed a course at the Bach Centre in the UK. Based on this course he uses different guidelines for their selection. He selects the flower essences by a combination of clinical interview mixed with assessment of the patient's behavior, condition, and environment. This involves observation and usually between 5 and 10 questions answered by patients or their parents. When the patient is at a verbally articulate age it is interesting to note the differences between the patient's responses and the parent's responses to the same question.

---

[19] You can see the short list and further explanations on the Bach Flower Centre website: http://www.bachcentre.com/centre/remedies.htm.

[20] See in particular the book that compiles several of Bach's publications: *The Bach Flower Remedies* (Bach, Wheeler 1979).

[21] See http://www.bachcentre.com/centre/remedies.htm.

Case 1
May, Girl Age 13 Years

Main complaints and history: She was born with a cleft palate. As a result she was unable to suckle and required a nasogastric tube to feed. She had surgery at age 1 to repair the cleft palate. After this she could start eating, but since she had also not developed a clear hunger reflex she has always had a very poor appetite. She has always eaten very slowly and in small quantities. Consequently she has always been below the normal growth curve for her age, smaller and thinner than most other children her age. At age 13 she is very small and does not gain weight easily.

She has also had problems with recurrent ear infections, requiring frequent use of antibiotics. She had tubes placed in both ears, but she can still have ear problems that sometimes affect her hearing. The last ear infection was 2 weeks earlier and was treated with herbal medicine rather than antibiotics. She had an infection on average once per 3 months.

She can become irritable easily. When hot and sweaty she easily develops patches of eczema. She has received a little acupuncture in the past.

Assessment: She is a bit nervous on this first visit. The pulse is difficult to read clearly; thus treatment was begun with the *enshin* and the pulses rechecked after that.

Treatment and diagnosis: Stroking with an *enshin* was applied lightly down the arms, legs, and abdomen. On rechecking the pulses it was now clear that she had a lung vacuity with liver repletion pattern.

Using the *teishin*, right LU-9 and SP-3 were supplemented. Left LV-3 and right TB-5 were drained.

Using the *teishin*, supplementation was applied to soft-feeling regions in the supraclavicular fossa regions and in the regions of the anterior-superior iliac spine on the abdomen.

Needles (0.12 mm) were inserted and retained a few minutes to reactions around bilateral TB-17.

Then using the *enshin*, stroking was applied down the back and back of the legs. Tapping was applied over the back of the shoulders.

Press-tack needles (0.6 mm) were placed to right BL-18 and left BL-20.

Second visit—8 days later

She had been a little more irritable this week, making her a little more tense, and she had had a discharge from the left ear but without pain.

She had managed the treatment all right and was less tense in the treatment room.

Treatment: Using 0.12 mm needles, in and out needling technique was applied to bilateral LI-4.

Using the *teishin*, right LU-9 and SP-3 were supplemented. Left LV-3 and BL-58 were drained.

Needles (0.12 mm) were then inserted to bilateral GB-20 and the reactive points around TB-17.

Press-tack needles (0.3 mm) were applied to GV-12 and on the back of the left ear behind *shen men*.

Comment: Stroking with the *enshin* had been applied on the first occasion to help her become more relaxed with treatment and as a simple aid to clarifying the pulses for the purposes of deciding the pattern for treatment. On this second treatment stroking was not applied, and 0.3 mm press-tack needles were applied instead of 0.6 mm to lower the dose of treatment in case the stronger dose of the 0.6 mm press-tack needles had caused the increased irritability during the week.

To finish treatment her mother was asked to select Bach flower remedies, choosing three of them. A set of Bach flowers was made up and given to the patient with instructions to take them under the tongue three to four times per day. I gave her a dose before she left the treatment room.

Third visit—55 days later

The previous treatment had had a remarkable effect. The patient and parents had to travel more than 1 hour to return home from the clinic. On the way May complained of being hungry so they stopped for her to eat. She devoured a large quantity of food. This was very surprising; she had never done this before.

Since that second visit she had had a much stronger appetite. She had eaten much more than ever before. She had grown more than 6 cm (outgrowing by far all her newly bought summer clothing). She was not as thin as before. Her parents were very pleased with this change. May was also very pleased with the change and appeared in the treatment room with more poise and confidence, and her mood had been much better.

During this time she also had a mild ear infection, but without pain, that did not need medical intervention.

Treatment: Using the *teishin*, right LU-9 and SP-3 were supplemented. Left LV-3, BL-58, and right TB-5 were drained.

Needles (0.12 mm) were then inserted to bilateral GB-21 and the reactive points around TB-17.

Press-tack needles (0.3 mm) were applied to GV-12 and on the back of the left ear behind *shen men*.

She was given more of the Bach flowers. Her mother selected the same three.

Fourth visit—28 days later

She had had no problem with her ears. Her appetite was still good; she was eating well and she had grown further. When she lay on the treatment table her abdomen now appeared slightly rounded, whereas previously she had been thin with a somewhat concave appearance of the abdominal wall.

Treatment: Using the *teishin*, right LU-9 and SP-3 were supplemented. Left LV-3, BL-58, and ST-40 were drained.

Light stroking was applied down the arms and across the shoulders using an *enshin*.

Light tapping was applied across the shoulders and around the ears using a *herabari*.

Needles (0.12 mm) were then inserted to bilateral GB-21 and the reactive point around right TB-17.

Press-tack needles (0.3 mm) were applied to GV-12 and on the back of the right ear behind *shen men*.

She was given more of the Bach flowers. Her mother selected the same three again.

Fifth visit—118 days later

She has been doing well continuously. Her ears have had no problem. Her appetite and eating remain improved, and she continues to grow. She has just been told that, due to the small size of her jaw, she will need to have some teeth removed and wear a brace to correct the position of the remaining teeth. She is slightly anxious about this.

Treatment: Needles (0.12 mm) were inserted bilaterally to the stiff region at the top of the sternocleidomastoid muscle, just below the attachment.

Using the *teishin*, right LU-9 and SP-3 were supplemented. Left LV-3, BL-58, and right TB-5 were drained. BL-13 and BL-20 were supplemented.

Needles (0.12 mm) were inserted bilaterally to GB-21.

Press-tack needles (0.3 mm) were applied to the stiff points just below the attachment of the sternocleidomastoid muscles and to GV-12.

Comments: The change after the second treatment was immediate. She had been given the first dose of the Bach flowers as she was leaving the treatment room. Thus it is not possible to say whether this sudden change was an effect of the acupuncture treatment or the Bach flowers. It was probably a synergistic effect of both. We do not know whether a child with this history of cleft palate and eating disorder would have started spontaneously eating better and gaining weight, growing more normally without the treatment, but it seems as if the treatment loosened a kind of emotional blockage she had had since infancy. On the last report she was happier, less irritable, more self-confident, and still growing to catch up with her peers!

For additional examples of the use of Bach flowers combined with *shonishin* treatment see the following: Karen, age 12, problem of bed-wetting, see Chapter 22, and Nellie, age 6, problem of anxiety and fearfulness, see Chapter 21.

Appendix

Glossary of *Shonishin* Terminology

Bachibari
Shonishin tool used for stroking (**Fig. 6.5f**).

Chinetsukyu
Warm moxa technique, developed by one of the early Meridian Therapists, Keiri Inoue, as a simple technique to help with *qi* regulation.

Chishin
The "retained needle" method: a technique by which the needle is inserted and retained for a while.

Chokishin
Flat-surfaced instrument used for stroking, tapping, or scratching (**Fig. 6.3d**).

Choto
Shonishin tool used for stroking (**Fig. 6.5g**).

Daishi hari
Tool used in the style of Masanori Tanioka of Osaka (**Fig. 2.13**).

Empishin
Press-tack needles, especially the new Pyonex type by Seirin.

Enrishin
Shonishin tool used for pressing, tapping, or stroking (**Fig. 6.11h**).

Enshin
One of the nine needles of the *Ling Shu*, the round-headed needle used for stroking or rubbing (**Fig. 6.5a, b**).

Herabari
Shonishin tool used for tapping (**Fig. 6.3a**).

Heragata
Shonishin tool used for tapping (**Fig. 6.3b**).

Hinaishin
Intradermal needles; these are placed obliquely and shallowly and then retained for awhile.

Honchiho
A well-performed Meridian Therapy root treatment (the Chinese term is *zhibenfa*).

Kakibari
Shonishin tool, an alternate name for the *herabari*.

Kan
The Chinese term is *gan*, which developed in pediatric medicine in China and encompasses many symptoms and different types, such as spleen *gan*, liver *gan*, lung *gan*, and so on. Each has a different manifestation. In Japan the term *kan* came to represent children's diseases in a more general sense.

Kan no mushi or kanmushi
A fusion of *kan* and *mushi;* the term came to refer in general to pediatric problems in Japan for awhile.

Kanmushisho or kannomushisho
Although originally the term had broader, more general uses and meanings, today it refers in a more limited way to an infant or young child who is distressed, sleeps badly, and is irritable.

Keiraku chiryo
Meridian Therapy: a traditional school or style of acupuncture that developed in the 1920s to 1930s from the efforts of a study group led by Yanagiya, Inoue, Okabe, and Takeyama. Today it refers to a number of styles following some basic core traditional principles.

Kyukaku
Cupping.

Muno
A treatment term from Toyohari, it refers to treatment of the inguinal region.

Mushi
A term that refers to different kinds of beings that were thought to inhabit the body, each responsible for both the normal physiology and the pathophysiology of its related system.

Naso

A special Toyohari treatment system; the word derives from Japanese Braille shorthand for cervicobrachial syndrome and refers to treatment of the region around ST-12.

Okyu

Direct moxa technique, in which small pieces of moxa shaped like a grain of rice are burned on the skin.

Oshide

This term refers to the structure of the supporting hand, where the index finger and thumb hold the needle at the skin.

Ryu

Press-sphere: a stainless-steel ball bearing, usually no bigger than 2 mm in diameter and secured to a circular piece of tape that can be placed on the skin.

Sanshin

The "contact needle" technique, where the needle is stroked across or held at the skin surface.

Shiraku

Bloodletting: there are several forms that can be used, in children it mostly refers to bloodletting of *jing* points.

Sho

The "pattern." In Meridian Therapy it refers to the underlying or primary patterns of vacuity, of which there are four types: lung, spleen, liver, and kidney vacuity.

Shonishin

A Japanese rendering of the older Chinese term *erzhen,* which literally means "children's needle" or "children's needling."

Shu ha ri

Refers to a concept about learning and development, which originates from the Japanese tea ceremony tradition. It means that first you must learn from and imitate what your teachers teach you, but then you need to free yourself of this restriction and move out in your own direction. This process naturally takes many years or several decades.

Sotai

A very gentle "exercise" system aimed at loosening tight muscles to create more symmetric muscle tonus throughout the body, developed by Keizo Hashimoto. On children the exercise consists of tickling the child, hence "tickle therapy," to provoke a lot of random movements.

Spring-loaded *teishin*

Invented by Keiri Inoue, one of the founders of *Keiraku Chiryo* (Meridian Therapy). The spring loaded teishin is a teishin placed inside a handheld tool that can be used for the shonishin methods of stroking and light scratching. The teishin backs up against a soft spring so that it can be applied in two ways: (a) with very light soft bouncing actions on the skin for Meridian Therapy root treatment; (b) more vigorously with pressure for the shonishin pressing technique.

Teishin

One of the nine needles of the *Ling Shu,* a blunt-tipped needle with a rounded millet-seed-like point used for pressing the body surface.

Tsumo-shin

Variation of, and more recent alternative to, the spring-loaded *teishin,* which comes with a variety of springs to adjust pressure.

Uranaitei

Extra point on the bottom of the foot, for acute gastrointestinal problems, including allergies.

Wakakusa

A type of Japanese moxa, termed "semi-pure," which is less purified than "pure" yellow moxa.

Yoneyama

Shonishin tool, used for tapping or stroking, and also pressing (**Fig. 6.3c**).

Yukoshin (large and small)

Shonishin tool, used primarily for tapping, but can also be used for stroking or scratching (**Fig. 6.3e, f**).

Zanshin

One of the nine needles of the *Ling Shu,* the "arrow-headed needle" used for lightly cutting the skin (much like a paper cut). Today the various *zanshin* instruments are not sharp and provide rounded surfaces that can be used for stroking or pressing (see the rounded surface of the *Yoneyama*).

Additional Information

Treatment Equipment

In order to use the treatment described in this book it is necessary to know where to buy the various tools described.

■ Shonishin Tools

Shonishin tools have been carried by Western acupuncture supply companies for a number of years. The following are a list of some (not all) supply companies.

Australia
Chinabooks: http://www.chinabookssydney. com.au/TCMProducts

Germany
Docsave: http://www.docsave.eu
Chinapurmed: http://www.chinapurmed.de

Netherlands
MAESC: http://maesc.nl/div-naalden-benodigd-heden/jap-kindernaalden-shoni-chin.html

Switzerland
ABZ: http://www.aarauabz.ch

UK
Dulwich Acupuncture: http://www.dulwichacu-puncture.co.uk/
Scarborough's: http://www.scarboroughs.co.uk/
Dong Bang: http://www.acuprime.com/en/prod-ucts/probes--accessories/children-needle

USA
LhasaOMS: http://www.lhasaoms.com
Kenshin: http://www.kenshin.com/shonishin.php

Japan
Maeda: www.needlemaeda.com

■ Seirin Needles

Seirin needles, Pyonex press-tack needles, and Spinex intradermal needles can be purchased in many locations.

3B Scientific GmbH (Hamburg, Germany) is the general importer of Seirin, Japan, and renowned European distributor of all Seirin products.

Press-spheres can be purchased in many locations. It is better not to use magnetized press-spheres. LhasaOMS in the United States and Dulwich in the United Kingdom have good selections.

Japanese pure moxa can also be purchased in many locations. Several have specialized in Japanese moxa products, among them Docsave in Germany, and Scarborough's and Dulwich in the United Kingdom.

Educational

■ Harikyu Museum Osaka

In Japan the Harikyu Museum in Osaka has a good collection of acupuncture and *shonishin* items: http://www.harikyumuseum.com. This collection started with one of the modern fathers of *shonishin*, Hidetaro Mori.

■ Toyohari Association

The Toyohari Iggakukai (Toyohari Association) promotes *shonishin* and various forms of combined Meridian Therapy and *shonishin* practice. To contact the Toyohari Association outside Japan, go to http://www.toyohari.org. You will find links for the various branches in the United States, Europe, and Australia listed here. For the European branch go to http://www.toyohari.eu. Training programs are run regularly in English in these three continents.

■ International Courses

Courses on *shonishin* can be found in the United States, Europe, and Australia. There are a number of teachers running courses in the United States (e.g., Brenda Loew), Europe (e.g., Stephen Birch), and Australia (e.g., Paul Movsessian).

Bibliography

Akabane K. Hinaishin Ho. 12th ed. Yokosuka: Ido no Nippon Publishing Company; 1986

Anon, ed. Tu Zhu Nanjing Mai Jue, containing Li Shi Zhen (1578). Qi Jing Ba Mai Gao. 2nd ed. Taipei: Shui Cheng Shuju Publishing Company; 1970

Bach E, Wheeler FJ. The Bach Flower Remedies. New Canaan, CT: Keats Publishing; 1979

Bensky D, Clavey S, Stoger E. Chinese Herbal Medicine. Materia Medica. 3rd ed. Seattle, WA: Eastland Press; 2004

Birch S. Keiraku Chiryo—Japanese Meridian Therapy: pragmatic in theory with clinical sophistication. North Am J Orient Med 1999;6(15):13–15

Birch S. Improving vitality—a case history. In: McCarthy M, Birch S, eds. Thieme Almanac 2007: Acupuncture and Chinese Medicine. Stuttgart, Germany: Thieme; 2007:80–87

Birch S. Filling the whole in acupuncture. What are we doing in the supplementation needle technique? Part 1.1. Eur J Orient Med 2009;6(2):25–35

Birch S. Filling the whole in acupuncture. What are we doing in the supplementation needle technique? Part 1.2. Eur J Orient Med 2009;6(3): 18–27

Birch S. A brief overview of the development of Keiraku Chiryo, Japanese Meridian Therapy [in Japanese]. Ido no Nippon 2010;69(11):96–l00

Birch S. Traditional needling techniques as practical constructions from reading historical descriptions. Eur J Oriental Med 2013;7(3)26–33

Birch S. Jingmai and qi—acupuncture perspectives. In: Birch S, Cabrer Mir MA, Rodriguez M, eds. Restoring Order in Health and Chinese Medicine: Studies of the Development and Use of Qi and the Channels. Barcelona, Spain: La Liebre de Marzo/ Jade Stone Group; 2014:183–266

Birch S. Historical and clinical perspectives on de qi: exposing limitations in the scientific study of de qi. J Altern Complement Med 2015;21(1):1–7

Birch S. Filling the whole in acupuncture. Part 2. The "treatment space"—modeling the treatment process in acupuncture. In preparation (a)

Birch S, Cabrer M, Rodriguez M, eds. Restoring Order in Health and Chinese Medicine: Studies of the Development and Use of Qi and the Channels. Barcelona, Spain: La Liebre de Marzo/Jade Stone Group; 2014a

Birch S, Cabrer M, Rodriguez M. Qi and the mind—explorations of the links between qi, the mind, mental and emotional states. In Birch S,

Cabrer M, Rodriguez M, eds. Restoring Order in Health and Chinese Medicine: Studies of the Development and Use of Qi and the Channels. Barcelona, Spain: La Liebre de Marzo/Jade Stone Group; 2014b:27–110

Birch S, Felt RO. Understanding Acupuncture. Edinburgh, Scotland: Churchill Livingstone; 1999

Birch S, Ida J. Japanese Acupuncture: A Clinical Guide. Brookline, MA: Paradigm Publications; 1998

Birch S, Ida J. Naso and muno—two of the supportive therapies unique to Toyohari. North Am J Orient Med 2001;8(21):10–12

Birch S, Ida J. An introduction to Keiraku Chiryo. Eur J Orient Med 2004;4(5):53–58

Brand E, Wiseman N. Concise Chinese Materia Medica. Taos, NM: Paradigm Publications; 2008

Cao JM, Su XM, Cao JQ. Essentials of Traditional Chinese Pediatrics. Beijing, China: Foreign Languages Press; 1990

Chace C. On greeting a friend: an approach to needle technique. Lantern 2006;3(3):4–7

Chace C, Bensky D. An axis of efficacy: the range of meaning in chapter one of the Lingshu. In: Birch S, Cabrer M, Rodriguez M, eds. Restoring Order in Health and Chinese Medicine: Studies of the Development and Use of Qi and the Channels. Barcelona, Spain: La Liebre de Marzo/Jade Stone Group; 2014:267–292

Chace C, Shima M. An Exposition on the Extraordinary Vessels. Seattle, WA: Eastland Press; 2010

Cheng XN. Chinese Acupuncture and Moxibustion. Beijing, China; Foreign Languages Press; 1987

Chiu ML. Mind, body, and illness in a Chinese medical tradition. PhD thesis, Harvard University; 1986

Ergil MC, Ergil K. Pocket Atlas of Chinese Medicine. Stuttgart, Germany: Thieme; 2009

Flaws B. A Handbook of TCM Pediatrics. Boulder, CO: Blue Poppy Press; 2002

Fukaya I. Kadenkyu Monogatari. Tokyo, Japan: Sankei Publishing; 1982

Fukushima K. Meridian Therapy. Tokyo, Japan: Toyo Hari Medical Association; 1991

Gu CF. Elementary pediatrics: an annotated bibliography. Int J Orient Med 1989;14(2):99–105

Harper D. Early Chinese Medical Literature: The Mawangdui Medical Manuscripts. London, UK: Kegan Paul; 1998

Hashimoto K, Kawakami Y. Sotai: Balance and Health through Natural Movement. Tokyo, Japan: Japan Publications; 1983

Hempen C-H, Wortman Chow V. Pocket Atlas of Acupuncture. Stuttgart, Germany: Thieme; 2006

Hyodo M. Acupuncture and therapeutic points suited to diseases and disorders. Japan J Ryodoraku Med 1986;31(4–5):101–152

Irie P. Fukaya Kyu Ho. Tokyo, Japan: Shizensha; 1980

Ishihara S. A case of children's asthma. Ido no Nippon 1971;2:30–32

Jiao Shude. Ten Lectures on the Use of Medicinals from the Personal Experiences of Jiao Shude. Trans. Mitchell C, Wiseman N, Ergil M, Ochs S. Taos, NM: Paradigm Publications; 2003

Jiao Shude. Ten Lectures on the Use of Formulas from the Personal Experiences of Jiao Shude. Trans. Damone B, Helme M, Kuchinski L, Mitchell C, Wiseman N. Taos, NM: Paradigm Publications; 2005

Jobst KA. Acupuncture in asthma and pulmonary disease: an analysis of efficacy and safety. J Alt Comp Med 1996;2(1):179–206

Kasumi H. Lecture on dose of treatment. Paper presented at Meridian Therapy Workshop, Amsterdam, May 2003

Katsuyoshi S. On the use of the point shitsumin. North Am J Orient Med 2006;13(37):20–21

Kudo K. Zusetsu Shiraku Chiryo. Tokyo, Japan: Shizensha; 1983

Lo V. Huangdi Hama jing (Yellow emperor's toad canon). Lecture, October 21, 2003. http://www.ihp.sinica.edu.tw/~medicine/ashm/lectures/Lo.pdf

Lu GD, Needham J. Celestial Lancets. Cambridge, UK: Cambridge University Press; 1980

Manaka Y. Okyu no Kenkyu. Tokyo, Japan: Goma Publishing; 1976

Manaka Y. Ika no tameno Shinjutsu Nyumon Kuoza. Yokosuka, Japan: Ido no Nippon; 1980

Manaka Y. Kyu to Hari. 8th ed. Tokyo, Japan: Shufu no Tomo Publishing; 1983

Manaka Y, Itaya K, Birch S. Chasing the Dragon's Tail. Brookline, MA: Paradigm Publications; 1995

Maruyama M, Kudo K. Shinpan Shiraku Ryoho. Tokyo, Japan: Seki Bundo Publishing; 1982

Matsumoto K, Birch S. Extraordinary Vessels. Brookline, MA: Paradigm Publications; 1986

Matsumoto K, Birch S. Reflections on the Sea: Hara Diagnosis. Brookline, MA: Paradigm Publications; 1988

Meguro A. Kyukaku Ryoho. 5th ed. Tokyo, Japan: Midori Shobo Publishing; 1991

Nakada K. Basic needling techniques. North Am J Orient Med 1995;2(4):24–26

Nakada K. Lecture on the treatment of children. Presented at Meridian Therapy Workshop, Amsterdam, April 2000

NICE, National Institute for Health and Clinical Excellence. Headaches: diagnosis and management of headaches in young people and adults. Issued September 2012, NICE clinical guideline 150. http://www.guidance.nice.org.uk/cg150

Okabe S. Specially effective points for night urination. Ido no Nippon J 1940;11(4):7–8

Ono B. Keiraku Chiryo Shinkyu Rinsho Nyumon. Yokosuka, Japan: Ido no Nippon; 1988

Rodriguez M. Pediatria en Medicina China. Barcelona, Spain: La Liebre de Marzo; 2008

Rodriguez M. Qi, jingmai, yaoyi: a study of their relationships. In: Birch S, Cabrer M, Rodriguez M, eds. Restoring Order in Health and Chinese Medicine: Studies of the Development and Use of Qi and the Channels. Barcelona, Spain: La Liebre de Marzo/Jade Stone Group; 2014:293–342

Rodrigucz M, Anton R. Cuidalos! Guia Practica de Cuidados Infantiles. Barcelona, Spain: La Liebre de Marzo; 2008

Saller-Fischbach A. Observational study of Dr. Manaka's treatment for elevated liver enzymes (hepatitis treatment). North Am J Orient Med 2009;47:24

Scheid V, Bensky D, Ellis A, Barolet R. Chinese Herbal Medicine: Formulas and Strategies. 2nd ed. Seattle, WA: Eastland Press; 2009

Scott J, Barlow T. Acupuncture in the Treatment of Children. 3rd ed. Seattle, WA: Eastland Press; 1999

Scott J, Barlow T. Herbs in the Treatment of Children. Edinburgh, Scotland: Churchill Livingstone; 2003

Shimada R. Jing-well point blood letting. North Am J Orient Med 2005;12(33):17–20

Shimizu C. Shonishin. Ido no Nippon J 1975;1:24–44

Shiroda BS. Kyuryo Zatsuwa. 6th ed. Yokosuka, Japan: Ido no Nippon sha; 1982

Shiroda BS. Shinkyu Chiryo Kisogaku. 16th ed. Yokosuka: Ido no Nippon; 1986

Shudo D. Japanese Classical Acupuncture: Introduction to Meridian Therapy. Seattle, WA: Eastland Press; 1990

Shudo D. Finding Effective Acupoints. Seattle, WA: Eastland Press; 2003

Sivin N. Traditional Medicine in Contemporary China. Ann Arbor: Center for Chinese Studies, University of Michigan; 1987

Tanioka M. Wakariyasui Shonishin no Jissai. Tokyo, Japan: Gensosha; 2001a

Tanioka M. Shonishin—paediatric acupuncture. Part 1. North Am J Orient Med 2001b;8(21):13–15

Taniuchi SH. Lecture on the treatment of children. Presented at Meridian Therapy Workshop, London, September 2007

Tian C, Wang Y. Clinical and experimental research on the antipyretic effects of moxibustion. In: Selections from Article Abstracts on Acupuncture and Moxibustion. Beijing, China: Association of Acupuncture and Moxibustion; 1987:221–222

Unschuld PU. Medicine in China: A History of Ideas. Berkeley: University of California Press; 1985

Unschuld PU. Nan Ching: The Classic of Difficult Issues. Berkeley: University of California Press; 1986a

Unschuld PU. Medicine in China: A History of Pharmaceutics. Berkeley, University of California Press; 1986b

Unschuld PU. Huang Di Nei Jing Su Wen—Nature, Knowledge, Imagery in an Ancient Chinese Medical Text. Berkeley: University of California Press; 2003

Valeriani M. Pharmacological and non-pharmacological treatment of pediatric primary headaches. Ital J Pediatr 2014;40(Suppl 1):A84. doi:10.1186/1824-7288-40-S1-A84

Wang JY. Applied Channel Theory in Chinese Medicine. Seattle, WA: Eastland Press; 2008

Wang Luo-zhen, ed. Qi Jing Ba Mai Gao Jiao Zhu. Shanghai, China: Shanghai Science and Technology Publishing; 1990

Wang Y, Tian C, Li Z. Preliminary observation on the treatment of fever due to the invasion of exogenous pathogenic wind cold with warm moxibustion. In: Selections from Article Abstracts on Acupuncture and Moxibustion. Beijing, China: Association of Acupuncture and Moxibustion; 1987:220–221

Wernicke T. Shonishin—Japanische Kinderakupunktur. Munich, Germany: Elsevier; 2009

Wernicke T. Shonishin—the art of non-invasive paediatric acupuncture. London, UK: Singing Dragon; 2014

Wiseman N, Ellis A. Fundamentals of Chinese Medicine. Brookline, MA: Paradigm Publications; 1985

Wiseman N, Feng Y. A Practical Dictionary of Chinese Medicine. Brookline, MA: Paradigm Publications; 1997

Yanagishita T. Lecture on children's treatment. Presented at Meridian Therapy Workshop, Tokyo, July 1997

Yanagishita T. Naso treatment. North Am J Orient Med 2001a;8(21):8–9

Yanagishita T. Muno treatment. North Am J Orient Med 2001b;8(22):19–20

Yanagishita T. Lecture on how to improve one's practice. Presented at Meridian Therapy Workshop, Tokyo, April 2003

Yang ZY. On presence of mind and subtle sensations. Lantern 2007;4(2):28–30

Yoneyama H, Mori H. Shonishin Ho—Acupuncture Treatment for Children. Yokosuka, Japan: Ido no Nipponsha; 1964

Young M, Craig J. Direct Moxa and Immune Response—A Review Study. Part 1. Eur J Orient Med 2009;6(3):54–60

Young M, Craig J. Direct moxa and immune response—a review study. Part 2. Eur J Orient Med 2010;6(4):53–60

Index

Page numbers in *italics* refer to illustrations; those in **bold** refer to tables